A WEED-LOVER'S CALENDAR

Secrets of those errant plants revealed

Rachel Fulcher

A Weed-lover's Calendar
Text © Rachel Fulcher 2024
Photos © Rachel Fulcher unless otherwise stated

The Author has asserted her rights under the Copyright, Designs and Patents Act 1988 to be identified as the Author of this Work.
All Rights Reserved.

No part of this book may be reproduced in any form by photocopying or by any electronic or mechanical means, including information, storage or retrieval systems, without permission in writing from both the copyright owners and the publisher of this book.

Published 2024 by Brambleby Books, Devon, U.K.
www.bramblebybooks.co.uk

Cover design Tanya Warren, Creatix
Front cover photo by Rachel Fulcher
Book design by JM InfoTech India
Printed by Short Run Press Ltd., Devon, U.K.

ISBN 9781908241740

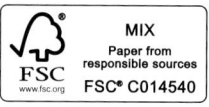

For my sister, Mary Pratt, biologist, teacher and author.
Remembered with warm affection.

Important Note

While information concerning the individual plants has been carefully researched, and scientific backup provided where appropriate, many of the remedies discussed are derived from folklore and are no longer prescribed by herbalists. Moreover, some weeds are poisonous. Please therefore heed all the warnings in the text.

If you suffer from any health condition or complaint, always seek professional advice in the first instance from your doctor or fully qualified medical herbalist. This is particularly important if you are taking prescribed medicines or if you are pregnant. Neither the author nor the publisher can be held responsible for any adverse effects if such precautions are not followed.

CLIMATE CHANGE

Since beginning research for this book several years ago, I have noticed how some wild plants are flowering earlier than usual. This can be by ten days, or, in some cases, as much as a fortnight. This is clearly due to global warming.

In 2022,, after a very sunny spell in the early spring, one or two plants opened their petals in March rather than April. Most noticeable has been the blossom of blackthorn. Others have appeared at unseasonal times: we even had primroses fully out at Christmas! However, as far as this book is concerned, I made the decision to keep the plants within their traditional month of flowering on the basis that this is when they can still be seen at their best – but do not be surprised if you find them in bud a little earlier.

Author

Daughter of a botanist, Rachel Fulcher learnt about wild flowers and came to love them from a very early age. This is an interest she has maintained through membership of the Botanical Society of Britain and Ireland. Passionate about the environment, Rachel spends much of her spare time campaigning on behalf of nature, mainly as an active member of Friends of the Earth and, until recently, through her environmental column for the *East Anglian Daily Times*.

She is also a specialist in the complementary health field and the author of several other books (under her former name of Rachel Charles), notably *Your Mind's Eye*, *Food For Healing* and *Mind, Body and Immunity*.

Rachel loves music and is an accomplished cellist. She lives in rural Suffolk with her husband and retired racing greyhound.

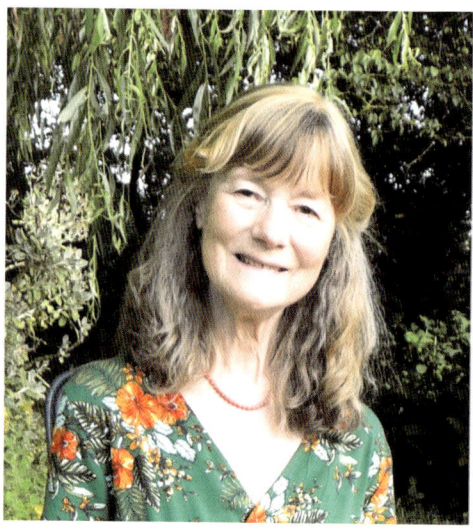

The author in her garden

Contents

Preface ix

Introduction 1

SPRING 5
- **March** 6
- **April** 31
- **May** 70

SUMMER 121
- **June** 122
- **July** 177
- **August** 247

AUTUMN 276
- **September** 278
- **October & November** 297

WINTER 316
- **December to February** 318

Postface 336
Acknowledgements 337
Glossary 338
Bibliography 347
Index 354

Preface

This book records the life, year-round, of a living garden in East Anglia in the United Kingdom. The plants selected happen to be those that have arrived here unbidden, carried by wind, bird or animal. They are the 'weeds', or plants in the wrong place, that have chosen to put down their roots in this particular garden. While they may be typical of common weeds, the list is not comprehensive nor has it tried to be. The reader may therefore find that other arrivals turn up in different gardens.

Generally, individual weeds are ascribed to this or that month according to the time of flowering. Occasionally, however, the month of fruiting has been selected if that is when the plant is of greatest interest. To find your way around the text, the best approach is to use the index. Here you will see all the plants listed under their common names.

As for the illustrations, most of the photographs have been taken by the author herself as part of her exploration of her own garden. If not, the name of the photographer is added to the appropriate caption.

It is hoped that the legends, stories and literary associations, together with the medicinal, culinary and wildlife benefits of the different weeds that have been collected here will inspire the reader to view these normally despised arrivals from a different perspective. It is also hoped that weeding will thereby become an enjoyable and absorbing pastime.

Rachel Fulcher

What would the world be, once bereft
Of wet and of wildness? Let them be left,
O let them be left, wildness and wet;
Long live the weeds and the wilderness yet.

Gerard Manley Hopkins (1844–89), from *Inversnaid*

INTRODUCTION

What are weeds and what are their associations? How do people generally regard them? Are they considered to be benign or malevolent? Unlike the heartfelt words of Gerard Manley Hopkins, quoted on opposite page, they are generally thought of as a nuisance, that they look a mess and spoil a beautiful garden or landscape. They are frequently despised. Underneath all of this there seems to be a chronic worry that they will take over and form an impenetrable jungle around us. Come what may, we must control them! This was the culture that surrounded me when I owned my first little green patch.

Leafing through any gardening magazine or book, we can see how we are encouraged to be ruthless, to exterminate the 'weeds' and even use poisons to eradicate them. I have a typical one on my shelf with a chapter entitled *War on weeds*, warning us that vigilance must be constant otherwise they will overrun the 'more desirable species'. It cautions us against trying to dig up perennial weeds for fear that this will cause them to spread even further. The author is adamant that these can only be controlled by chemicals and lists the ones that should be applied. While pulling up or hoeing is accepted as a possibility for annual weeds, the many hours of unnecessary labour and the back-breaking work is emphasised.

Instinctively I have never used weed killers, despite the exhortations of the magazines, as a garden has always seemed to me to be a peaceful haven, somewhere to unwind after a busy day, where nature can flourish, indeed the very last place to wage any kind of war. Reading up on the harmful effects of herbicides left me appalled by the dangers of chemicals frequently recommended for garden use. These included such phrases as 'potential to contaminate ground water', 'harmful in contact with skin', 'toxic if swallowed – may be fatal', 'dangerous to livestock and wild animals'

– and so on. From then on, I committed myself to organic gardening only. The prime motivation was to care for my own small green space in a calm and gentle way, and to work with nature, not against it.

Now I am the co-owner with my husband of a very large garden. When we first saw it we were so captivated by its beauty that we bought the house standing in its midst, even though at that time it was something of a wreck! We were enthralled by the variety and maturity of the plants and the obvious thoughtfulness with which they had been laid out. On one side of the house there was a small woodland of mostly native trees, with lawn areas beyond and curving flowerbeds and borders filled with shrubs and perennials, carefully chosen so that there were always colours, shapes and perfumes to entice the senses. The other side was quite different, reminiscent of the former farm, with the remains of a meadow sloping down to a pond, presumably used at one time for fish and to supply drinking water for cattle. It had since become a wildlife haven, inhabited by frogs and newts and a great many other creatures, iridescent mayflies and dragonflies patrolling above it on warm, sunny days: altogether a little paradise!

Initially, after moving in, our spare time was spent renovating the house so that the garden was often left to take care of itself. There came a point, though, when we needed to pay considerable attention to it otherwise it was likely to get out of hand. One day I was on my knees by one of the flowerbeds, despairing about the amount of work to be done, when an idea struck me. If I was to spend a great many hours weeding, then it needed to be interesting rather than a chore. I decided to find out more about the plants that gardeners seemed to dislike and reject, and to think of them not as weeds but as wild flowers. Feeling suddenly inspired, I made a tour of the entire garden, identification guide and camera in hand. What I discovered was truly astonishing. Around the pond and meadow, I identified 25 different plant species. Next, it was the turn of the more formally laid-out side of the house, where I expected to find some kind of repetition. Amazingly, however, there were 27 more entirely different species. None of them had been deliberately planted, yet here they were flourishing, seeds apparently blown here by the wind or brought from elsewhere by birds or ants, or other creatures. The resilience of nature and the variety of its products was truly impressive.

INTRODUCTION

'Weeds' were now to be an adventure of discovery. The aim was no longer to try and get rid of them but rather to find out as much as possible about them. Then to make an informed decision whether to keep them, to transplant some, or conclude that they were redundant. What was the history of these plants? Were they native to this part of the world or had they been brought here from elsewhere? Maybe some had healing properties, others might perhaps be edible. What other benefits could they have? Which species might be poisonous? What part do they play in the ecology of the garden? Do birds or bees or any other creatures rely on them? Could they indicate which garden species might best thrive in this location? There were so many questions to ask, so much to discover!

As each month went by, I made extensive notes of the life in the garden, illustrated by many photographs. Moreover, the urge grew to pass on my findings to others and these ultimately became the basis of the present book. Who would have thought that weeds could be so utterly absorbing? Any idea of weeding being a chore has long since been banished. Some of our wild plants are to be treasured, either for their beauty, their ecological benefits or therapeutic value.

SPRING

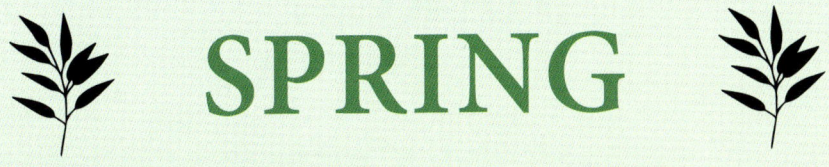

The year's at the spring,

And day's at the morn;

Morning's at seven;

The hillside's dew-pearled;

The lark's on the wing;

The snail's on the thorn;

God's in his Heaven –

All's right with the world!

From *Pippa Passes* by Robert Browning (1812–89).

MARCH

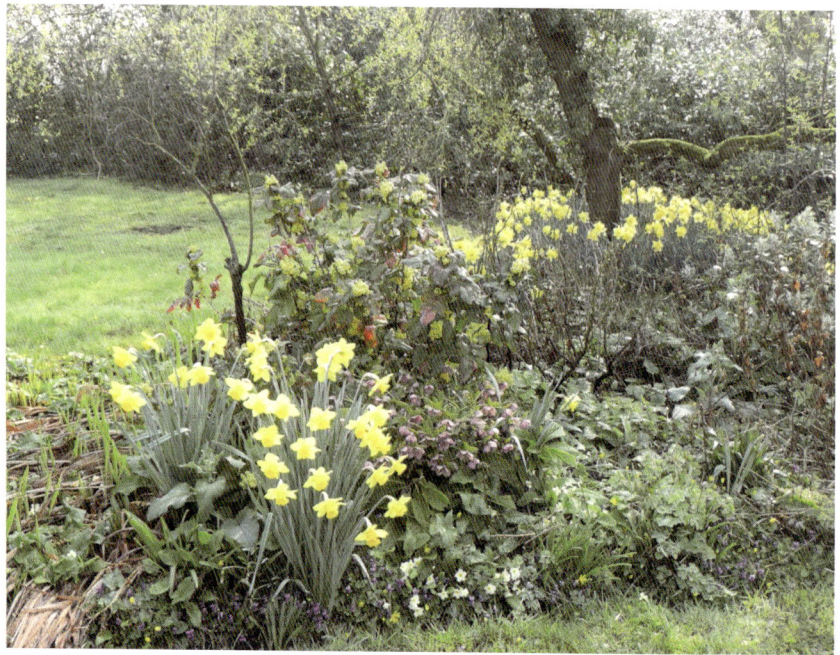

You can just see the wild primroses and violets, both surprise arrivals, which have been left to develop at the front of the border.

This is a month full of contradictions. One day can be perishingly cold, with driving sleet and howling gales, while the next can be reassuringly warm and sunny, an encouragement to the spring flowers, and the 'weeds' of course, to raise their heads and open their petals. Today is the 19th: the sky is overcast and gloomy, and there is a finger-freezing breeze. Yet, as I look back to last year's diary, I read that this same date was like summer, with the sweet perfume of daffodils on the air, the sound of tennis rackets batting a ball next door and laughter and idle chat drifting over the hedge. This year, however, the weatherman tells us that more snow is on the way.

Despite its wintery aspects, March was the first month of ten in the very earliest Roman calendar. This seemed a good enough reason to begin this book with the same month. It was named after Martius, the god of war, and indicated the start of the season for both warfare and farming. Sometimes this month seems to be truly war-like in character, with strong gales bending the trees almost to breaking point. No one captures this characteristic better than American poet and educator Henry Wadsworth Longfellow (1807–82):

> I Martius am! Once first, and now the third!
> To lead the Year was my appointed place;
> A mortal dispossessed me by a word,
> And set there Janus with the double face.
> Hence I make war on all the human race;
> I shake the cities with my hurricanes;
> I flood the rivers and their banks efface,
> And drown the farms and hamlets with my rains.
>
> 'March' from *The Poet's Calendar* (1882)

Despite these sometimes violent outbreaks, the month nevertheless offers hope for new beginnings with the birds already busy with nest-building. A tiny wren has taken up residence in our carport, well sheltered from the March winds, and is remaking the old mud nest of a swallow. Each day a little more moss is added to the sides and top, thus creating a snug round home. We look forward to the arrival of the babies.

The 'weeds' that appear this month are as mixed as the weather. Some we welcome gladly as they brighten our patch, but others we decide have no place in our garden and will have to go. My husband has started regular hoeing of the allotment as he wants to avoid any competition with the vegetables in order to give them the best of the nutrients and light and air.

Lesser Celandine (*Ficaria verna*)

Buttercup family (Ranunculaceae). Perennial. Pollinated by flies, beetles and bumble bees. Propagated by tuber, bulbil and seed. Mildly toxic and irritant.

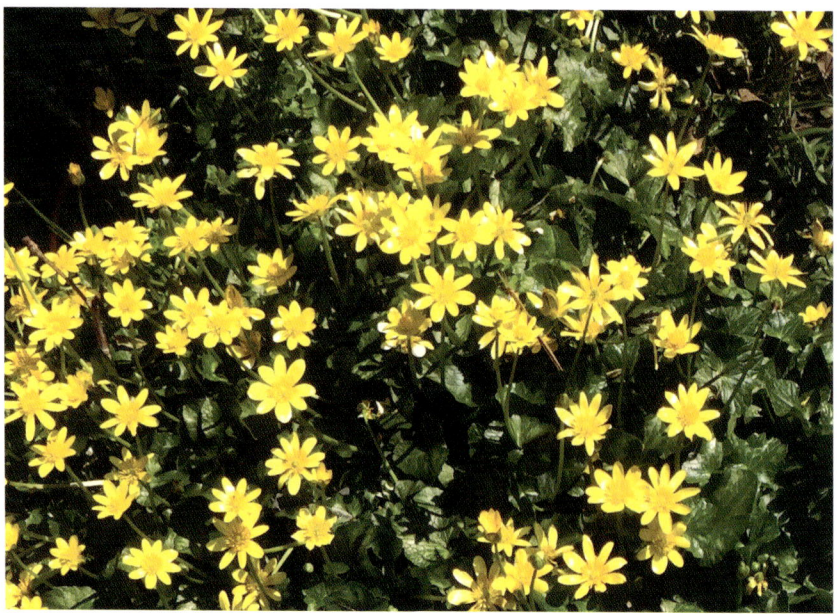

This humble little plant, often despised by gardeners, was greatly admired by the poet William Wordsworth. *Photo © H D Loxdale*

What could be more joyful than this messenger of spring as it opens its gleaming yellow petals towards the first warm sunshine of the year! In the late 18th century, Gilbert White recorded it in flower in his Hampshire village as early as 21st February, although in our East Anglian garden we have to wait a little longer. The name 'celandine' comes from the Latin for swallow, *chelidonia*, referring to the arrival of this bird from warmer places. However, in the UK we do not generally see swallows until the end of April. There seems to have been some confusion with another, unrelated plant, the greater celandine, which flowers later in the year.

Its former scientific name was *Ranunculus ficaria*, denoting its relationship to the buttercup. *Rana* is the Latin for frog, perhaps indicating that this genus thrives in damp places, on pond or ditch banks, in low-lying meadows or shady woodland. It is certainly quite content on our damp clay, especially wherever I have been turning over the soil in the borders.

Ficaria stems from *ficus*, the Latin for fig, because of the knobbly tuberous roots that are thought to resemble this fruit. Lesser celandine can spread very rapidly via its tiny 'bulbils', rather than by seed, which form at the leaf axils, quickly creating new plants. Dark green carpets of the low-growing, shiny, heart-shaped leaves can soon colonise favourable situations. If you really do not want so many, then a dressing of ash, either wood or coal, can discourage their proliferation.

The starry, golden-yellow flowers may have any number of petals between seven and twelve, each of which is backed by three sepals. The colour fades to white as the flower ages. In the centre are many stamens. The petals have the knack of closing up just before the arrival of rain and, as they are greenish on the underside, seem to disappear. At the end of the flowering season the vanishing act is complete as the plant dies back. During winter, energy is stored underground in the tuberous roots.

Folklore

In former times it seems that the bulbils attached to the roots of celandine were associated with the teats of cows. For this reason, farmers used to hang the roots in the byre in the hope that the cows would thereby produce creamier milk and more of it.

The lesser celandine emerges every now and again in English literature. Indeed, this modest little plant seems to have captured the imaginations of several writers. As far as William Wordsworth is concerned, it is widely assumed that the daffodil was his favourite bloom, because his poem about this flower is so well known. However, it was the unassuming lesser celandine that he most admired.

> There's a flower that shall be mine,
> 'Tis the little celandine.

From *To the Small Celandine*

After his death a celandine was inscribed on to his tombstone, but unfortunately the artist depicted the wrong one, the greater celandine which is related to the poppy!

Wordsworth wrote three poems about the lesser celandine. 'The Small Celandine' is particularly charming as it gives a true picture of its special characteristics. The opening verse refers to its canny ability to respond to the weather:

> There is a flower, the lesser celandine,
> That shrinks, like many more, from cold and rain;
> And the first moment that the sun may shine,
> Bright as the sun itself, 'tis out again!

This glowing little flower is not just restricted to poetry. D.H. Lawrence's main character in his novel *Sons and Lovers*, Paul Morel, has a special feeling for these 'scalloped splashes of gold', perhaps reflecting the writer's own regard for the flower. He particularly likes them 'when their petals go flat back with the sunshine' and the way in which they 'seem to be pressing themselves at the sun'.

Uses

A very long-standing common name for lesser celandine is the somewhat unlovely 'pilewort' on account of its traditional usage as a remedy for haemorrhoids. The visual similarity between the knobbly tubers of the plant and this uncomfortable condition doubtlessly prompted herbalists to prescribe it, in line with the Doctrine of Signatures. This theory was proposed by Paracelsus in the 16th century in which he states that each plant gives us a sign of its medicinal use that can be 'read' by a physician. There may be a resemblance with a part of the human body needing to be healed or, alternatively, with the symptoms of a specific disease which it might cure. Amazingly, lesser celandine really does contain therapeutic properties helpful in the curing of piles: the saponins are naturally anti-haemorrhoidal and the tannins enhance this effect. No doubt, herbalists combined the ideas of the Doctrine of Signatures with their own practical knowledge. Nicholas Culpeper (1616–64), an English botanist, herbalist, physician and astrologer, says that 'it is certain by good experience that the decoction of the leaves and root doth wonderfully help piles and haemorrhoids'. Herbalists may still prescribe it in the form of an ointment for topical application.

The plant needs to be used with care, however, as it contains a toxin, protoanemonin, but when dried or heated the poisonous effect is nullified. Despite this, the raw young leaves were eaten as a prevention against scurvy. The German name is *Scharbockskraut*, which means scurvy herb. It is now known that the leaves are rich in vitamin C. It seems that the toxin becomes increasingly potent as the plant matures, so newly emerging leaves are relatively safe.

Wildlife

Like the nectar of other early blooms, this can be a life-saver for bees and other insects when there is so little nourishment available. In particular the red-tailed and buff-tailed bumble bees benefit, along with various flies and beetles. Although pollinated in this way, the seeds rarely set. The plant relies rather on its creeping tubers and bulbils for propagation, which can cause it to be invasive. For this reason gardeners tend to want to eradicate it. Please think again and consider allowing it to flourish in a spare patch where it can easily be restricted.

Cherry Plum (*Prunus cerasifera*)

Rose family (Rosaceae). Deciduous shrub. Self-fertile; also pollinated by insects including bees. Propagated by seed or suckering. Edible fruit.

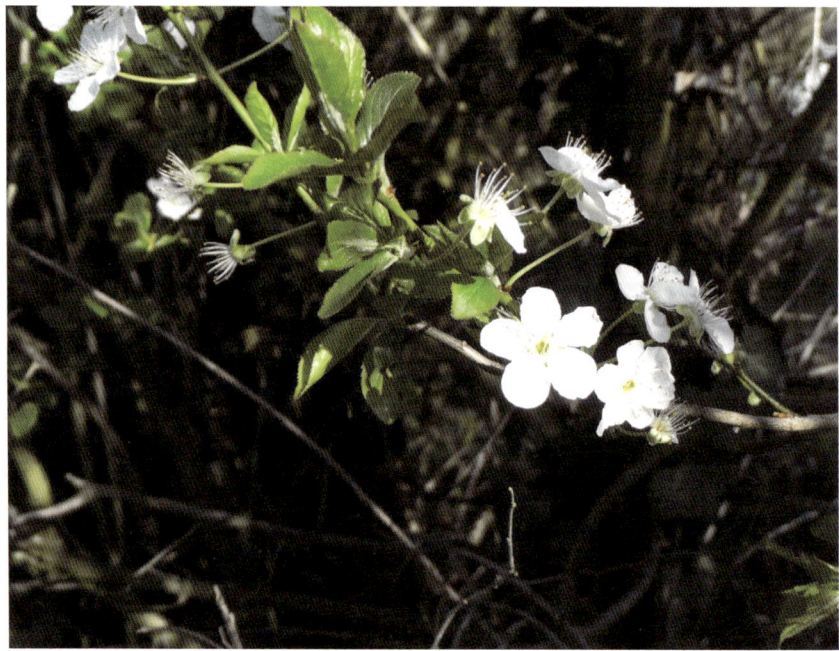

Brought on by the spring sunshine, the blossoms of cherry plum can tolerate the cold of early March.

THE LEAVES AND FLOWERS

Out before the fresh green leaves and even before blackthorn has made a showing, these plucky little five-petalled, snow-white flowers burst open with the very earliest spring sunshine. In some areas this can be as soon as mid-February, but in our cool garden it is generally March.

I may be cheating a bit by including this shrub as a weed as I am not entirely sure how wild it is. Even if it had originally been planted as a hedge or shelter belt, by the time we arrived here it had turned into a sprawling mass of branches up to a good 7.5 m/25 feet along part of our western boundary. It most certainly needed to be tamed.

The plant was not in fact originally a native of the British Isles, having been introduced, perhaps in the 17th century from somewhere further east, the Balkans or Central Asia, but it is now well naturalised. No doubt the delicious fruit was a great attraction.

The flowers are hermaphrodite, in other words they contain both male and female organs. Bees and other insects make the most of the early spring nectar and thereby pollinate the shrub.

The leaves, when they finally appear, are slender and oval, situated alternately on reddish stalks. Close inspection reveals downy hairs on the underside of the veins. The bark is a distinctive dark grey.

Folklore

In Christian art a flowering *Prunus* often symbolises independence. It may also signify the virtue of fidelity. Because it flowers so early, the Chinese regard it as the harbinger of spring and forthcoming fruitfulness. If, however, it happens to flower too early, in December, this forewarns of a death in the family, according to Welsh tradition.

Uses

Both the leaves and seeds are very bitter, the result of toxins which in large quantities can cause poisoning. All members of *Prunus* in fact contain amygdalin and prunasin, which, when broken down in water, produce hydrocyanic acid (cyanide or prussic acid). This sounds very alarming, but in small doses they have been shown to help improve the digestion and encourage respiration. Excess, however, could cause respiratory failure, so remedies from the leaves and seeds are not recommended here.

That said, if you have ever taken RESCUE Remedy® then you will already have used the plant therapeutically as it is one of the five ingredients that make up this restorative. By checking *Prunus cerasifera* in the Bach™ Flower Remedies, you will see that the treatment phrases are 'Desperation', 'Fear of losing control of the mind' and 'Dread of doing some frightful thing'. This seems to indicate that it earned a reputation for boosting confidence.

Other than its potential for healing, another reason for bringing the plant to the British Isles could have been its usefulness for making dyes. In the past a green dye has been obtained from the leaves and a dark grey-green colour from the fruit.

As for enjoying the intense flavour of the wild cherry plums, you will need to turn to the pages of August where you will find a recipe for a delicious jam (p. 255).

Wildlife

If you notice roundish, brown blotches appearing on the leaves in the summer and autumn, then these will be the 'mines' or marks left by the feeding larvae of the moth *Stigmella plagicolella*. The adult, mainly dark greyish-brown, has a distinctive white mark on each wing that, when folded, connect to form a continuous band. The moth is small, with a wingspan of just 4-5mm.

If, on the other hand, the leaves are mined along the edges, then these are likely to be caused by the feeding larvae of the moth *Phyllonorycter spinicolella*. The adult has striking brown and white markings with hairy tufts at the base of the wings. Its wingspan is 6-8mm. It flies in May and then August.

Otherwise, the blossoms of the plant provide crucial early spring nectar for those insects that are already out and about. Bullfinches will also devour the buds. Fortunately, they only take those at the very top of the shrub which we cannot reach.

Dog's Mercury (*Mercurialis perennis*)

Spurge family (Euphorbiaceae). Perennial. Pollinated by wind or small flies. Propagated by rhizome or seed. Poisonous.

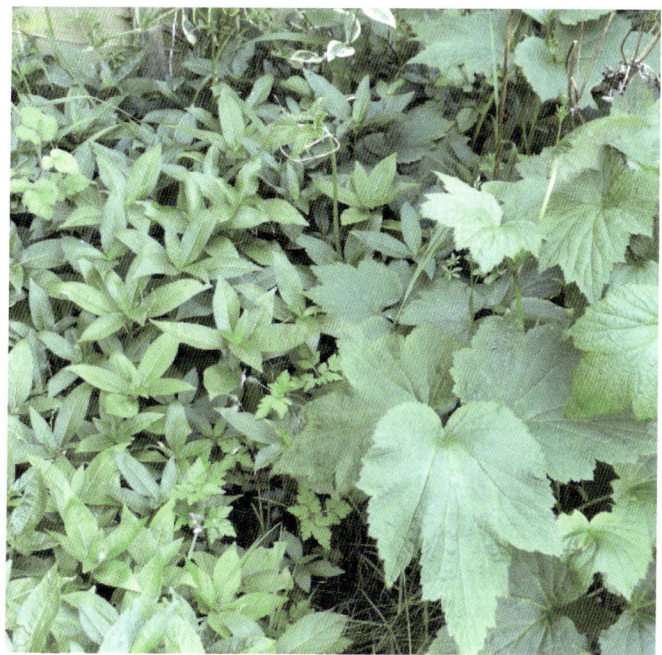

Invasive and poisonous, dog's mercury is here a nuisance as it has invaded the border where our lovely Japanese anemones grow (right).

One year I had noticed a few plants with dark-green leaves appearing on the northern, cool and shady side of our front boundary fence but, despite my curiosity, had paid them no further attention. As it happens, there had been little time for gardening that year, so the weeds had proliferated. By the following spring, a sturdy patch had established itself and it was time to find out what the plants were. Searching through botanical guides was not immediately productive as the flower was so insignificant it was hard to identify. It was my husband who suggested that I check it for dog's mercury. He was right! It fitted the description exactly.

A lover of damp, shady woodland, this member of the spurge family (Euphorbiaceae) is a perennial and can quickly carpet the floor by sending out underground stems which put down new roots. Each plant can grow to 40 cm/16 inches, although ours tend to be somewhat shorter. The leaves, which appear in pairs on small stalks either side of the upright stem, are softly hairy with an attractive elliptical shape, pointed at the end and with rounded teeth. If you press them between your fingers, however, the smell is quite odious. It has been compared to rotting fish – but I cannot say that ours are quite that revolting.

The flowers, which grow in clusters, are unusual in that they are either male or female. The green female flowers have three tepals (i.e. the petals and sepals are indistinguishable), while the male, catkin-like flowers are noticeable by their yellow stamens.

Folklore

Scandinavian mythology features dog's mercury as a sacred herb of the god Odin or Wotan in the Germanic tradition. He crept into Old English as Woden. If the magic of the herb is to be productive, it must be picked only on Woden's day, therefore *Wödnes daeg* or Wednesday. It is interesting that Roman writers identified this god as the equivalent of Mercury.

The common name of dog's mercury may simply signify an herb that is of little worth. Culpeper was markedly dismissive describing it as 'a rank poisonous plant' and that 'there is not a more fatal plant, native of our country, than this'. Indeed, when eaten in large quantities, in the mistaken belief that it is some other herb, fatalities have resulted. On the other hand, there are many anecdotal reports that dogs find it irresistible, devouring the leaves then vomiting profusely. Is this some instinctive way of clearing out the system? From a scientific perspective, the chemical constituent of tri-methylamine seems to be the culprit that causes the poisoning.

Uses

The Roman messenger to the gods, Mercury, was reputed to have discovered the healing properties of this plant – hence the scientific name. Indeed, it was used with therapeutic intentions in ancient times, and its purgative and diuretic effects were well known. Hippocrates recommended it for female complaints. However, as it is extremely poisonous it is difficult to know whether it did more harm than good, although the prescriptions seem to have contained small quantities well mixed with other ingredients such as chicken. It was also used as an anti-syphilitic. Was this because the handsome Mercury did so much travelling around, one wonders?

Wildlife

Dog's mercury is an outstandingly successful survivor. The poisonous leaves fend off nibbling from browsers, such as deer and, given the right shady, damp habitat, it will spread very rapidly. Unfortunately, it can out-compete other more delicate woodland species, some now rare, such as oxlip. Overall, it seems to have little obvious benefit for wildlife, apart from some passing small mammal or bird taking a snack from the seeds. They evidently come to no harm from these. Some ecologists consider dog's mercury to be a problem plant.

It is thought that former coppicing kept it under control, the extra light allowing other species to flourish. It is now so common, however, especially in East Anglian woods, that I have no compunction about removing it from our garden.

Ground-ivy (*Glechoma hederacea*)

Dead-nettle family (Lamiaceae). Perennial. Pollinated by insects, including bees. Propagated by stolon or seed. Edible. Medicinal.

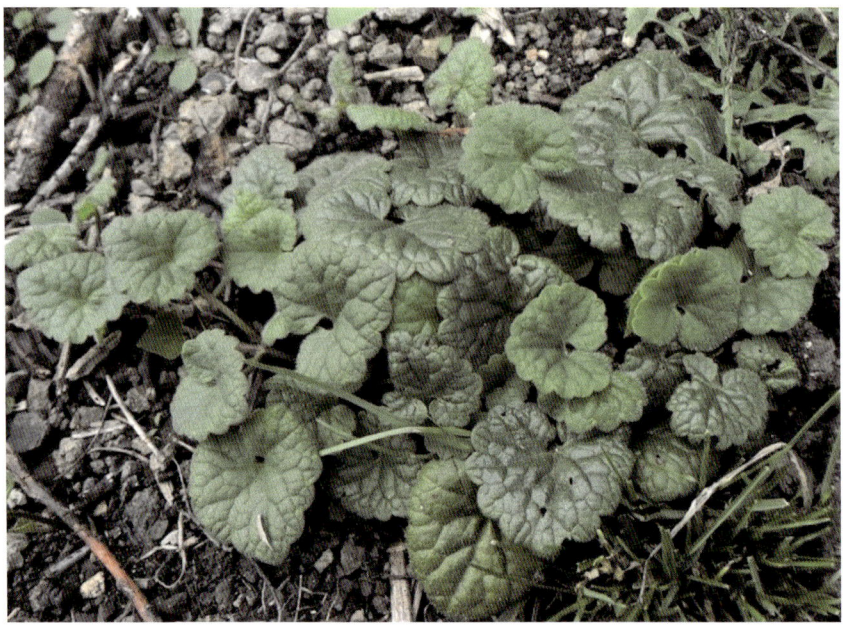

The kidney-shaped leaves of ground-ivy are distinctive and easily recognisable.

By the end of March, the violet-blue flowers of ground-ivy will be appearing, the kidney-shaped, scalloped leaves and long, creeping stems having survived the winter very well. This plant particularly likes our rich, heavy soil and readily appears anywhere, but mostly favouring the many damp, shady places.

Although insects are attracted to ground-ivy, doubtless on account of its pungent aromatic smell, and will pollinate it, the main form of regeneration is via the long stolons. Each node can produce new roots and shoots wherever it touches the ground. So, after a spell of weather that has been too wet or cold for gardening, I can wander outside and discover that the ground-ivy has already formed something of a carpet.

MARCH

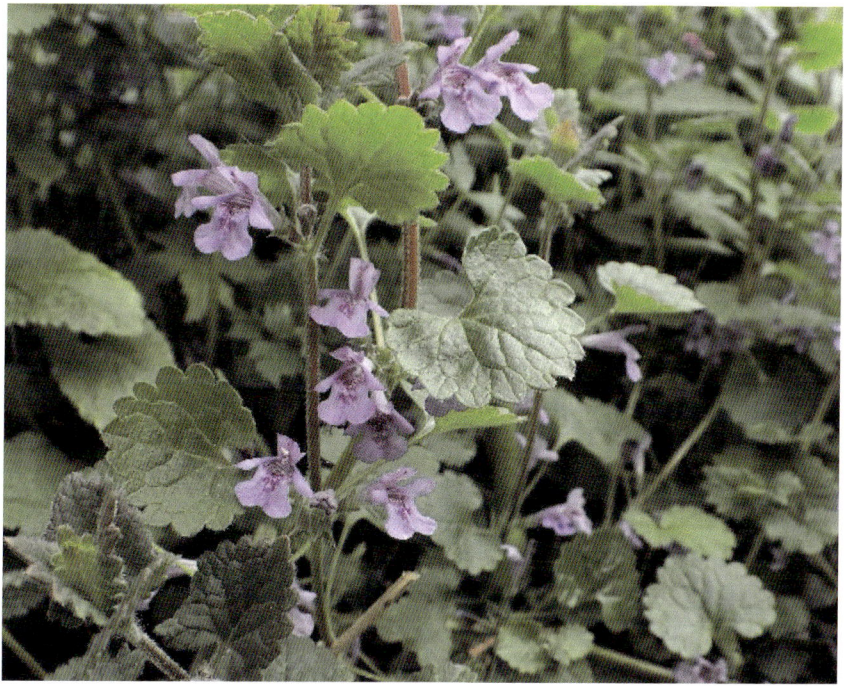

Although small, the flowers of ground-ivy have interesting markings.

Along the square, hairy stem the leaves are in opposite pairs and are dark green or even reddish brown. The hooded flowers appear in small whorls at the leaf axils. Close examination will reveal purple striations on the outside of the tube-like corolla and also within the 'throat'. The lower lip is slightly divided into two 'skirts', with a couple of winged arms either side. If you look very carefully into the hood you will see that it is marked by a white cross. On the outside, the sepal tubes are reddish green with pointed, curved teeth, prickly at the end.

Folklore

According to legend, if you carry ground-ivy in your hand, it will give you protection against assaults from bad fairies! Otherwise much English folklore surrounding this plant has to do with the brewing of beer, as mentioned below.

Uses

Knowing that ground-ivy was once considered to be a valuable medicinal herb, I was surprised not to be able immediately to find it listed in my copy of Culpeper's *Complete Herbal*. After persevering I eventually discovered it under 'alehoof'. Until the reign of Henry VIII, one of its main uses was as a clearing agent and flavouring for beer, hence the common name. At the same time, the plant was often recommended for healing a variety of ailments. John Gerard (1545–1612), an English botanist and author of *Herball*, wrote in the 16th century that it was a good cure for headaches: 'It purgeth the head from the rheumatic humours flowing from the brain.' More recently the flowering tops have been dried and made into snuff for the same purpose. Culpeper prescribed it for tinnitus and deafness: 'The juice dropped into the ear doth wonderfully help the noise and singing of them, and helpeth the hearing which is decayed.' Like many other herbalists, he noted its effectiveness in the healing of wounds and other skin problems: 'It helpeth the itch, scabs, weals, and other breakings out in any part of the body.'

During the 19th century it was promoted as the best herbal remedy for consumption. As it is rich in vitamin C, it may indeed have been helpful. At any rate, there was very good reason to recommend a ground-ivy tisane for coughs and bronchitis. Mrs Maud Grieve (1858–1941) suggested in her book *A Modern Herbal* (1931) that it is not just for coughs and nervous headaches but also for kidney problems and indigestion. The tisane, referred to as 'Gill tea' by country folk, was made from 1 oz/25 g of the herb and 1 pint/570 ml of boiling water, with the addition of a little honey. When cool, the tea could be taken up to four times a day in wine-glass doses.

Although some modern herbalists may still prescribe ground-ivy, there remains a query about its safety as it is known to contain the volatile oil terpene, which, while an antiseptic, is also an irritant. Moreover, if horses have eaten too much of the plant in hay they have become unwell. It is best, therefore, to err on the side of caution and use it only externally. I have discovered that it works even better than dock to soothe nettle stings simply by rubbing in the crushed leaves.

Wildlife

Occasionally large red galls may appear on ground-ivy. These form when a particular species of a tiny ant-like creature, known as a gall wasp, lays its eggs on the plant. The larvae live and feed inside the gall, well protected during their vulnerable stages of development.

Ground-ivy has a clever strategy to persuade bees to visit many flowers, rather than just one or two. An American researcher, E E Southwick, discovered that the amount of available nectar contained in each flower varies greatly, so that the bees keep looking for those that offer the most. In the afternoon they will have to search even more thoroughly for those 'lucky hits' as by then overall quantities will have become reduced. The main reason for this is that nectar is mostly produced at night or in the early hours, so it is easier to find good sources in the morning. By being lured to search for that satisfying supply of nectar, pollination is thereby enhanced.

Primrose (*Primula vulgaris*)

Primrose family (Primulaceae). Semi-evergreen perennial. Pollinated by flies; may self-pollinate. Propagated by seed or division. Edible.

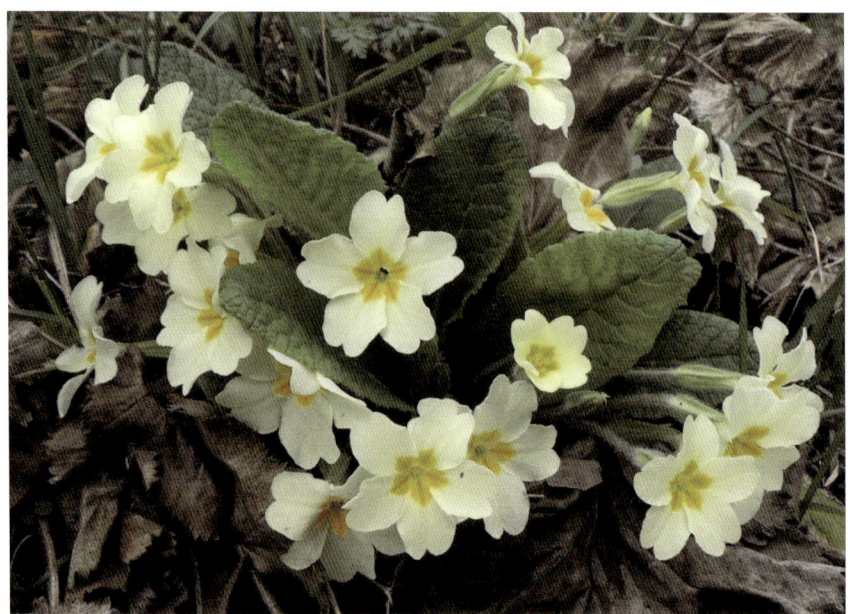

Primroses grow in ready-made posies, adding to their charm.

It is early in the month and already little groups of soft-yellow flowers are opening beside our pond. This is a perfect location for them as the plant thrives well on damp, grassy slopes, although they can also favour open woodland. As I look carefully among the greenery, I see a great many more rosettes of crinkly leaves with tiny buds rising on short stems from the centre. Soon there will be spring's favourite show – a whole bank of primroses. Sadly, this is a rare sight now in the countryside due to excessive picking and, most particularly, digging up of roots. We are truly fortunate that this pretty charmer has decided to establish itself in our garden.

Part of the appeal of the flower is the 'notch' in each of the five petals, giving a frilly effect to the posy. Beneath the flower head you will see that the sepals are joined into a long tube, while further close inspection will reveal the hairs on the flower stalks.

Botanically this is a somewhat unusual plant for there are two distinct kinds of primrose. One has five stamens, known as 'thrum-eyed', while the other has a single stigma, 'pin-eyed'. If you peer into the centre of the flower where the colour deepens you will notice the difference. For fertilisation to occur, there is generally cross-pollination between the two kinds. Since new plants appear very readily in our garden, insects must be busy flying from one type to another, no doubt attracted by the delicate fragrance. Later, each capsule will produce a great many seeds. As an herbaceous perennial, patches of primroses can become well established, flowering year after year.

Cultivated primulas are very popular spring flowers, garden centres showing off their range. However, do spare a thought for their wild cousin. Should it appear unexpectedly, then treasure it. You will be well rewarded.

Folklore

The name 'primrose' comes from the Latin *prima rosa* or first flower of the year, often considered to be the herald of spring as in Beaumont and Fletcher's *Two Noble Kinsmen (Act I, i)*:

> Primrose, first-born child of Ver,
> Merry Spring-time's harbinger.

It is not quite clear why it has been connected with wantonness, but Shakespeare certainly thought of it that way. Laertes advises Ophelia not to take Hamlet's affections too much to heart, but she responds by telling him not to lecture her and to heed his own advice:

> Do not, as some ungracious pastors do,
> Show me the steep and thorny way to heaven,
> Whiles, like a puff'd and reckless libertine,
> Himself the primrose path of dalliance treads …

(Act I, iii)

Perhaps it was simply that young couples would begin to walk out together in spring wandering through country lanes hand in hand. No doubt, a romantically inclined young man would pick a posy of primroses to give to his sweetheart. Otherwise 'wantonness' could be a description of the behaviour of the plant, distributing itself freely here, there and everywhere. Certainly, primroses were used as love charms. Yet at the same time, if they bloomed in winter, this was thought to be an omen of death. It is just as well that my husband and I are not superstitious as we nearly always have one or two plants blooming from November through the coldest days without apparent harm.

The centre of the flowers often contains small orange-brown marks. The story goes that St Peter lost his keys to the gates of Heaven and they dropped to Earth among the primroses. It took him so long to find them that they rusted away, leaving these marks!

For a long time, on the 19th of April, primroses were left by Disraeli's statue in front of Westminster Abbey in London, in remembrance of this famous Prime Minister and in the belief that these were his favourite flowers. The custom was, however, based on a mistake. Queen Victoria had sent a wreath of primroses for Disraeli's funeral with a note attached saying 'his favourite flower', but the 'his' referred not to the Prime Minister but to Queen Victoria's husband, Prince Albert.

Uses

If you want to cheer up a salad with something rather different, then both the leaves and flowers of primroses are edible. Indeed, they are thought to be helpful to people with arthritis.

If a man were to cut himself while working in the fields, he would find a primrose leaf and rub it on the abrasion. At home, the flowers and young leaves would be chopped, heated in lard, allowed to cool and then used to soothe both cuts and chapped hands.

A remedy local to us here in the East of England, made from the dried leaves, has been the one of choice to cure burns.

Soothing a minor burn

Handful primrose leaves, fresh or dried
¼ pint/150 ml linseed oil

Crush the leaves, then thoroughly steep them in the oil until they are soaked through. – Apply to the burn, cover with lint and fix with tape as necessary. Leave for 2 to 3 hours. Repeat until the burn is healed.

Wildlife

Apart from providing nourishment for those insects brave enough to fly during the chilly days of early spring, primroses, along with cowslips, are the main caterpillar food plant of a most beautiful, now rare butterfly – the Duke of Burgundy. Those readers who live near chalk downs or limestone grasslands may have the privilege of spotting these fragile creatures with their characteristic orange, brown and white markings. A sunny, sheltered spot with a profusion of flowers is a likely place.

Common Dog-violet (*Viola riviniana*)

Sweet Violet (*V. odorata*)

Violet family (Violaceae). Herbaceous perennial. Pollinated by flies and bees. Propagated by stolon or seed. Edible.

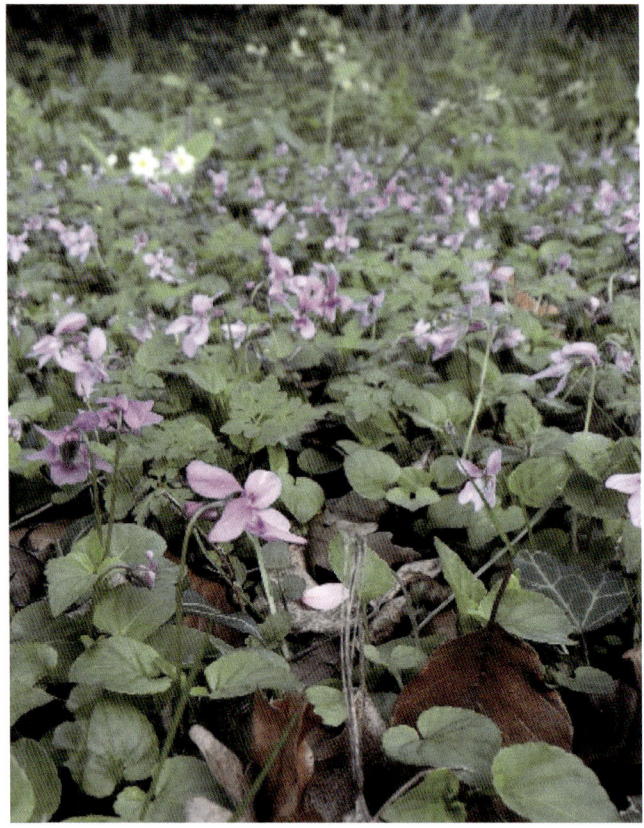

Dog-violets carpet the floor of our small woodland area, where sunlight can filter through the bare branches in the early spring.

There are several native species of violet, difficult to distinguish one from another. The most common is the dog-violet, which spreads itself freely in the dappled shade of woodland and along hedgerows and is a frequent inhabitant of gardens, ours included. The most distinctive feature of the sweet violet, however, is its heady perfume. This is the one which is used in confectionary and cosmetics. It is also noticeable for its long runners which will root themselves at a distance from the parent plant.

There can be slight difference in the colour of the flowers between these two species, the dog-violet tending towards blue rather than violet. Each is occasionally white. The five petals are unequal, two of which are uppermost with the other three pointing downwards. Both have romantically heart-shaped leaves, although you will see that the upper leaves of the sweet kind are often kidney shaped.

The seed-case is an angled, pointed capsule, which when fully ripe splits open into three. Drying may cause it to eject the seeds, often casting its contents widely into the surrounding area.

There is something very curious about the scent of the sweet violet. It contains a chemical that desensitises the nerves in the nose so that the

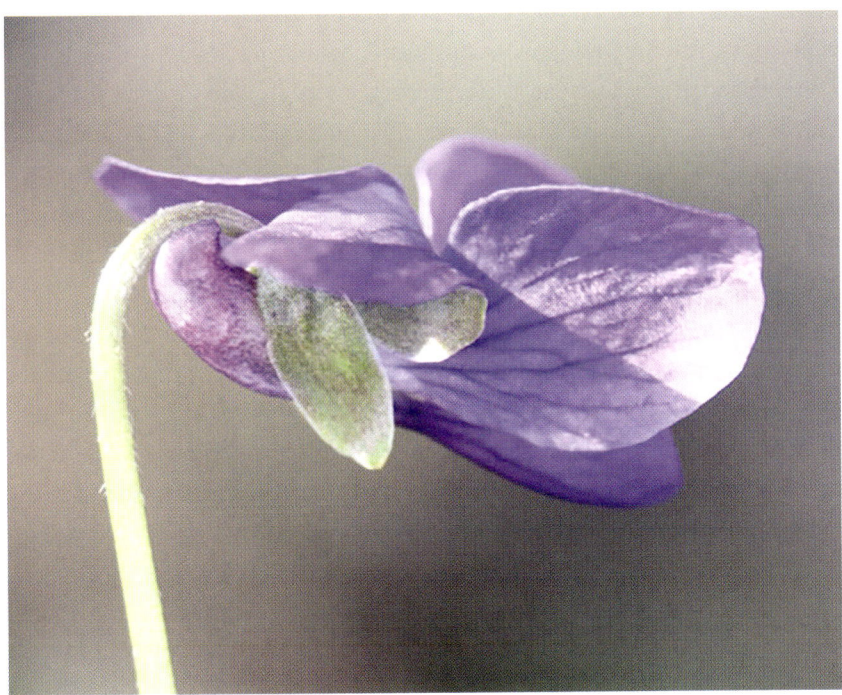

Sweet violet has characteristic blunt sepals. *Photo © NatureSpot/David Nicholls*

perfume can no longer be detected until the receptors recover. It is difficult to imagine the biological purpose for this, except that it could be a way of encouraging pollinating insects to move on to another flower.

Folklore

The Ancient Romans and Greeks considered violets to be the flowers of love. Indeed, the aroma compound in the plant with the name of ionone is derived from *ion*, the Greek word for violet, which in turn comes from Io, a seductive young woman in mythology whom Jupiter transformed into a cow because his wife was so jealous of her – a rather catastrophic way of preserving one's marriage!

In the Middle Ages, the violet was favoured as a strewing herb to keep odours and illnesses at bay. In more recent history, violets have been strongly associated with the French general and emperor Napoléon Bonaparte. When banished to the island of Elba, he promised to return in the violet season. As a result, this became the secret symbol of his supporters. After escaping from the island, he was greeted with violets and was subsequently known as *le père de la violette.* His wife Josephine adored the flower. A locket was found after Napoléon's death that contained a strand of her hair along with a pressed violet. Later in the 19th century during the reign of Queen Victoria, posies of violets became the fashion. Thousands were grown in glass houses at Windsor so that they could be worn at court for formal evening occasions.

Violets also became the gift of choice to present to one's parent on Mothering Sunday. Cards commemorating this day often depict bunches of violets. Rather oddly, towards the end of the 19th century, the perfume of sweet violet was thought to have a deleterious effect on one's voice to the extent that singers would refuse to have them in their dressing rooms. This belief still lingers among some musicians.

Uses

Perhaps on account of the fleeting nature of the scent of the sweet violet, the herb has traditionally been thought to enable sleep. The Greeks made an infusion of it as a cure for insomnia and also to soothe outbursts of anger. The tradition of the calming effect continued for a very long time. The 16th-century herbalist and courtier Roger Ascham recommended the flowers for deep slumber: 'For them that may not sleep for a sickness seethe violets in water and at even let him soke well hys temples, and he shall sleepe well by the grace of God.'

In *The Diary of a Farmer's Wife*, written between 1796 and 97, Anne Hughes relates how on 20th March the first violet was found – 'so later we must get some for the drying for puddings.' These were made if a man came home from market in a bad mood: 'it being a good cure for cross husbands.' To make the pudding, you will need a great many violets, so do not take from the wild. They are easy to grow and make a pleasurable addition to any garden. If you dry them you can use them all year.

Drying the violets

Pick the flower heads as soon as the buds have opened. Stretch muslin over a cake rack and lay the flowers on this, without any overlaps. Put in a place where warm air is freely flowing, but out of sunlight. This will prevent mould from forming. Check frequently until the flowers are crisp and papery. Store in a dark-coloured, air-tight glass jar. If you notice any condensation, remove the flowers and allow to dry for longer. The leaves can be dried similarly, but pick them just before the buds form, on a warm, sunny morning.

Calming violet pudding

This is Anne Hughes's very rich recipe, no doubt successful in sending any irate husband to sleep.

6 handfuls dried sweet violet blossoms

6 eggs

1 tbsp clear honey

juice 1 lemon

cream

'You take of the dried blossoms 6 handfuls and boil gently till verrie tender, then chop verrie fine; next mix with 6 eggs whipt to a froth with a big spoonful of bee honey and the juice of a lemon. Put in a greased dish and bake till set, then chop some of the dried violets verrie fine and sprinkle atop, and eat it with plenty of cream.'

Soothing violet tea

Violet flowers have traditionally been thought to be good for all inflammations, especially of the lungs. This rather seems to contradict the belief that the perfume was bad for the voice. However, Gerard says in his *Herball*: 'They take away the hoarseness of the chest, the ruggednesse of the winde-pipe and jaws, and take away thirst.' This time-honoured practice continued into the 20th century. As recently as 1977, Godfrey Baseley in his *Country Compendium* lists violet tea as a remedy for bronchitis and catarrh. It is very easy to make a quick tisane, especially if you have some dried flowers to hand. Besides coughs, this tea can also soothe headaches.

1 heaped tsp dried sweet violet flowers
275 ml/½ pint water
1 tsp honey

Put the violets into a mug, boil up the water then pour over the flowers. Allow to steep for 5 minutes. Stir in the honey.

Wildlife

Violets are crucial to the survival of the elegant fritillary butterflies as their caterpillars use them as their main source of food. These beautiful insects are becoming increasingly rare due to loss of suitable habitats – especially the high brown, lover of hot sunshine, whose caterpillar is almost exclusively dependent upon the common dog-violet. The delicately spotted pearl-bordered fritillary is also on the red endangered list, but at least its caterpillar has the choice of several violet species, all of which provide it with essential nutrients.

APRIL

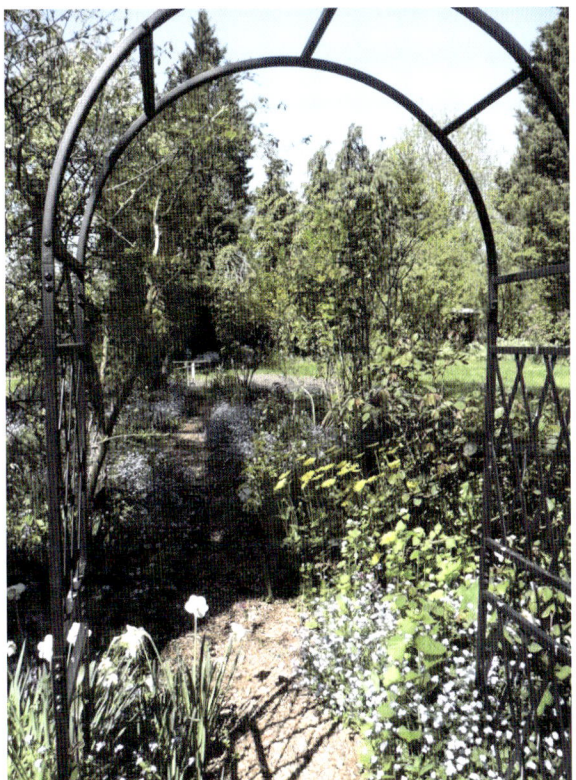

Self-planted forget-me-nots mingle freely with garden plants alongside this path.

The drabness of winter is now only a distant memory as April brings with it an explosion of life and colour. The wild blackthorn bushes in our hedges, until recently just uninspiring prickly sticks, now produce a dazzling display of white blossom along the bare branches. How fresh the perfume is!

The early bees are relishing the new abundance of nectar from our flowering shrubs and small plants. We have a cultivated dead-nettle, *Lamium maculatum*, with pretty, mauve-pink flowers and a silvery stripe down each leaf, now fully out, which provides excellent ground cover. This is a particular favourite of our bees and they spend much time crawling methodically into each hooded flower head. The wild dead-nettle, or 'weed', is also especially attractive to them and I allow these to flourish here and there in patches by hedges. Bees are suffering a dramatic decline due to habitat loss and pesticides. How important it is, therefore, to provide for their needs in our gardens!

By the middle of the month our little meadow is a real picture, the cowslips nodding their heads with each gentle breeze, now making a better show than the primroses. When we arrived here some twenty-five years ago there were only three. By staking them out with protective sticks as soon as the leaves appeared and mowing round them, they have been able to reproduce and now number well over 150. In early April we tread carefully over the grass, also watching out for the glossy leaves of pyramidal orchids that thrive in the damp places by the pond. Here again we indicate their presence with a stick. I must confess that I helped them to arrive here. In the late summer, the grass in the village churchyard is mown, and one year I noticed that some of the orchids, which are normally left to flourish, had been accidentally cut. I picked them up and placed them in a bucket of water on our meadow, optimistically hoping that their seeds might disperse. The following year we were excited to see that this had been a success, just a few pink pyramids appearing in the grass. It is surprising how little help nature needs to flourish.

By leaving areas of the meadow unmown in spring, simply creating pathways where we can walk, many other wild flowers have now joined the cowslips and orchids, including quite a carpet of blue speedwell, which, along with the self-seeded honesty in our flower borders, is a real magnet to the orange-tip butterflies. This led me to wonder what in our garden had fed the caterpillars of this unmistakable, cheerful insect, and some research indicated the importance of 'the flowers and seed pods of tall crucifers', or flowers with four petals, such as lady's smock. Indeed, this plant also flourishes on our meadow, in the same damp area as the orchids, liking our heavy clay soil. Boggy meadows are now extremely scarce, so all the more reason to care for ours and not be tempted to turn it into a lawn. Another food plant, along with honesty, is hedge mustard, a summer-flowering weed which I am now caring for in my new wildflower garden, although modest in appearance with its somewhat straggly stems and insignificant yellow petals. More attractive, with its heart-shaped leaves and starry white flowers, is jack-by-the hedge, or garlic mustard, which favours shady corners (see May p. 90). Now that I understand the importance of these members of the cabbage family for the orange-tip butterfly, it is well worth encouraging them.

With the mixture of sun and showers, other weeds are now pushing up at a phenomenal rate and I can scarcely keep up with them. It is difficult deciding which to pull up and which to keep, bearing in mind the needs of our garden plants as well as those of the wildlife – not to mention human aesthetics! What I try to achieve is a good balance.

Blackthorn (*Prunus spinosa*)

Rose family (Rosaceae). Deciduous shrub or small tree. Pollinated by insects. Propagated by sucker and seed. Sour edible fruit.

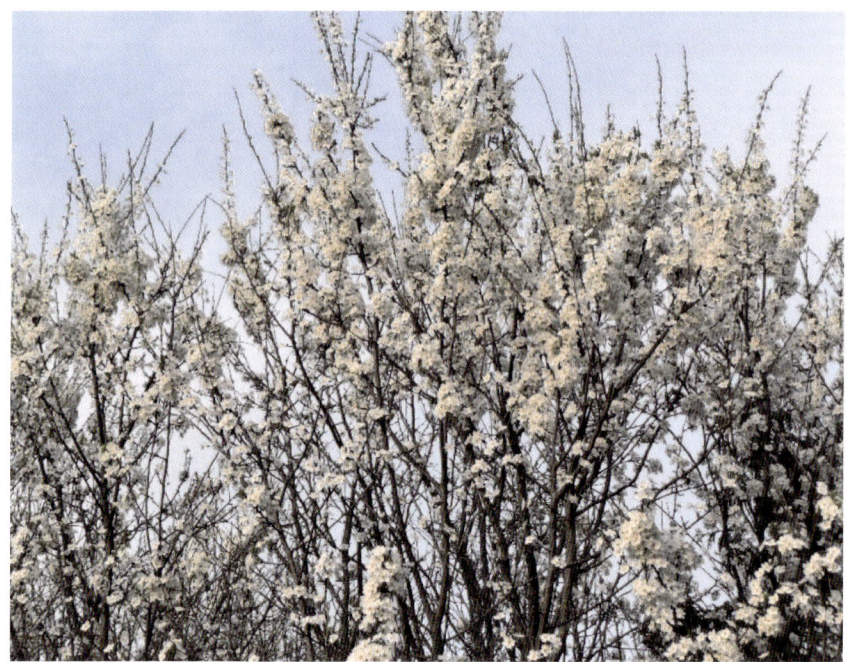

Blackthorn flowers adorn the bare branches.

THE FLOWERS

These early hedgerow flowers of spring, brought on by a warm spell, look almost surprised to be here, appearing along the spiny branches of blackthorn shrubs well before the leaves push through. Having planted themselves around the far side of our pond, the startlingly white blossom is reflected in the water, justifying the country name 'lady of pearls'. Despite its beauty, I have to classify blackthorn as a weed, simply because it propagates itself most effectively by sending suckers under the ground which then pop up as new plants. If these are not dug out a thicket will quickly form. From a wildlife perspective it is a much-valued shrub as small birds can find safe nesting places among its prickly branches.

If you have a blackthorn you wish to keep, check regularly within several metres of its base. You might notice first of all an insignificant stick poking up from the ground, which might be brown if already established or green if new. In winter you will see the alternate bud points of the leaves, which, when out, are oval with toothed edges. Give it a tug and you will be aware that the base runs off at a right-angle just below the soil towards the nearest blackthorn shrub. You can now dig it up or not.

Folklore

Although a harbinger of spring, our weather, especially here in East Anglia, can still be chilly as the 'blackthorn winds' blow from the north-east. Country folk talk of the 'blackthorn winter', a cold snap that invariably follows as the flowers fade. Do not put away winter clothes just yet.

It is very unlucky to bring blackthorn blossom into the house or wear it in a buttonhole. It is a mystery why exactly this superstition has evolved. One recent theory is that a scratch from the sharp thorns could conceivably cause blood poisoning. There is a story of a small child innocently bringing a posy of blackthorn blossom into the school room, only to be met by an irate teacher who immediately threw it out of the window much to the child's distress. Here in East Anglia it is supposed to provoke a death in the family or, in Lincolnshire, somewhat less calamitous, foretell of broken limbs. Perhaps it is an example of preventative superstition: if you do not bring the flowers indoors, then such disasters will not occur.

It is true that the thorns are long, sharp and extremely hard, and can cause a nasty gash. These are known to puncture tyres quite easily if branches are left on the ground after pruning. The Crown of Thorns placed on Jesus' head was reputed to be made of blackthorn. The thorns were certainly used in black magic to stab wax images, and a witch's walking stick was very likely made from the wood.

Yet, in Wales the thorns had a more positive aspect as objects to foretell the future. A young woman in love would throw the sharp points into the

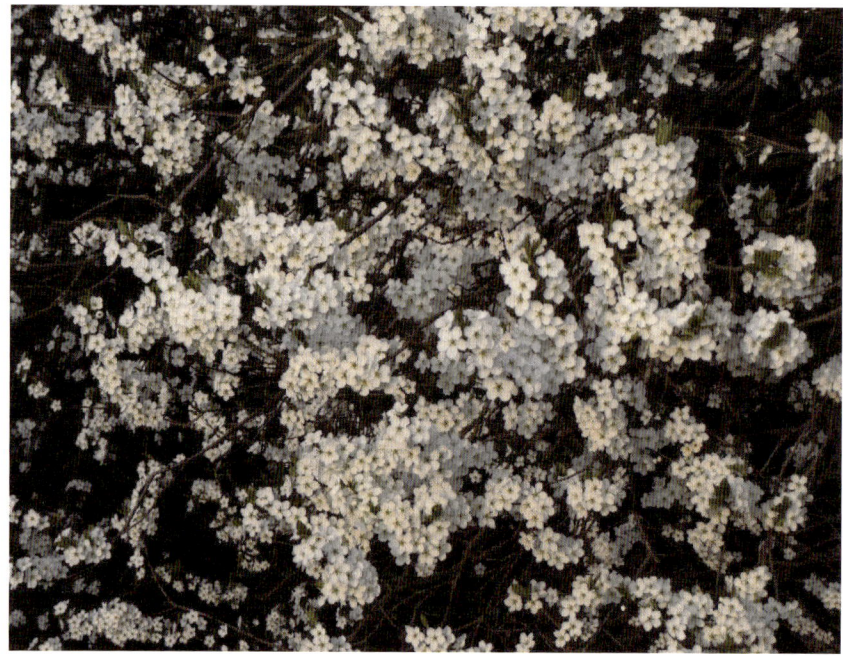

The pearly white blossom of blackthorn is a real joy in the spring.

Silver Well at Llanblethian in Glamorgan. She would wish fervently that they would float for this would indicate that her lover would be faithful. Moreover, if they whirled around a cheerful nature was most likely. Stubbornness, however, would be suggested if the thorns sank a bit, and if they sank totally then, alas, that would mean infidelity. I could not resist testing this out myself by throwing some thorns into our pond and watching carefully. Unfortunately, they all sank without trace!

Uses

Blackthorn makes an excellent protective hedge and can be seen lining a great many roads and lanes. The wood of the shrub is very dense and therefore has traditionally made fine walking sticks and riding crops, looking splendid when polished to bring out the grain and knots. The thorns were sometimes hardened further by heating in the oven to make into fishhooks.

Infusions from the flowers have a mildly laxative and diuretic effect. In *A New Family Herbal*, published in 1810, Robert Thornton describes this tea as 'a safe and easy purge'. However, such remedies no longer feature in modern herbal medicine. The deep-blue, bitter fruit on the other hand is famous for its medicinal properties and is well known for the making of sloe gin (see 'October' for recipe, p. 302).

In the 19th century, dishonest merchants would dry the leaves and use them as a cheap way of filling out packets of tea. *Punch* magazine in the 1870s jokingly made a pun on the common name of the fruit describing this practice as 'sloe poison'! The Irish in some desperation smoked the leaves as a substitute for tobacco, but it is unclear whether there was any narcotic effect.

Wildlife

Blackthorn is an extremely important native shrub for the survival of a wide variety of insects. Well over 100 macro-moths and more than 50 micro-moths, also sawflies, beetles, bugs and aphids, use it as a food plant. Sadly, the unsympathetic flailing of hedges in the countryside has led to the loss of many of these insects. The brown hairstreak butterfly, for example, is now reduced to small areas of Devon and Wales.

One truly spectacular survivor, however, is the emperor moth. When extended, its wings reach to 60 mm/2¼ inches. Strangely, the female flies at night and the male by day and can be observed during April and May. There are two prominent 'eyes' on both the forewings and hindwings of each, but the female is mainly grey, while the male has bright orange hindwings. The caterpillars are green with yellow spots within black bands.

Another attractive moth that might find its way into your garden if you have any blackthorn is the brimstone. As its name implies, it is mainly yellow with reddish-brown markings on the edges of the forewings. In favourable habitats there can be up to three generations in a season, with adults flying any time between April and October.

While blackthorn can be difficult to keep under control, do think twice before cutting it down and you will find that many interesting invertebrates will have a chance of thriving in your garden.

Cowslip (*Primula veris*)

Primrose family (Primulaceae). Perennial. Pollinated by bees and butterflies. May self-pollinate. Propagated by seed. Edible leaves and flowers.

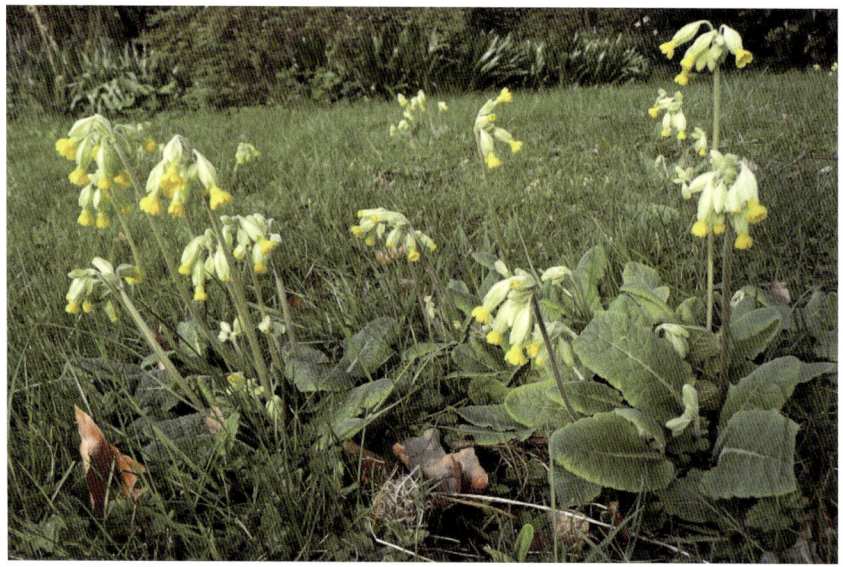

By carefully mowing around the leaf rosettes in the lawn, we are rewarded with a joyful display of cowslips.

'Surely, you can't include cowslips in a book on weeds!' I hear you exclaim, the belief being that the appearance of this flower would be a very welcome addition to any garden border. However, the fact remains that, should a rosette of the leaves establish itself in certain lawns in the early spring, it would be forked out or sprayed to extinction straight away by certain zealous gardeners, without any questioning as to what it might turn into. A 'perfect' lawn is seen to be one composed of grass only, without any intruders at all. If such a person had owned our lawn, there would be no display of those deep-yellow, nodding heads, one which we enjoy every April. We were delighted when the seeds travelled there from our small meadow, my husband carefully mowing around them. It is my job to place a marker by the leaf rosettes, so he knows which areas to avoid.

At first, the wrinkly leaves are tightly coiled before unrolling and flattening out. They are very similar to those of primroses but a little shorter and more rounded. As the plant matures, the stalk pushes up from the centre, the flowers forming at the top from a single point to create a cluster falling mostly to one side. There can be as many as thirty, or more.

The five petals are united together to create a tube, which fits into a long, green, pouched calyx. Each petal is notched, giving the edge of the flower an appealing, frilly appearance, while the delicate perfume adds to its charm.

Folklore

The Latin name *veris,* from *ver* for spring, reminds us how much the plant is associated with that season. As for the common name of 'cowslip', this may be derived from the unlovely Old English term for cow dung, *cuslyppe*, perhaps because the plants tended to establish themselves in meadows inhabited by cows. Mrs Grieve had a different idea in her *Modern Herbal* of 1931. She thought it was a corruption of 'cow's leek' from the Anglo Saxon *leac*, or plant. At any rate, it has nothing whatever to do with a cow's lip. In fact, cows dislike the plants as they can cause colic.

Other common names were in general use when this perennial used to grow in great profusion. The clusters of flowers were likened to a bunch of keys, hence 'key flower' or 'keys of heaven' and 'herb Peter'. The story underlying such ideas is that St Peter accidentally dropped the keys of heaven and the place where they fell was the spot the first cowslips grew.

At the base of each of the five yellow petals is an orange-red spot. In literature these were sometimes likened to freckles and the belief was that they held magic powers that were good for the complexion. Such a tradition was alive in Shakespeare's day as we see from *A Midsummer Night's Dream*, (*Act II, i*):

> The cowslips tall her pensioners be;
> In their gold coats spots you see,
> These be rubies, fairy favours
> In those freckles live their savours.

At a time when the plant grew in profusion in meadows, children used to pick them and make the flower heads into balls called 'tisty-tosties'. A rhyme would be chanted:

> Tisty-tosty tell me true
> Who shall I be married to?

A child would then toss a ball in the air and chant the names of boys and girls. When it touched the ground, the name being called out at the time would become the future marriage partner. Such games can no longer be played as, sadly, the ploughing up of ancient meadows and intensive use of herbicides in fields and along verges, especially between the 1950s and '80s, caused this once common plant to become a rarity. It used to be said that you'll only hear a nightingale where there are cowslips. Nowadays you will neither hear the one nor see the other, except perhaps in reserves. Is this really the countryside that we wish to leave for our descendants?

Uses

Cowslips once grew in such profusion that the flowers were used to make a popular country wine. This is no longer possible, but there is no reason why you should not make use of some of the young leaves, picked carefully from your garden so as not to destroy the rosette. They have traditionally been added to salads, as were the flowers, both being edible. The leaves have a slightly bitter taste due to saponin. Indeed, the leaves are thought to have sedative properties, having a calming effect, so the tisane is still recommended to reduce stress and as a painkiller.

As for the fairy power of the 'freckles', Culpeper certainly believed in it as an aid to the complexion: 'The ointment or distilled water of it adds beauty, or at least restores it when it is lost.' He thought that the flowers were more effective than the leaves and suggested that an ointment be made from them when dried. For wrinkles and sunburn, he prescribed a salve by mixing the leaves with hog's grease. Today, an unguent for the complexion from the juice together with linseed oil is still thought to be effective. The leaves can also be used to make a tisane.

A tisane for the nerves

A few fresh young cowslip leaves
a little honey

Tear the leaves and place in a mug, then pour on boiling water. Allow to infuse for at least 5 minutes. Stir in the honey. ♦ Take when feeling stressed or overexcited, and as an aid to refreshing sleep. Alternatively, allow to cool and pat on to the face to assist with a lovely complexion.

Wildlife

Like most wild flowers and 'weeds', cowslips are a very valuable food source for bees and butterflies. Along with primroses, the plants provide nourishment for the caterpillars of the Duke of Burgundy butterfly, now very scarce and found only occasionally on chalk downland. If you are in such an area on a sunny day in spring and where cowslips are growing, look out for the aerial displays of this attractive insect, with its brown, yellow and white markings.

Daisy (*Bellis perennis*)

Daisy family (Asteraceae). Perennial. Pollinated by insects; or may self-pollinate later. Propagated by seed. Edible leaves. Medicinal.

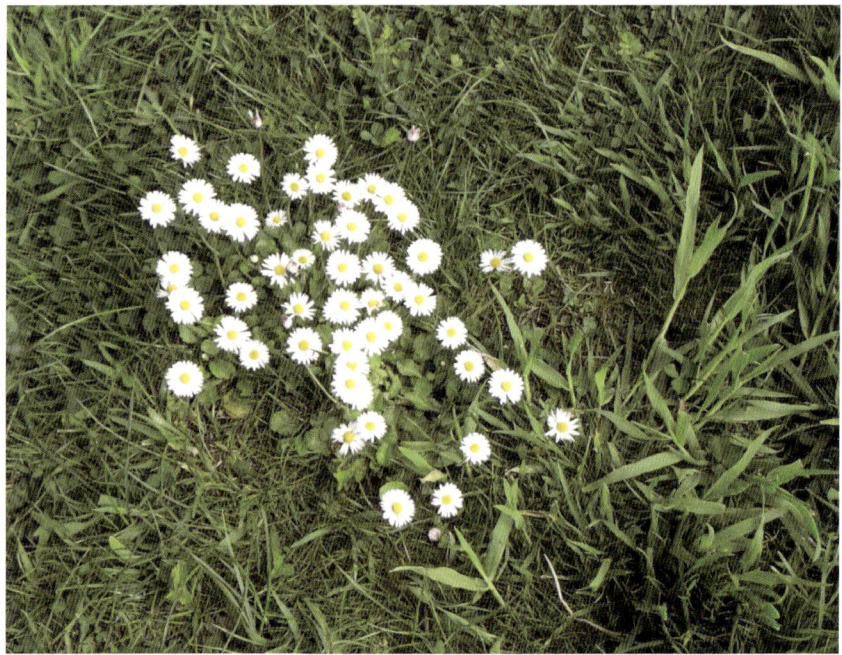

Daisies may be ubiquitous, but they can brighten up an otherwise dull lawn and provide nutritious seeds for birds.

This plant, the bane of those who insist on a perfect grass lawn, preferably mown into stripes, was nevertheless given the name *Bellis* on account of its striking beauty. To my mind, a lawn that sparkles with this pretty 'weed' is infinitely more interesting and attractive than a carpet of plain green. Yet many gardeners insist on waging war on daisies.

It is in fact two flowers in one on a single sturdy stalk. The white, sometimes pink-tinged, petals form the outer flower, while the inner one is composed of a cluster of bright-yellow, minute tubular petals. The flat rosette of leaves is familiar in any lawn. The roots will creep out to form new plants, each suppressing the grass beneath. The leaves are spoon shaped and slightly hairy.

Folklore

The common name daisy is derived from the Old English *daes eage*, or 'day's eye', referring to its habit of opening at dawn to welcome the day, the pinkish tinge redolent of the sky at sunrise. Geoffrey Chaucer (1343–1400) wrote fervently about this ordinary little plant in his Prologue to 'The Legend of Good Women', saying most touchingly: 'That blissful sighte softeneth al my sorwe'. I have to agree! A lawn dotted with daisies most certainly lifts the spirits.

The Celts associated the daisy with the innocence of new-born babies. In Scotland it was strongly connected with children and their habit of making daisy chains and thus given the name 'bairnwort'. In other parts of the country, especially the South West, these chains were considered to be protective; as long as children were wearing them, they would not be kidnapped by fairies! I clearly remember slitting daisy stalks with a fingernail and pushing another one through, and so on, to form necklaces or tiaras. A game played by older children was to pull off the petals one by one, each time chanting '*He loves me*' followed by '*He loves me not*', the final petal giving the verdict.

Another traditional name was 'bruisewort' after the ointment made to heal the wounds and bruises of Crusaders. Herbalists still recommend a healing salve made from the leaves and flowers.

Uses

The leaves contain bitter agents, flavonoids and essential oils, which, when eaten fresh, will stimulate the metabolism and give one a welcome boost. Equally, a tea made from the leaves will have a similar effect. This can also be used as a gargle to alleviate coughs, catarrh and sinusitis or, if dabbed on the skin, will help to cure any blemishes. Even more effective is to steep the flowers and leaves in water, as follows:

A clear skin

2 daisy plants
1.25 litres/2 pints water

Chop the leaves and flowers and stir into the water. Leave to steep overnight at room temperature. Strain and bottle. ♦ Dab the skin three times a day with the flower water until the blemishes disappear.

Daisy salve

This is a traditional recipe for soothing cuts, bruises and stiff joints.
100 g/4 oz fresh daisy leaves and flowers
275 ml/½ pint sunflower oil
25 g/1 oz beeswax, grated

Chop the leaves and flowers and put in a pan with the oil. The oil should cover the daisies. Add more if necessary. Cook gently over a low heat for about 20 minutes until the oil becomes coloured with the plant material. Stir in the beeswax and allow to melt fully, then scoop out the plant pieces. ♦ Pour into a clean jar. The mixture will solidify into a salve as it cools. Tip: To test the required consistency, spoon a drop or two of the melted mixture into cold water. If it forms into balls, then you have a thick salve. If it spreads over the surface, it will probably be too thin and you need to add more beeswax.

Wildlife

Unlike other members of the Asteraceae family, or flowers with multiple petals, the seeds of daisies are not carried away on 'parachutes' but simply drop nearby. However, being rich in oil, they are much sought after by ants and birds, both of which disperse them efficiently.

Dandelion (*Taraxacum officinale*)

Daisy family (Asteraceae). Perennial. Pollinated by insects, especially bees; or may self-pollinate later. Propagated by seed and root cuttings. Edible leaves.

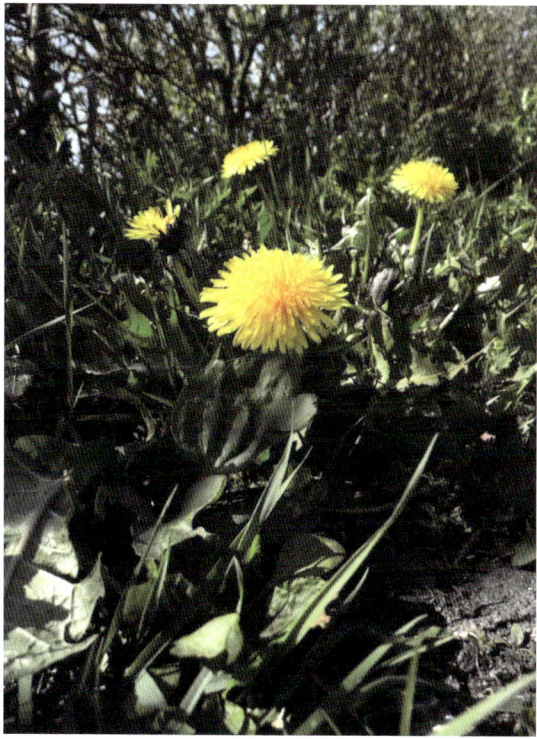

Dandelions can look very cheerful on a sunny spring day and make an attractive addition to a garden.

Its golden, multi-petalled flower heads are a joy in spring, brightening the verges on dull days. However, in many gardens it is not welcome. In fact, it is my husband's most unwanted weed. If he sees one anywhere near our garden, he will immediately dig out the long tap root with his penknife. There is some justification for his personal vendetta against this plant, as, like the daisy, the leaves form into a basal rosette discouraging the growth of the lawn grass underneath and, moreover, if you fail to remove the entire root, any small piece will produce yet another plant. In addition, seed production is prolific with around 180 per head, each attached to a minute parachute which will be blown by the wind, giving it the opportunity to plant itself elsewhere. As long as the weather is mild, it can carry on flowering and producing seeds for many months, ultimately establishing itself as a perennial.

In fact, its method of reproduction is curious. While bees and other insects enjoy its nectar, they do not act as fertilisers as the seeds are formed without the need for this. This means that there is no intermingling of genetic material from two plants, so that if there are any changes to the DNA, i.e. by mutation, they will be passed on to all the offspring, leading to many different strains of dandelion. Generally, however, distinctive features are the multitude of fine yellow petals, the downturned bracts and the jagged leaves with deeply cut edges. The smooth stem will yield a milky sap if broken. Interestingly, dandelions exhale ethylene gas that will stunt the growth of other plants nearby.

Folklore

The common name appears to come from the French *dent de lion*, 'tooth of lion', most probably because of the teeth-like indentations of the leaves. At any rate, it was the plant of the spring goddess, Brigid, who later became St Bridget in Christian tradition. The connection seems to have been the milky sap as she was sometimes believed to have tended cattle.

Children who have grown up in the countryside, or with a garden, will be familiar with the dandelion's 'clock' seed head. The number of puffs it takes to blow the fluffy seeds away will tell you the time! You should note which way the seeds fly as they are indicating to you the route to take to seek your fortune. The flowers also act as useful weather vanes as the petals close before rain and open with the sun.

Uses

Despite dandelion's reputation as a persistent weed, the plant is in fact extremely valuable medicinally and safe to use. The folk names of 'pissabed' or 'tiddlebeds' are candidly descriptive of its diuretic properties and it is therefore advisable not to take the plant before going to sleep! However, for patients with some sort of oedema, such as swollen ankles, it is the ideal remedy. Diuretic drugs tend to deplete potassium from the body and, as a result, can exacerbate any current heart problems; but dandelion is abundant in this mineral and therefore naturally replaces any loss. Other minerals present in the plant include copper and iron, which are helpful to people suffering from anaemia.

Vitamin content is also rich. Indeed, vitamin A is higher in dandelions than in carrots, contributing to good vision. Vitamins B, C and D are also present in useful amounts. Both the leaf and root, if made into a tea and drunk regularly, or dabbed on to the skin, will help to relieve complaints such as eczema.

The milky sap offers further healing ingredients and is well known for its ability to remove warts and age spots. Simply apply directly to the area needing treatment.

The inulin available in the root, particularly in the autumn, is a soluble fibre that will help to increase the beneficial bacteria in the gut. It is thereby good for the health of the colon. The bitter glycocides of taraxacin, mostly present in the spring, will stimulate the digestive system and give a boost to the appetite. The root has also been used for the treatment of jaundice and gall-stones and to prepare a tonic for the liver.

So next time you dig up this tenacious weed, rather than throw it away, just think about how you might use it profitably. Here are some pointers.

Salade de pissenlit

Despite this rather unlovely French name, salads made from the young dandelion leaves, preferably picked before flowering, are extremely health giving. The taste is slightly bitter, rather like chicory, but these salads were very popular in Victorian times. Indeed, dandelions were specially grown in glass houses in winter for use as a lettuce substitute. Adding parsley will increase the iron and vitamin A content still further, while the lemon juice will add to the vitamin C.

Handful young dandelion leaves
2 tbsp olive oil
1 tbsp lemon juice
sprig parsley, finely chopped

Wash the leaves and arrange on a plate. Make up the dressing by whisking together the oil and lemon juice. Dress the salad and sprinkle on the parsley.

Dent-de-lion stew

We are not always as efficient with shopping as we would like to be, and sometimes the fridge is bare of vegetables, with nothing ready on the allotment. Dandelion leaves are therefore a good standby, especially in spring, and are very tasty cooked like spinach in a little butter. Mrs Beeton appreciated their value as a vegetable and recommended the following 'stew'.

225 g/½ lb dandelion leaves
25 g/1 oz butter
1 round tsp flour
3 tbsp vegetable stock (you can use the dandelion water)

Wash the leaves carefully, then chop. Put into a steamer and cook until soft. ♦ Melt the butter in a pan, stir in the flour, then gradually add the stock to make a sauce. Add the dandelion leaves and heat through.

Detox tea

This tea, made from fresh, young dandelion leaves, through its diuretic action, is marvellous for clearing the blood and lymph. It also benefits the eyesight and the skin and will help to alleviate urinary tract infections.

2 tsp chopped young dandelion leaves
275 ml/½ pint boiling water
honey

Pour on the water and allow to infuse for at least 5 minutes. Sweeten with a little honey.

Wildlife

A special delight of my childhood was the discovery of hairy caterpillars. I would keep them in jam jars as pets and watch their progress with fascination. These days, sadly, it is rare indeed to find a hairy caterpillar. However, you can increase the chance of this by allowing dandelions to flourish along the bottoms of walls and hedges. With luck the white ermine moth will set up residence and lay its eggs here. In summer you may spot the caterpillar feeding. It has brown hairs and a distinctive reddish stripe along its back. You can boost the odds by allowing dock, sorrel and stinging nettles to grow as these are all good food sources for the caterpillars.

As soon as dandelions come into flower, they will attract both honey and wild bees. The *Andrena* species, those that nest in holes in the ground, are particularly fond of dandelion nectar. Strangely, you may see goldfinches attack the flowers and tear them up. This is particularly odd because they love the seeds. It is as if they are unable to wait long enough for the seeds to form!

Red Dead-nettle (*Lamium purpureum*)

White Dead-nettle (*L. album*)

Dead-nettle family (Lamiaceae). *L. purpureum*: annual. Pollinated by insects, especially bees. Propagated by stolon and seed. Medicinal. *L. album*: perennial. Pollinated by insects, especially bees. Propagated by rhizome and seed. Edible flowers. Medicinal.

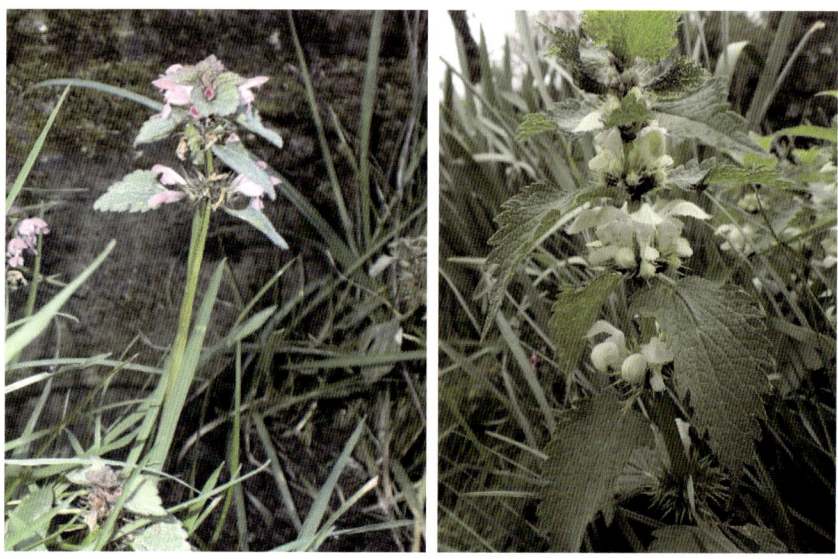

Both white and red dead-nettles are very attractive to bees. The edible flowers of white dead-nettle have sweet nectar, enjoyed by country children and bumble bees alike.

It is the white dead-nettle which seems to favour our garden, although the red dead-nettle is also common. Country folk often refer to the white variety as 'archangel', but it is unclear how the plant acquired such an exalted name. It may have something to do with the colour, white being associated with angels, or the shape of the flower, which has a hooded upper lobe, a lower one bent backwards and two smaller side lobes. The image of an angelic figure looking down from heaven could perhaps be created from these elements. Therapeutically it has a number of protective qualities, further reasons to connect the plant with a guardian angel.

The flowers encircle the square stem just above the leaf axils. Although they first appear in spring, they continue into the autumn. The leaves are very nettle-like – heart-shaped, pointed and serrated – but without the stinging hairs, hence the name 'dead-nettle'. Indeed, it is often found intermingling with stinging nettles. Could this be one of nature's clever defensive ploys? Certainly, it seems that this edible plant manages to protect itself successfully in this way. Despite this, children have often plucked the flowers to suck out the sweet nectar.

White dead-nettle is a perennial with creeping underground stems which readily form other plants. It favours semi-shade and likes disturbed ground. Therefore, if you have been digging over a border, you may well find this plant establishing itself.

If either plant has arrived, this could be an indication for the mat-forming garden plant *Lamium maculatum*, which is most attractive with its silver-striped leaves and purple flowers. Moreover, it gives excellent ground cover. It will also reduce the time you need to spend weeding!

Should you find that you have to pull up some of your dead-nettles, then put them on your compost heap as they will add significantly to the nutrients and help to enrich it.

Folklore

Perhaps because white dead-nettle was believed to have angelic qualities, it then became associated with protection against evil spirits and witchcraft. At any rate, the root was chewed during the Great Plague in an effort to fend off the disease. There was a further belief that an angel had appeared in a dream telling of the plant's efficacy.

Uses

On a more realistic level dead-nettle can be considered to be one of the most precious herbs for women. As long ago as in the 17th century, the herbalist Nicholas Culpeper had discovered that the flowers could 'stay the whites' or help to control vaginal discharge brought on by infection. The tannins contained in the plant, which have a beneficial astringent action, are also responsible for keeping bleeding in check and can therefore ease heavy periods or promote their regulation. Modern herbalists still find dead-nettle therapeutically useful in these ways.

This ability to keep loss of fluids under control can be applied equally to disorders of the intestine, alleviating diarrhoea and the cramps associated with that. The herb is also suitable for respiratory ailments, especially if these involve streaming colds and catarrh.

If people accidentally hurt themselves while out in the countryside, dead-nettle might well come to the rescue in the form of a poultice quickly made from chewed-up leaves placed on the cut, bruise, sting or splinter. This is quite safe as both the flowers and leaves of either variety can be eaten in salads, and the leaves, cooked like spinach, are good as a stand-by vegetable. A dead-nettle salve may also be prescribed for piles or varicose veins. You can make this in the same way as Daisy Salve (see p. 44).

Fortunately, dead-nettle has a long-flowering period. You can also dry the herb for use in winter by hanging up the bunches in a warm and airy place until they become brittle. Then remove the leaves and flowers from the stems and crumple them up before storing in air-tight jars.

Dead-nettle douche or compress

For the best effect, make this good and strong.
1 large handful flowering dead-nettle tops
570 ml/1 pint boiling water
Pour the water over the herb and leave for at least 10 minutes. Allow to cool, then strain before applying as a douche. ♦ This also works well as a compress. Soak a cloth in the hot liquid and lay on the affected area. Repeat frequently.

Note: If the condition fails to improve within a few days, then see a physician.

Archangel jelly

This is a very special children's treat which employs the naturally sweet flowers of white dead-nettle. Heating the wine will of course burn off the alcohol!

20 white dead-nettle flowers

5 gelatine leaves (or 3 level tsp crystals)

570 ml/1 pint sparkling white wine

125 g/4 oz caster sugar

1 tbsp rosewater

cream to serve

Wash the flowers carefully and spread out to dry. Meanwhile soak the gelatine leaves in cold water for a couple of minutes. ♦ Heat a quarter of the wine with the sugar in a pan over a medium heat, stirring throughout. When the sugar has dissolved add the gelatine allowing it to melt. Take off the stove and stir in the rest of the wine, the rosewater and the flowers. ♦ Pour the mixture into a pretty mould that is sparingly oiled. Put in the fridge until set (several hours). Turn out and serve with cream.

Wildlife

Country children not only love to suck the sweet nectar of the flowers, they may also in springtime search among dead-nettle leaves under a sunny wall or hedge in the hope of finding a 'woolly bear', the hairy caterpillar of the garden tiger moth. This has long dark hairs along its back, with a red patch at the front, continuing underneath to cover its many feet. *Lamium album* is one of the food plants of this caterpillar. The spectacular moth itself has mottled brown and white upper wings and is red beneath with black spots. You are fortunate indeed if you have this marvellous creature living in your garden! The leaves are also liked by the wolf spider for sunning itself.

Long-tongued insects, especially bumble bees and mason bees, eagerly seek out dead-nettle flowers for their sweet nectar. While these assist in pollination, it is the ants that scatter the 'nutlets', or fruits, so ensuring that the plants will take root elsewhere.

Field Forget-me-not (*Myosotis arvensis*)

Borage family (Boraginaceae). Annual/biennial. Pollinated by flies and bees. Propagated by seed. Formerly medicinal.

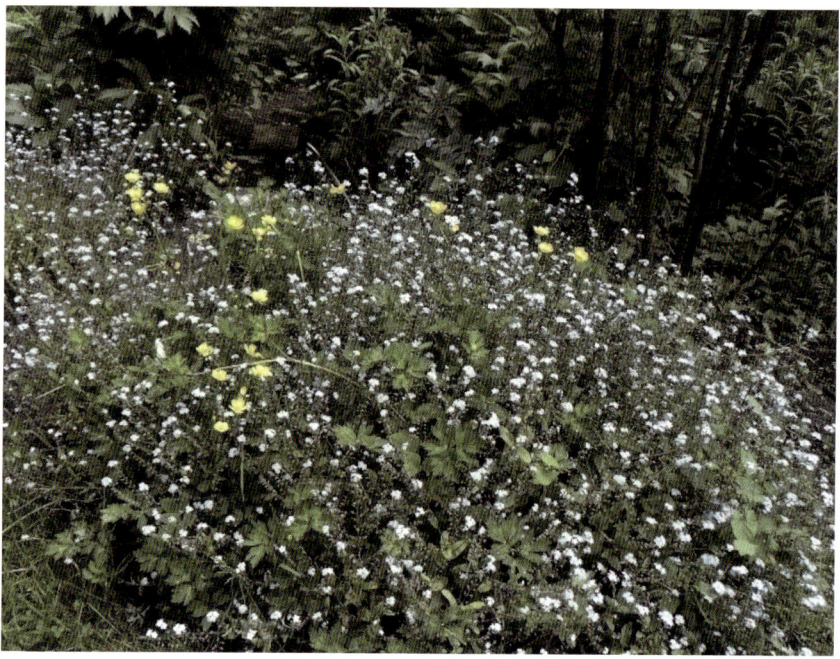

We allowed a few buttercups to spread through the forget-me-nots temporarily as the colour combination was so striking.

You may well have deliberately planted these popular flowers in the front of a border as their gentle blue petals offset stronger colours most pleasingly. The forget-me-nots that arrive in our garden, however, are the smaller 'field' variety (*arvensis* is from *arvum*, Latin for 'field') brought here by natural means, later seeding themselves very freely. It could be that we humans unwittingly act as transporters as the hooked hairs on the seed pods readily attach to clothing, or indeed to the hair of animals. I have often picked the pods off my trousers as well as from my dog's ears! Obligingly, the seeds seem to plant themselves generally, but not always, in suitable places. Once I see their soft, green, oblong leaves in the early spring, I decide whether to leave them *in situ*, transplant them or pull them up. This way they give a splendid showing from April for several weeks in just the right part of our borders. The term *Myosotis* comes from the Greek, meaning 'mouse's ear', an apt description of the downy leaves.

Occasionally pink petals are produced on the delicately branching stem, each flowering stalk being curled initially but then straightening. Whatever the hue, the five petals open more or less flat but remain joined at the yellow centre to form a narrow tube beneath.

Folklore

Most of the ancient legends concerning this plant come from continental Europe. In Germany it was said that God named all the plants but accidentally missed out this little blue one. A tiny voice cried out: 'Forget me not, oh Lord!' – hence the German name *Vergissmeinnicht*.

Another folk tale, from both medieval France and Germany, said that a knight and his lady were walking by a river. The knight stooped down to pick a posy of the blue flowers, but his armour was so heavy it unbalanced him and he fell into the water. Unable to swim, he threw the posy to his lady crying 'Forget me not!' before drowning. Ever since, the flower has had romantic associations.

Indeed, Henry Bolingbroke, later Henry IV of England, adopted the flower as his emblem, again for romantic reasons. In 1399 he was banished by Richard II for his political activities and spent some time with the Duke and Duchess of Brittany. As he left for England the following year to raise a rebellion, he gave his hostess a bunch of the flowers with the message '*Souveigne vous de moy*'. Clearly, she did remember him as she later became his second wife.

In Victorian Britain, when floriography became very popular, the gift of forget-me-nots was taken to mean 'true love'. This was a time when social convention made the expression of strong feelings difficult; posies of flowers could say everything safely. There was even an annual called *Forget Me Not*, devoted to the topic of 'talking bouquets', which was very popular from 1822–34.

It may have been Coleridge who helped to establish the common name through his poem 'The Keepsake' of 1802. During a lonely walk he writes:

> That blue and bright-eyed floweret of the brook,
> Hope's gentle gem, the sweet Forget-me-not!

The following century, Freemasons in Germany used the flower as an emblem to keep in mind the poor and sick. Later it became a secret signal in place of the original Square and Compass symbol, whereby members could recognise each other without risking persecution by the Nazis. Today it is still worn in memory of those who have suffered in the name of Freemasonry.

Uses

As for folk remedies, it seems that the plant was considered to be of little value. The Greek physician Dioscorides had recommended it as a cure for a scorpion sting, no doubt because of the curling flowering stems, likened to this creature's tail. One wonders how many of his patients survived! Until the name 'forget-me-not' came into common use, the plant was referred to as 'scorpion grass'.

Wildlife

Nature has the most remarkable and cunning means of ensuring regeneration and survival by inviting assistance from other creatures. It was the yellow 'eye' in the centre of each forget-me-not flower, along with the fine, radiating white lines, that inspired the 18th-century German naturalist Christian Konrad Sprengel to investigate the way in which these floral patterns guide pollinators to the nectar. He referred to them as 'honey guides'. I have often noticed how our wild bees are attracted to these flowers. This way, both the plants and the insects benefit.

Honesty *(Lunaria annua)*

Cabbage family (Brassicaceae). Biennial. Pollinated by insects; may self-pollinate. Propagated by seed. Edible.

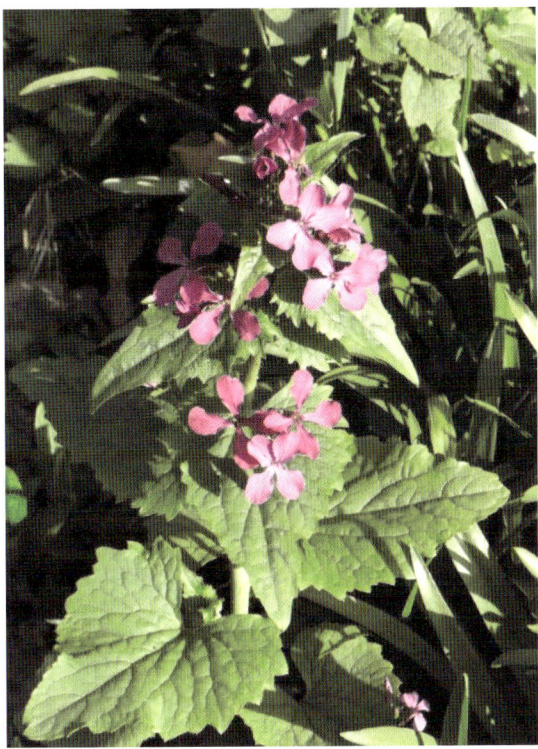

Honesty will freely seed itself around the garden.

The rich deep-red of honesty's four petals provides welcoming warmth to a shady hedgerow in spring. In our garden this plant seeds itself freely, so we are never quite sure where it will appear next. Generally, we let it decide for itself on the most inviting locations as these are invariably where little else flourishes. Some readers may argue that honesty is not really a weed, being originally a garden escapee. However, it is now widely naturalised and is included in wildflower guides. As it may decide to plant itself in the 'wrong' place, there is some justification for allowing it an entry here.

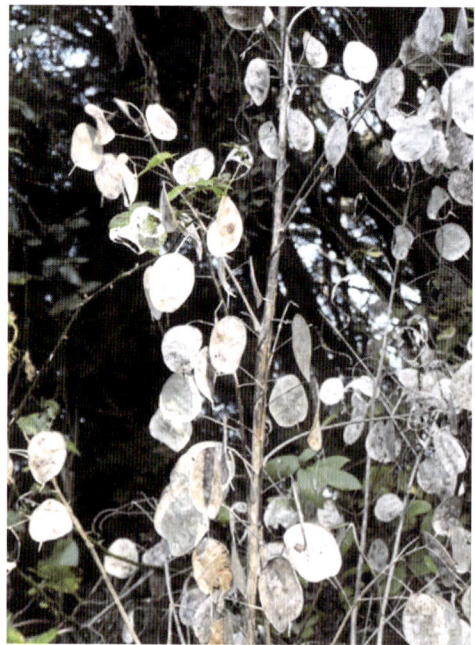

Often likened to coins, the silvery pods of honesty will last all winter and make an attractive decoration.

Wild honesty generally grows to a height of 1 to 1.5 m (3 to 4½ ft) and is a biennial, flowering the following year. Gardeners can choose to grow the plant as a hardy annual, but it will be smaller. The stem is densely hairy, branching out towards the top. Somewhat similar in shape to jack-by-the-hedge, the leaves are beautifully heart shaped and pointed, and toothed along the edges.

Most distinctive of all are the seed pods, which are large, round and flattened, and green to begin with. As they dry, they take on a silvery, translucent appearance. They can remain on the plant all winter and are highly prized by flower arrangers.

Folklore

The 16th-century herbalist John Gerard gives the seed pods a most poetic description. First he mentions the three films, the two outer being 'of an overworne ash colour', while the innermost 'whereon the seed doth hang or cleave, is thinne and cleere shining, like a shred of white Sattin newly cut from the piece'. What could be more evocative! Indeed, the name he gives to honesty is 'white satin floure'. Yet, he refers to further country names of 'penny floure', 'mony-floure' and 'silver plate'. People from various countries have likened the pods to coins: in America the names given are 'silver dollars' or 'Chinese money', while in Holland it is *Judaspenning* from the 30 pieces of silver that Judas Iscariot was paid by the chief priests for pointing out Jesus. What about the common term of honesty though? It is the women folk, says Gerard, who call it 'honestie'. Perhaps it was the transparent quality that gave them this idea. Others have likened the pods to the moon – hence the Latin name of *lunaria*.

Uses

Although listed in his *Herball*, Gerard does not recommend honesty as a remedy except to mention that it is sometimes used as a cure for the 'falling sickness' or epilepsy. Thankfully there are effective modern drugs that can help keep this debilitating disease under control.

Wildlife

Another bird which has suffered disastrous declines is the bullfinch. One problem is that it has a liking for the buds of fruit trees and has therefore been systematically persecuted. However, it is also partial to honesty seeds which it will devour greedily, much to the annoyance of flower arrangers! The solution is to collect some of the seed pods for replanting, allowing the rest to self-seed, so that there are plenty next year for both you and the bullfinches. The males are very colourful with their red chests and blackcaps and are a joy to have in the garden. Do give them a chance.

Field Horsetail (*Equisetum arvense*)

Horsetail family (Equisetaceae). Perennial. Self-fertile. Reproduced by spore. Toxic unless boiled. Poisonous to horses and other animals.

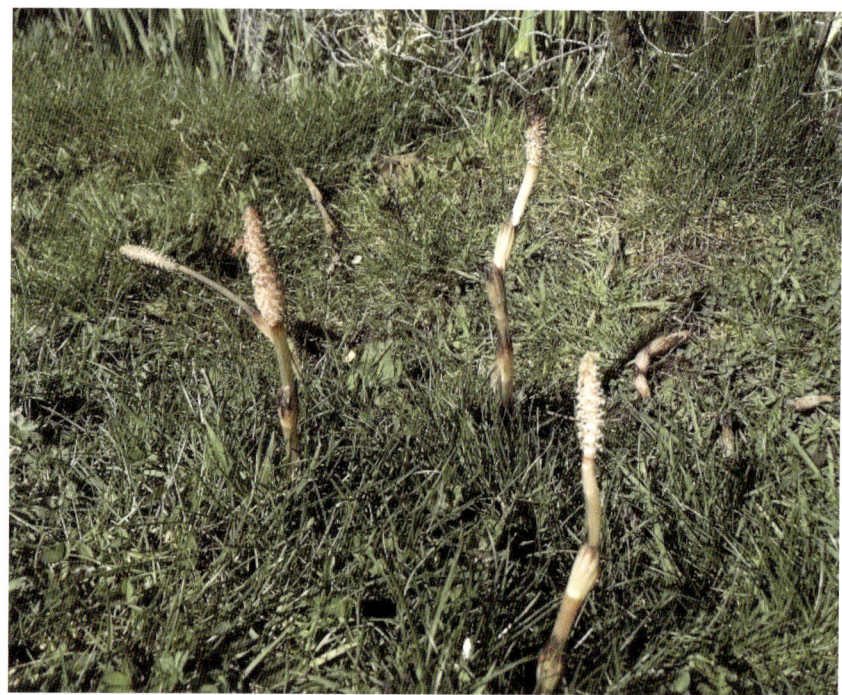

The photo shows the first stages of this ancient plant before the 'horse's tail' appears.

One April the weirdest plant I had ever seen pushed up through the grass close to our pond. It was brownish and distinctly phallic shaped, about 30 cm/1 ft tall. Shortly afterwards more of its friends appeared until there was quite a clump. I searched through our botanical guides but without success. Whatever was it? It was only when my husband suggested that I try horsetail that I realised that what I had witnessed was the first stage of its growth above ground. These were the fertile stems, bearing at the top a cone-like structure, which, like ferns, produces spores. The second and instantly recognisable stage we had never seen in our garden due to mowing of the meadow in this particular place. Hence my bewilderment.

Gardeners and farmers alike loathe this weed, describing it as a pernicious pest impossible to get rid of. This is due to the network of underground rhizomes that grow near the surface and spread very quickly and roots that can be up to 2 m/7 ft deep, making them extremely difficult to dig out. Even a tiny piece left behind can produce a new plant. You will not want horsetail in your borders. If one appears, nip it off quickly and repeat every year until it gives up. You can, if you like, cook and eat these tender shoots. In fact, Romans enjoyed them as a delicacy, rather like asparagus.

The second stage of growth arrives some two months later, now dark green with a hollow, segmented main stem and whorls of upward-pointing,

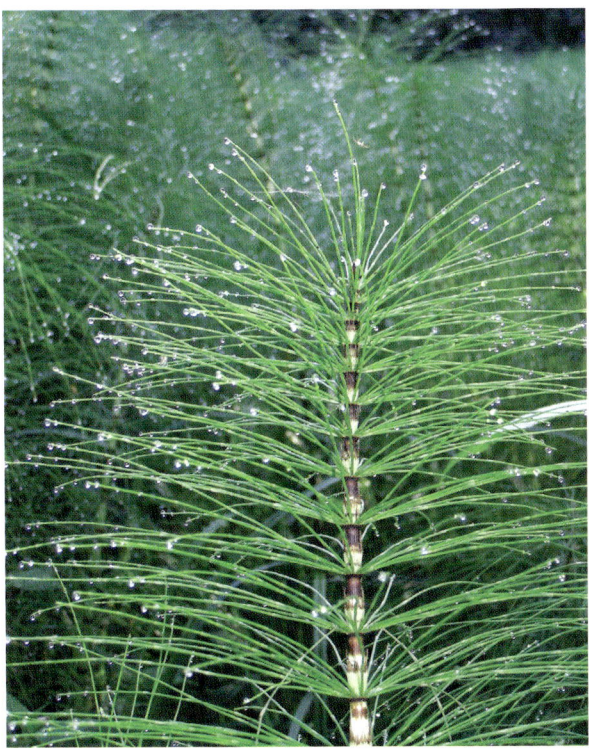

The 'horse's tail' only appears when the plant is mature. *Photo © Pixabay*

fir-like shorter ones around each node. It is now obvious where the name comes from, the whole giving the impression of a horse's tail. There are no leaves as such nor are there any flowers.

Often referred to as a living fossil, this extraordinary plant has a very ancient lineage, being descended from a much bigger variety which existed some 500 million years ago. Somehow it managed to survive the mass extinctions at the time of the dinosaurs.

Folklore

Country children love to pull horsetail to pieces as each segment can be refitted back into its socket. For this reason, it is sometimes called the 'Lego plant'!

Uses

Many common names given to horsetail reflect a special property that it has. Close inspection will reveal the tiny crystals of silica attached to the second-stage stems, which, if you run a hand along the plant, will feel scratchy. Indeed, silica is its main constituent at about 30 per cent. People have used horsetail since time immemorial as a natural sandpaper or wood polisher, calling it 'shave-grass'. Another name 'pewterwort' indicates its usefulness for shining pewter, yet without causing damage to the metal. It was regularly sold in the streets of towns for just this purpose. 'Bottlebrush' suggests how effective it was for cleaning and polishing glass. When horsetail is burnt, the resulting ash is some 80 per cent silica. It is said that when powdered and mixed with a little water this is the best possible cleaner of silver.

Gardeners will be pleased to know that the plant makes an excellent treatment against mildew and black spot.

Horsetail garden spray

Just boil up a couple of horsetail plants in water, then simmer for 20 minutes or so. Leave to infuse overnight. Strain and dilute two parts to one before spraying your rose bushes and other plants.

Horsetail has earned a bad reputation, not only because of its invasiveness but also because it can be toxic to horses and other animals. A constituent of the plant is the enzyme thiaminase, which if ingested can cause a deficiency in vitamin B1 (thiamine). However, the poisonous enzyme is easily destroyed by heat, so the plant is quite safe if taken as a tea or syrup. To be sure, it needs to be boiled for at least ten minutes.

The silica is soluble in water and can therefore be absorbed by the body. It is a useful remedy for brittle nails or thin hair when drunk as a tisane. It is also mildly diuretic due to the silicic acid, so it can be helpful in cases of cystitis.

Horsetail tisane

This is best made from the dried plant. To dry, cut the green stems in summer, then to speed up the process, bruise with a rolling pin to let out some of the moisture. Hang the bunches in a warm airy place. When dry cut into small pieces.

1 tsp dried horsetail

275 ml/ ½ pint water

½ tsp clear honey

Put the horsetail and water in a pan and bring to the boil. Turn the heat down and simmer to reduce by about a half. Stir in the honey.

♦ Drink from time to time for maintenance of hair and nails and for keeping the teeth strong. It is also good for healthy skin and all connective tissue. **NB: Not suitable for diabetics.**

Wildlife

The tiny, brown-green horsetail flea beetle relies on this plant as its main food source, both the adults and larvae feeding on the stems. The peak time for spotting these minute visitors is in the spring through to the summer. They are distinguished by the brown-green wing case with golden rear.

Wild Pansy (*Viola tricolor*)

Violet family (Violaceae). Annual/biennial. Pollinated by flies and bees; may self-pollinate. Propagated by seed. Edible. Medicinal.

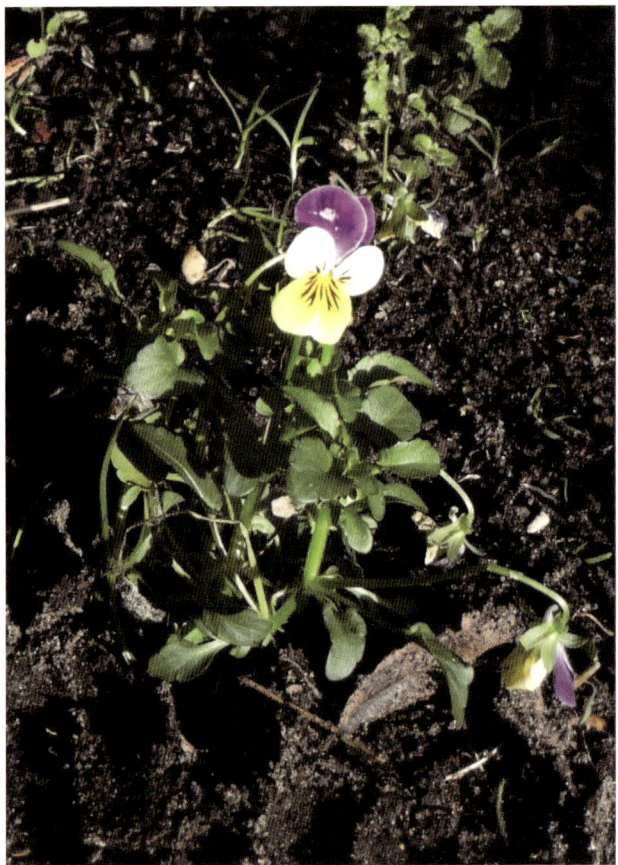

Even though a shy little flower, wild pansy, or heartsease, is said to have the power to bring you a happy love life!

This most pleasing of little flowers generally inhabits cultivated or waste ground. Before our fields were sprayed with herbicides, it favoured arable land, especially corn fields, but now is found much more in our gardens. So if a few appear spontaneously in your flower beds, do give them a chance. As the forebear of the garden pansy, it may be less showy, but a group at the front of a border will certainly add charm. It will also grow quite happily dotted here and there among other flowers. Moreover, you will have the pleasure of their dainty blooms for a long period until the end of summer.

The Latin name *tricolor* is of course descriptive of the three colours of the petals. Classically, the upper two petals are a deep purple (but may also be a paler violet), the middle two a creamy white and the lower lobe a rich gold. So, colouring apart, what is the difference between the wild pansy and the violet? If you look closely, you will see that the middle pair of petals of wild pansy is swept upwards, while that of the violet points downwards. The leaves of these two plants are also different: rather than heart-shaped, those of the wild pansy are narrow with rounded teeth along the edges, some of the upper ones being quite deeply cut.

Bees and other insects are attracted to wild pansy and thereby help to pollinate it. As an annual, it has the most effective way of propagating itself. The seed capsule splits open into three parts. The drying process causes the seeds to be expelled with considerable vigour, so there is a good likelihood that some at least will land in a favourable position.

Folklore

If you do decide to let wild pansy grow, then perhaps this will bring good luck to your love life! For centuries it has been regarded as a love charm, perhaps because the broad, lower petal is both golden and heart shaped. Most famously it was the juice of this plant laid on the eyelids of Titania in *A Midsummer Night's Dream* that caused her to fall in love with the grotesque Bottom. Shakespeare considered it to be 'Cupid's flower':

> Yet mark'd I where the bolt of Cupid fell:
> It fell upon a little western flower,
> Before milk-white, now purple with love's wound,
> And maidens call it love-in-idleness.

(Act II, i)

Uses

Apart from its reputation as an aphrodisiac, Culpeper believed it to be 'an excellent cure for the venereal disease'. Fortunately, there are more reliable medications for this condition nowadays. However, herbalists still recommend heartsease for sore throats and skin conditions, especially acne and eczema. Scientifically there is good reason for this as the plant is rich in vitamins C and A. It also contains the antioxidant anthocyanin. The simplest method is to make a tisane from the leaves and flowers. It's best to use them very fresh.

Wild pansy tisane

2 tsp finely cut wild pansy leaves and flowers
honey
boiling water

Put the chopped flowers and leaves in a cup, pour on the boiling water and stir in a little honey. Leave to infuse for 10 minutes. Strain before use. ♦ You can drink two or more cups a day, as well as pat the tisane on to the skin.

Wildlife

Wild pansy is the favourite food plant of the beautiful Queen of Spain fritillary butterfly. However, you will be very lucky to see this as it is a rare visitor from continental Europe. The best time to find this elegant butterfly, with its orange-yellow colouring and black spots, is in the autumn, when it occasionally appears along the southern or eastern coasts. She will lay her eggs on heartsease, and the dark, hairy caterpillars will eagerly devour the plant when they hatch.

Being edible, many wild creatures will take a nibble out of wild pansy, including slugs and snails. You may not want these in your garden but be aware that they are the staple diet of thrushes, which have suffered a dramatic decline in numbers in recent decades. Please, never ever put down poisonous slug pellets; instead encourage their natural predators, which include frogs and toads as well as birds.

Germander Speedwell (*Veronica chamaedris*)

Heath Speedwell (*V. officinalis*)

Slender Speedwell (*V. filiformis*)

Speedwell family (Veronicaceae). Perennials. Pollinated by hoverflies and butterflies; may self-pollinate. Propagated by stolon. Edible flowers. Medicinal.

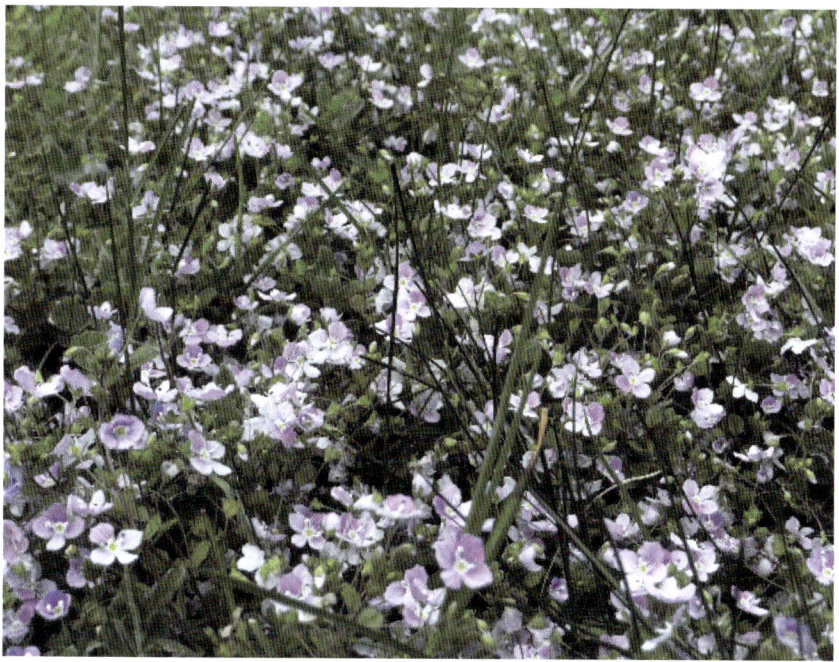

The striking blue of the petals is attractive to butterflies and other pollinators. Speedwells are rich in antioxidants and have been important medicinally in the past.

We have in our garden two sorts of speedwell: one that pops up along the edges of flower beds or around our mini-woodland, the germander or bird's eye speedwell, and the other that nestles among the lawn grasses, with smaller, more rounded leaves, the slender speedwell, sometimes dense enough to form a mat. The first has exquisite, sky-blue flowers with four petals and a white 'eye' in the centre, and loose clusters of blooms ascending to the top of each stem; the second has just a single flower on each slender stalk, mauvish-blue in colour. Both are perennials. Over on our meadow, groups of the flowers create a gentle, blue haze on a spring morning, outdoing the grasses which have yet to catch up.

Like the slender speedwell, the heath has creeping stems that will root to form new plants. The leaves are oval and much less toothed than the germander, while the colour of the flowers tends more towards lilac. As its name implies, it is more likely to be found in heathland areas.

Folklore

Supposedly, the flower resembles a bird's eye – hence the common name. The badge of the RAF 541 Squadron features this blue flower which is considered symbolic of the unit's functions of photographic reconnaissance, referring to the camera above and 'speedwell' to the ground crew who see the pilot on his way. 'Speed well' is the shortened form of 'God speed you well' or 'goodbye' as the dainty petals will fall off at the slightest touch. As for 'Veronica', this name is derived from *veron eikon* or 'true image'. It was Saint Veronica who wiped Jesus' face as he carried his cross to Calvary, his likeness being forever impressed in the cloth.

Uses

There is some confusion about which of the many species of this genus was used medicinally and therefore regarded as 'official' giving it the Latin name of *Veronica officinalis*. Some sources say it is the common field speedwell, others give this title to the heath speedwell, the most authoritative pointing to the latter. It does seem that the heath is the richest in active constituents and therefore the most efficacious, containing vitamins E, K and C, antioxidant polyphenols, the glycoside aucubin, which is anti-inflammatory, astringent tannins and the glycoside scutellarin known to be naturally tranquillizing. Yet, the herb fell out of favour in the early 20th century and is currently little used medicinally.

In the 16th century germander speedwell was used by the Emperor Charles V of Spain, a gout sufferer, known to have benefitted greatly from it. Two centuries later, the plant was so highly prized as a remedy that there was a rush to pick the leaves and flowers, so much so that it became hard to find for many miles around large towns.

A tea made from the flowering tops was popular on the continent, known in France as the *tée d'Europe*. The blue flowers also make an attractive addition to a salad and help digestion. Rather than trying to eradicate the plant from flower beds and lawns, how about collecting and drying them for later use? Simply hang them upside down in a warm, airy place. The tea can be made from either fresh or dried flowers. Apart from a remedy for gout, this can soothe a sore throat as a gargle or, if patted on the skin as well as taken internally, can assist in the healing of eczema.

Tée d'Europe

Use either germander or heath speedwell.
4 tsp flowering tops
275 ml/½ pint boiling water
Chop the tops finely, place in a mug, pour on the boiling water and leave to steep for 10 minutes. ♦ Drink one mugful daily until the condition improves. Also apply topically as appropriate.

Wildlife

Hoverflies are frequent visitors to the open flowers of speedwell and readily pollinate these plants. It is very useful to attract these mimics of bees and wasps to your garden as the larvae of several species eat aphids. Be reassured: although they may look like bees or wasps, they do not sting!

Butterflies are also drawn to speedwell. Indeed, it is one of the food plants of the rare heath fritillary. However, it is extremely unlikely that you will see this lovely insect in your garden, unless it is very close to coppiced woodland in the south-east or south-west of Britain. More common is the orange-tip, which may choose to lay its eggs on speedwell.

MAY

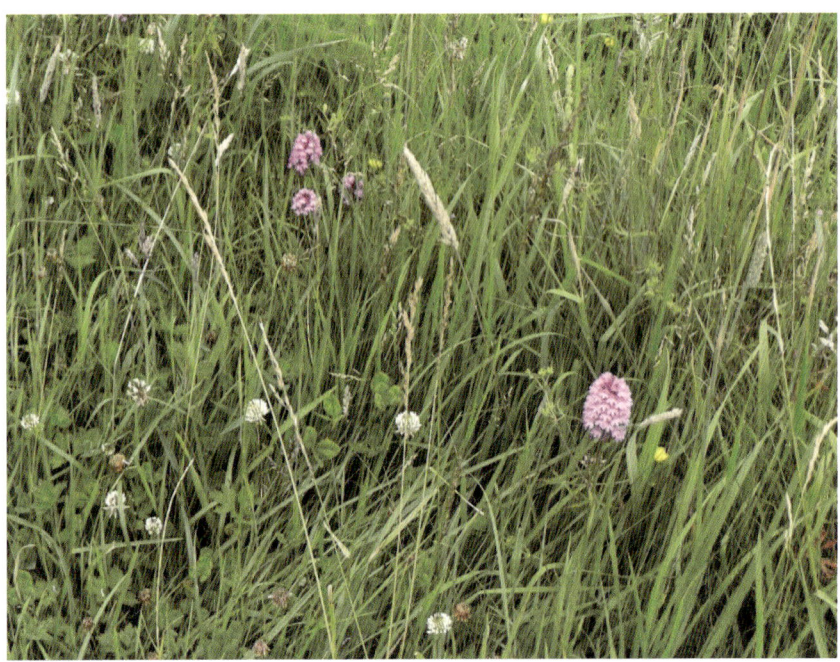

Pyramidal orchids have established themselves amid the clover and buttercups of our meadow.

May was always my mother's favourite month. Although a scientist and botanist by profession, she would eulogise in a positively romantic fashion about the glories of the month. As I survey our garden with its profusion of blossom, I can only agree. Normally lush after the showers of April, the green of grass and leaves is at its most intense, offsetting the whites, yellows and blues of the flowers.

This year, however, at the time of writing, we have had here in East Anglia less than ten per cent of our normal rainfall. Last month was the hottest on record and farmers describe their crops as standing in dust. They have long since given up arguing about climate change.

What of the 'weeds'? Ground-elder has been as aggressive as ever, apparently unaffected by the unseasonal heat, but at least we have had a useful crop of their leaves that have added interest to our salads and, when cooked, have been an agreeable substitute for spinach. Other wild plants, however, have been badly affected, most notably our pyramidal orchids which enjoy the damp grass beside our pond. Last year we counted over 30, but this year, by the end of May, only two were flowering. We searched in vain for their pointed, glossy leaves which we had carefully staked out early in spring, but they were no longer to be seen, presumably having dried up in the drought. Clearly, some of our native species are extremely sensitive to any unfamiliar changes and can only survive when conditions are just right.

Fortunately, the water level in our pond remains reasonable and the flag irises are standing tall and proud making an impressive display with their golden yellow blooms. The starry white flowers of the hawthorn form a distinctive contrast and soften an otherwise prickly hedge.

Indeed, I am struck by the different textures in the garden. The catkins of the self-planted goat's willow recently became covered in a dense white fluff and, having matured, dropped off, now forming a downy carpet on the lawn. Close inspection shows that they are composed of hundreds of minute seeds, each attached to a tiny 'parachute'. Whenever there is a breeze, many thousands are lifted up and wafted along in search of a suitable place to germinate and put down roots. Not far from the willow is a beech tree. Its nuts are protected by an outer husk with rough, curled bristles. Nature has many ways of ensuring its progeny.

Creeping Buttercup (*Ranunculus repens*)

Buttercup family (Ranunculaceae). Perennial. Pollinated by rain or insects. Propagated by stolon. Caustic.

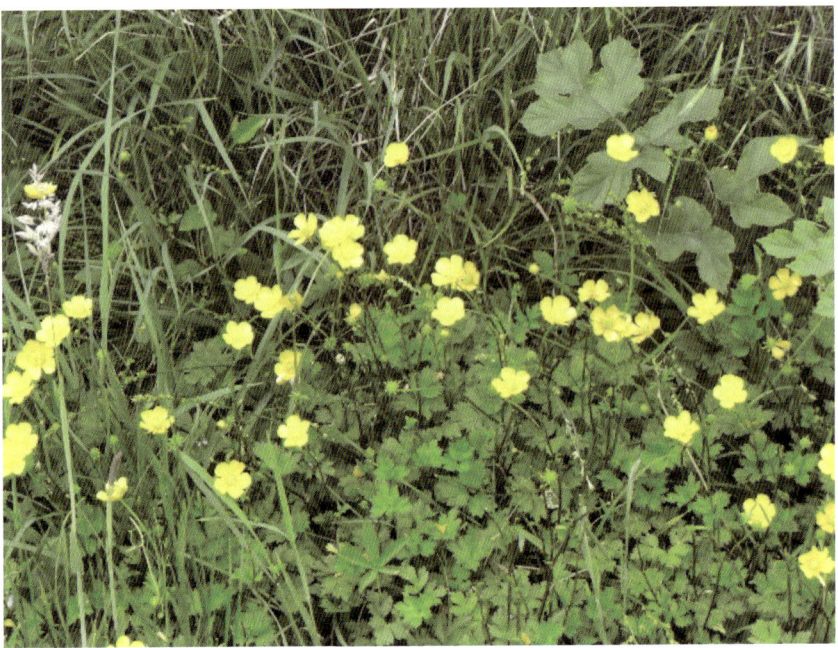

Buttercups are unusual because they are generally pollinated by rain.

It was my husband's decision to cut our grass long to give the wild flowers a chance to push through. By May, areas of our bottom lawn are a truly joyous sight, with the lustrous, bright-yellow petals of buttercups mingling with the meadow grasses. It is sad indeed that so few pastures remain today, but John Clare, writing in 1827 in the poem 'May', evokes for us the natural beauties of unploughed land:

> …
> How lovly now are lanes and balks
> For toils and lovers sunday walks

> The daisey and the buttercup
> For which the laughing childern stoop
> A hundred times throughout the day
> In their rude ramping summer play
> So thickly now the pasture crowds
> In gold and silver sheeted clouds....

There are a great many species within the Ranunculaceae genus. Here in the east of England, our moist, heavy clay supports the creeping buttercup and indeed this is the one most commonly found in British gardens. Botanically, the creeping buttercup is unusual because its flowers can be pollinated by rain. It therefore thrives in Britain's damp climate. Water collects in the 'cup' and is drawn to the stigmas by capillary action. On cold days the flowers have an ingenious way of capturing any available warmth by tracking the sun. This in turn promotes the ripening of the pollen.

This is a hairy perennial that is easily recognisable with its somewhat triangular-shaped, green leaves, each with three deeply cut lobes, the centre one stalked. The first leaves push up straight but then spread out into a rosette. When the buttercup is established, it produces runners which creep along the ground and root at the joint to produce another plant. In my county of birth, Cumbria, the 'weed' is sometimes referred to as 'Meg many-feet', a most apt description!

Fortunately, the plants are easy to prise out of the ground by placing a fork under the base of the main stem and levering them up. Generally, I leave them in the long grass but remove them from the vegetable plot. They are not good plants to have here as they have a habit of depleting the surrounding soil of various elements, including potassium. Moreover, the roots send out a secretion which deprives the area of nitrogen. Your legumes and strawberries will certainly not like this. It is best to allow them to flourish in a meadow, out of harm's way.

Folklore

Children still delight in holding a shiny buttercup under someone's chin and watching carefully for any yellow reflection. If there is one, then the

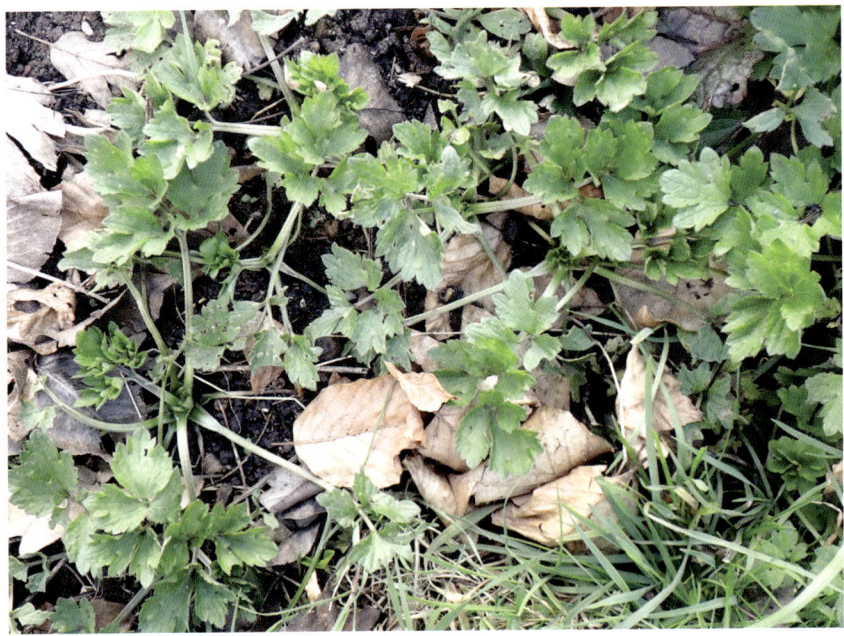

The rooting runners of buttercup establish new plants, which soon form a mat.

person likes butter. In fact, the shine is caused by layers of air just beneath the yellow pigment in the petals which reflect the light in the way that mirrors do.

Traditionally, dairymen used to place garlands of buttercups round their cows' necks on midsummer's eve in the belief that their milk would be blessed. Yet, despite the strong link between cows and buttercups, the herds dislike the acrid taste produced by the chemical ranunculin and will generally avoid eating them, unless they are dried in hay. Indeed, the fresh sap can cause blistering and inflammation of the digestive system.

Uses

As the juice is caustic, the plant is rarely found in herbals, except as a remedy for warts or occasionally for other skin complaints. John Pechey, in his *Compleat Herbal* of 1694, describes how beggars would rub buttercup leaves into their feet deliberately to produce blisters, thereby to elicit greater sympathy from people and no doubt more generous offerings: 'Beggars make Soars upon their Flesh with this Plant, to move Compassion.' However, such comments most probably refer to the bulbous buttercup (*Ranunculus bulbosus*) which is considerably more caustic than the creeping variety.

I did discover one remedy in *A Country Compendium*, written by Godfrey Baseley and published in 1977, providing a recipe for 'buttercup ointment'. This is reputed to be good for a variety of unspecified skin disorders, but it is noticeable that only the flowers are used and not the stems, thereby avoiding the caustic juice.

Buttercup ointment

225 g/½ lb pure Vaseline
buttercup flowers

Melt the Vaseline in a pan, then add as many of the flowers as it will hold. Bring to the boil then simmer gently for ¾ hour. Strain, pour into a jar and allow to cool. **NB: For external use only.**

Wildlife

The seeds of buttercup are a useful source of nutrition for many birds. In particular, house sparrows and wood pigeons will peck at them. Small rodents will also search for the seeds and carry them off for safe storage and later use.

The shiny petals will lure various insects to the yellow flowers, including butterflies. In particular, the grizzled skipper and marsh fritillary use buttercups as a source of nectar. Sadly, you are very unlikely to have the pleasure of seeing these scarce butterflies as they are both red-listed and now confined to small areas.

Cleavers (*Galium aparine*)

Bedstraw family (Rubiaceae). Annual. Pollinated by insects. Propagated by seed. Medicinal (but can cause dermatitis).

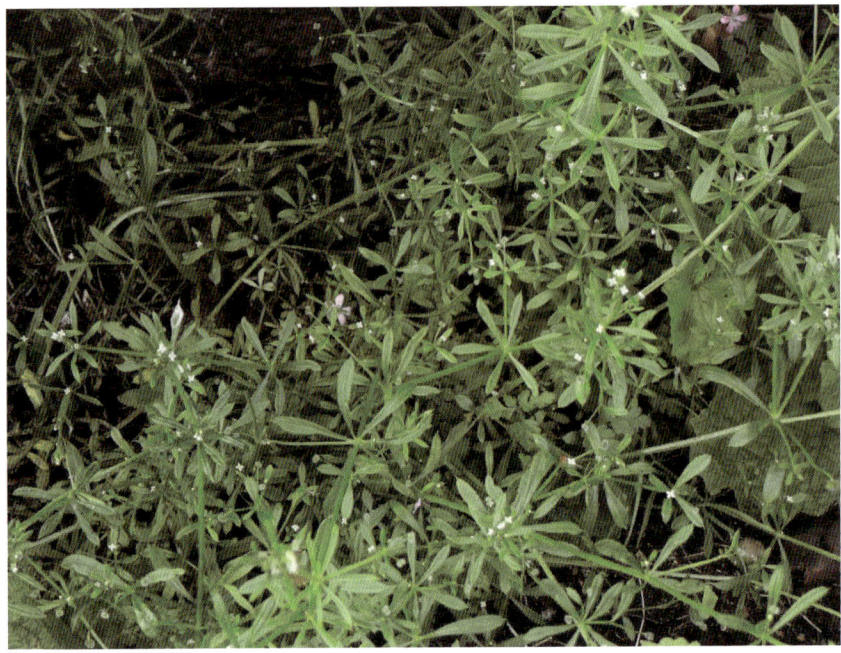

Cleavers, also known as goosegrass, has tiny, white flowers.

Two idyllic years of my childhood were spent in a country village in the north of England. We had a huge, semi-wild garden, with trees that my brother and I could climb and plenty of space for imaginative games. How fortunate we were! Among many activities, we loved to play practical jokes on people. I have memories of creeping up behind adults and sticking pieces of cleavers that we called goosegrass onto their backs, then running off and hiding behind a bush trying to suppress our giggles as we watched their reactions.

Intrigued by the sticky nature of cleavers I decided to look at a piece under the microscope. This showed clearly that the whole plant is covered

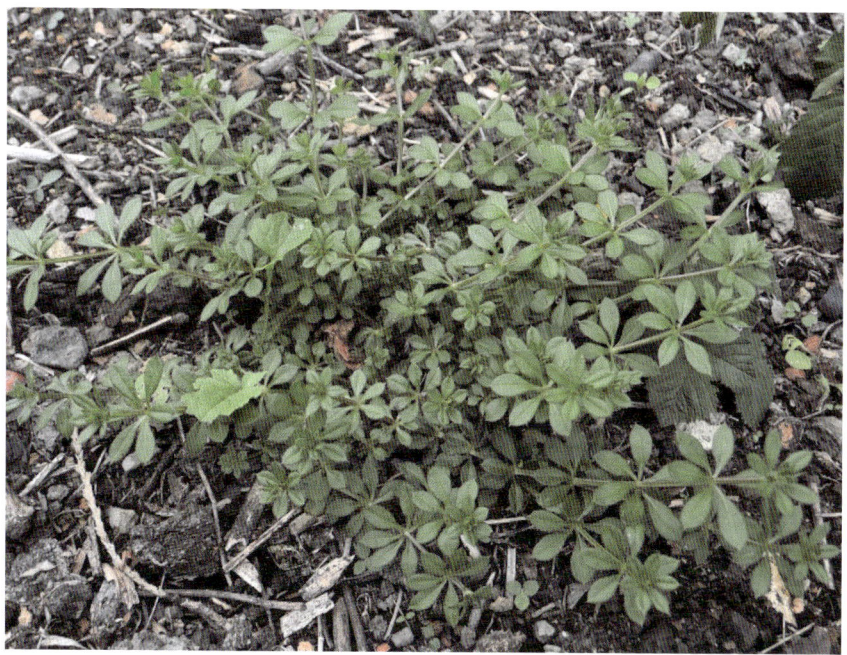
A cleavers seedling will quickly produce several stems from a central point.

in bristly hooks. Not only does it cling to the clothes of humans but, of course, will attach itself to animals which transport the seeds to other destinations.

These days I spend much time in May and June pulling up armfuls of the stuff before seeds start to set. Even though I have done this every year for the past two decades, it still grows in great profusion, especially in shady places under shrubs and alongside hedges. I have discovered that it is best to leave the plant until it is fully grown and in flower as the bottom of the stalk starts to die off, which makes it very easy to pull out. No doubt this is nature's way of ensuring that it will readily detach and stick to the fur of any passing animal, thereby spreading its seeds as far and wide as possible. If it has planted itself among tall perennials, as mine invariably does, then you can give it a tug from the top. This also gives you the opportunity to appreciate the minute white flowers with their four dainty petals that grow out on individual stalks from the whorls of leaves at intervals up the stem.

Folklore

Perhaps because of the plant's ability to stick and cling, and the way in which the seeds were difficult to pick off clothes, it is sometimes referred to as 'sweethearts'. The common name of goosegrass, however, comes from the folk practice of collecting it in the spring, cooking it and feeding it to goslings, which they clearly enjoyed. Other names I have come across are equally descriptive: 'sticky-willy', 'grip-grass' or 'catchweed'.

Uses

My husband, who is an archaeologist, was fascinated to learn that seeds of cleavers have been found in Neolithic settlements. It is thought that stone age people used the seeds to curdle milk for the making of cheese. The seeds can also be roasted to make a sort of coffee. It is easy enough to collect them when they occur in profusion during July. I counted 113 on a single stem!

Culpeper, the 17th-century physician, recommends cleavers as a spring tonic to return the body to sound health after the rigours of winter. Modern herbalists still believe that it has useful detoxification properties, in particular being a cleanser of the lymph. This important part of the immune system picks up the body's wastes and any foreign material which is then dealt with by the white cells carried in the lymph before being returned to the blood stream.

It is also well known that cleavers is strongly diuretic and therefore helpful in relieving the burning sensation caused by cystitis. Another Culpeper remedy involves making it into a poultice for the healing of wounds, and Gabrielle Hatfield in her *Herbal* reports that this was still common folk practice early in the 20th century.

Culpeper's gruel

Do not be put off by the tiny hooks which cover cleavers as they will rapidly melt away when cooked.
1 small cup organic porridge oats
3 cups boiling water

1 handful young cleavers
honey to taste
Wash and chop the cleavers into small pieces. In a pan, pour the water on to the oats to make the porridge, stir well and add the cleavers. Boil up for 5 minutes, continuing to stir. Sweeten with the honey.

Spring detox

Fresh young plants of cleavers
Put the young plants into a juicer. Alternatively chop finely and strain through a sieve or muslin. Take 1–2 tsp three times daily. ♦ To preserve the juice for later in the year, mix equal parts juice with clear honey. Cover securely and store in a dark place.

A remedy for cystitis

In addition to this tisane, make sure that you drink plenty of water to help flush out the bacteria. The remedy has a pleasant, slightly pea-like taste and can also be used as a detox.
2 tsp finely chopped leaves and stalks of cleavers
275 ml/½ pint boiling water
Pour the water on to the cleavers and allow to infuse for 5 minutes. Drink 3 cups per day

Cleavers poultice

Make a tisane following the above recipe for cystitis. Soak a lint pad in the infusion and apply gently to a wound or bruise. **Caution: Do not use this plant if you are pregnant or breast-feeding**.

Wildlife

I have often noticed the foamy 'cuckoo spit' lodged in a leaf axis of cleavers. This hides the plant-sucking nymph, the tiny 'spittle bug', of the frog hopper. The foam protects the nymph from predators, prevents it from drying out and controls the temperature. A frog hopper can jump as high as 70 cm/2ft 4in, which, bearing in mind its minute size, is even more than a flea.

Other sap feeders are also attracted to cleavers, especially greenfly and blackfly. You may not want these in your garden, but please consider their ecological importance. They provide food for both birds and insects, including ladybirds and parasitic wasps, also the larvae of lacewings, hoverflies and aphid midges. These will also devour the aphids on your rose bushes!

The larvae of seven moths depend on *Galium* for nutrition, four of which have the common name of carpet, i.e. silver-ground, common, water and green. Of these the common carpet is the one most likely to appear in your garden if you have cleavers present. In the south of Britain there are two generations, so you will see the adults flying in May to June, then again in August to September. This moth has a beautiful brown and white, or beige, zig-zag pattern across the forewings. Its tiny, pale-green eggs are laid singly along the edge of a leaf.

Other moths that depend on *Galium* are the brightly coloured yellow shell, the early flying mottled grey and the barred straw, which is easily recognised by its extended forewings when resting. You can see from the above how important it is to allow some cleavers to flourish in a spare corner of your garden.

Common Comfrey (*Symphytum officinale*)

Borage family (Boraginaceae). Perennial. Pollinated by bees. Propagated by seed. Medicinal. Root toxic.

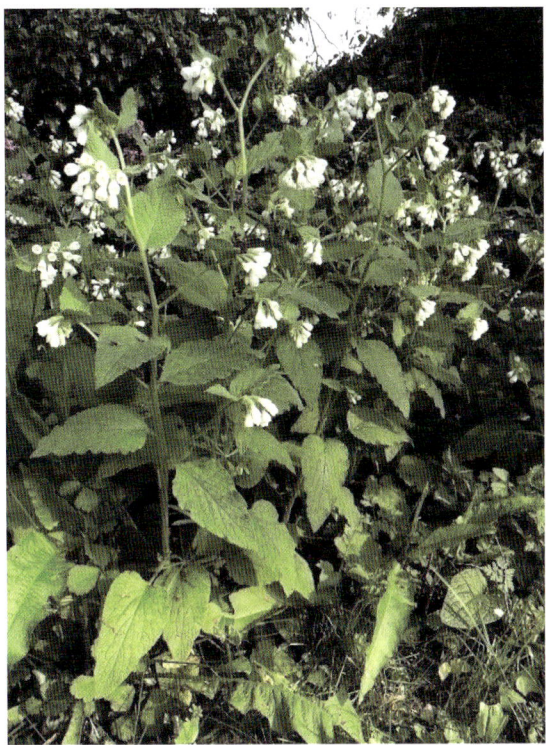

Comfrey is not only attractive, it makes an excellent fertiliser.

What a delightful surprise it was when I noticed the sprays of creamy, bell-like flowers unfurl themselves under a damp hedge early one May! One of the joys of having a large, rambling country garden is that we are not always aware of what is happening in each corner, especially after a period of rain. Walking afresh around the lawn or meadow often produces these little discoveries. The flowers of comfrey are extraordinarily pretty, with frilly edges to their nodding heads. While ours are the creamy white of common comfrey, they can also be the pinky purple of rough comfrey

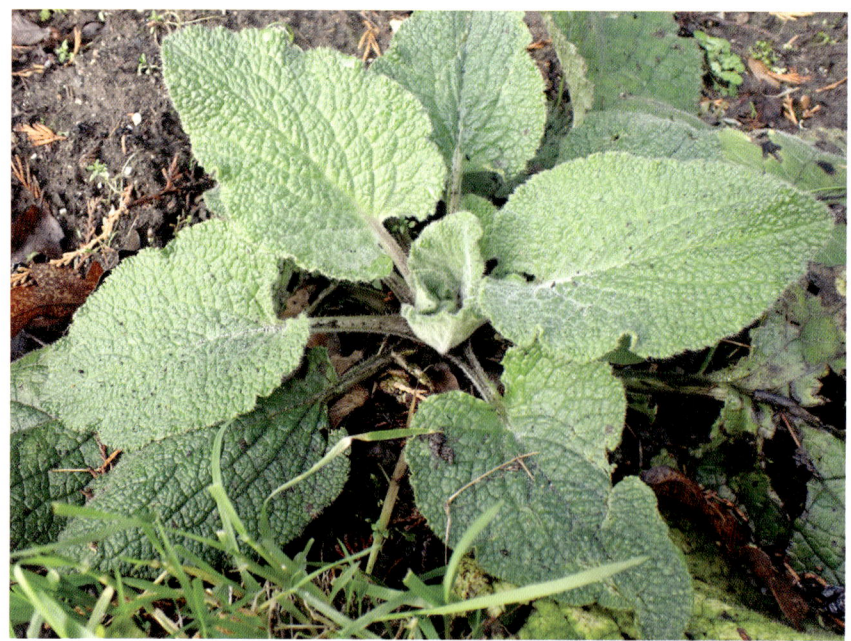

A nourishing plant feed is easily made from the leaves. Be careful of identification as emerging foxglove leaves can often look similar.

(*Symphytum asperum*), originally introduced to Britain as a fodder plant but now naturalised.

You will notice the soft, hairy leaves of this herbaceous perennial pushing up in early spring after which they grow vigorously to produce a plant a metre/3 ft or more tall. The leaves closest to the ground can be up to 25 cm/1 ft long, while those further up the stem are shorter. All are pointed with slightly wavy edges and their bases running down into the stem, giving this a 'winged' appearance.

Uses

Comfrey has been sought after as a medicinal plant since at least 400 BC. The scientific name comes from the Greek *symphuo*, to unite or make whole, while the common name is thought to derive from the Latin *conferre*, to gather or come together, which later merged into the Anglo-

Norman *cumfirie*. Both give a clue as to its traditional usage: comfrey has the ability to assist with the healing of broken bones as well as sprains, wounds, bruises and ulcers – hence the old names of 'knitbone' and 'bruisewort'. Crusaders knew of its value as a healing plant and carried it with them.

It is interesting that these traditional therapeutic qualities are borne out by scientific research as the plant contains allantoin, which stimulates the growth of epithelial cells and thereby promotes healing within connective tissue. It is also naturally anti-inflammatory. However, pyrrolizidine alkaloids are found in the root and to a lesser extent in the leaves, which are toxic to the liver and linked to cancer in some animal studies. For this reason, internal consumption of comfrey is not recommended here. Nevertheless, the plant can be used externally to great effect. Even so, it is best to restrict application to no more than 10 days concurrently or up to six weeks in a year.

Kneebone poultice

Use this to speed up the healing of fractures, sprains or bruises.
Comfrey leaves and root in equal proportions
water
Scrub the roots and cut them into small pieces. Put these together with the leaves and a little water into a blender. Switch on and blend into a paste. ♦ Spread this on a piece of muslin, folding the cloth over into a parcel. ♦ Apply to the affected part, leaving the herb to penetrate deep into the skin. Repeat until the condition has eased.

A remedy for boils, wounds and ulcers

In medieval times the roots of comfrey would be lifted and grated, then allowed to set. The resulting gel would be placed on cuts to keep the edges together and promote healing. Today, modern sticking plaster is a helpful addition.

Dig up one of the tuberous roots, wash well and scrape it vigorously or grate it to produce a creamy mush. Place this on some lint and lay over the boil or wound, fixing it with sticking plaster. Boils should vanish within a day or so.

Comfrey for gardeners

It is well worth allowing comfrey to grow in your garden, especially if you cultivate vegetables as it is a wonderful fertiliser. The extensive root system draws out nutrients from the soil, storing them in the plant. In particular it is a rich source of potassium, containing up to three times the amount found in farmyard manure. This mineral is vital for the production of flowers, seeds and fruits.

It is possible to harvest the leaves several times a year. It is best to cut them just before flowering when the nutrients are maximised. The plant will quickly re-grow.

The easiest way to use the leaves is simply to lay them around your crop to a depth of around 5 cm/2 inches. They will gradually break down and release their nutrients into the soil. They are also of value on the compost heap, but not too many at once as they lack fibre and therefore become slimy.

A potassium feed

Be warned! This fertiliser has a strong smell. If you can stand the stench, then it is unbeatable as a tomato feed or for the production of excellent soft fruit.

Fill a bucket with the leaves and press well down. Cover with rain water and leave for at least one month to produce a thick black liquid. When ready, dilute 15:1.

Wildlife

Honey bees and bumble bees simply adore comfrey flowers and will crawl repeatedly into the tubular bells to reach the nectar. Bearing in mind the worrying loss of our pollinators, do leave space for comfrey, especially if you have some damp areas as they will grow well here.

Cow Parsley (*Anthriscus sylvestris*)

Carrot family (Apiaceae). Biennial/perennial. Pollinated by small beetles and other insects, especially hoverflies. Propagated by seed. Edible.

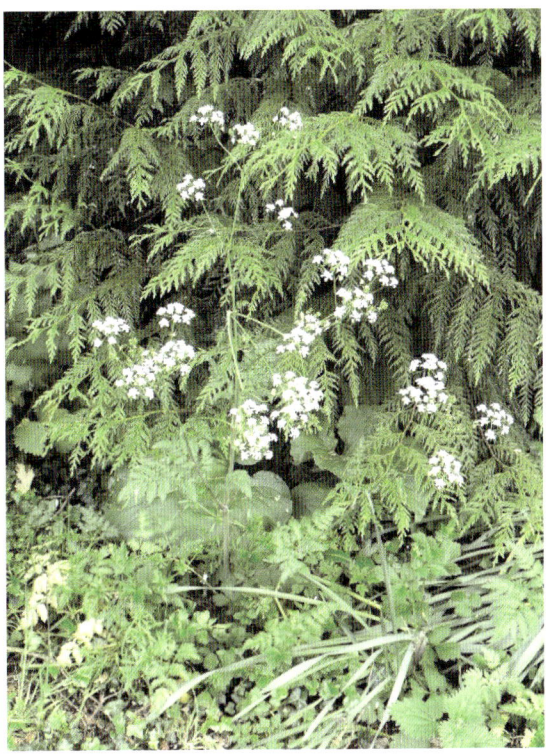

Cow parsley can provide an interesting lacy texture against a dark green background.

Always a welcome sight in the hedgerows, the delicate white flowers, clustered together and fanning out to form pretty parasol shapes, give off a sweet fragrance which can linger in country lanes, providing a special springtime pleasure. The bright-green, attractive leaves are soft, downy and fern like. Cattle apparently relish the taste, farmers describing how they will rush towards a clump and devour it eagerly – hence the name.

Folklore

The dainty flower heads have also earned picturesque country names: 'Queen Anne's lace' or 'lady's needlework'. At the same time the plant has sometimes been referred to by the alarming term of 'mother die'. The only explanation can be that children might confuse the plant with the similar-looking, deadly poisonous hemlock. To prevent any possible accident, children were warned never to touch anything resembling cow parsley; if they did, mother would die. Despite this terrifying threat, cases have been reported of children – and indeed adults and animals – dying of hemlock poisoning. The most famous case in history was of course that of Socrates who was condemned to death in this way.

Uses

At first it seemed very odd to me that such an attractive, sweet-smelling plant as cow parsley should be almost entirely excluded from herbals. One explanation is that it is not particularly rich in nutrients. However, I suspect that the real reason is the fear of confusion with hemlock. You may indeed find both appearing close together in your garden, although hemlock generally flowers later. Nevertheless, it is well worth describing the differences as clear identification is important.

In the early stages, both plants produce leaf rosettes, but those of cow parsley are slightly more bluish in colour and tend to have pink stems. Cow parsley leaves are not quite so finely divided as hemlock and are slightly downy. The most distinctive feature of hemlock is its smooth stem, which later becomes marked with deep-red spots and blotches, especially on the lower half. By contrast, the stem of cow parsley is ridged vertically and may develop a purplish hue. Moreover, at the base of the flower heads (i.e. where the small stalks join together at the top of the main stem) there are no bracts, whereas hemlock has small, leaf-like bracts in this position.

Be aware that both plants have hollow stems. Here again any children wishing to make pea-shooters must be extremely careful about identification as even the aroma from hemlock is poisonous. Fortunately, the smell is quite unpleasant, being described by some as 'like mouse piss'.

While cow parsley, with its lacy flower heads, can be a pleasing addition to a garden border, you will almost certainly want to get rid of hemlock. **Warning: do not touch without wearing gloves!** Any attempt to pull it up with bare hands will leave you suffering from the alarming sensation of being stabbed by hundreds of red-hot needles.

Wildlife

Most plants classed as Apiaceae, with flower clusters at the top of a single stalk, are very attractive to insects, especially hoverflies. You may see many of these yellow and black, or white and black, striped wasp mimics on your cow parsley. You should welcome them into your garden as their larvae feed on aphids!

Cow parsley is also the food plant of the moth *Agonopterix heracliana*, the caterpillars consuming the seeds and flowers. These live within spun or rolled leaves, which you may notice. The moth is on the wing in the autumn and again in the spring.

If you notice that cow parsley grows abundantly in your area, then the chances are that the conditions are just right for *Anthriscus sylvestris* 'Ravenswing', a decorative form of cow parsley. The name describes its leaves, which are a striking deep purple.

Garlic Mustard (*Alliaria petiolata*)

Cabbage family (Brassicaceae). Biennial. Pollinated by insects. Propagated by seed. Medicinal.

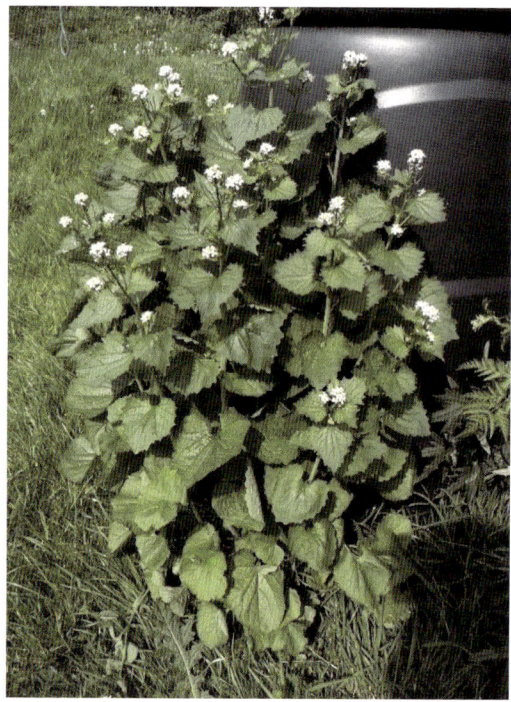

Here, the heart-shaped leaves of garlic mustard help to hide our compost bin!

At the back of our house is an ancient, hand-made shed supported by a framework of worm-eaten tree trunks and clapboarded on the outside. It is large and extremely useful for storage. Moreover, it has such character that we do not have the heart to pull it down and replace it with a flat-pack model looking like millions of other sheds. It is partly disguised on the north side by a rather straggly box hedge. In front of this are a dozen or so garlic mustard or Jack-by-the-hedge plants, each tall and erect as if standing to attention. The way in which they show off their heart-shaped leaves has me wondering whether a certain Jack once waited patiently for his sweetheart in such a fashion. The tiny white flowers are alert little points of light against the dark hedge. I leave them where they are as I cannot think of any garden plants that would look so splendid at this time of year and that would do so well in such a difficult position.

Folklore

It seems that the name 'Jack' refers to no person in particular. Rather it indicates everybody. This may be because the plant rarely appears in isolation, seeming to like its companions. The implication, therefore, is that this is a common plant found anywhere and available to all.

Uses

The name of garlic mustard gives a clue as to its flavour, which is pleasantly tangy. The garlic-like savour of the young leaves lingers behind as a distinctive aftertaste. In fact, they are rich in provitamin A and vitamin C, and make very welcome additions to salads.

Jack's green salad
This is a vitamin-rich salad. Pick heart-shaped leaves when young.
1 small crisp lettuce
2 tbs alfalfa sprouts
handful of fresh garlic mustard leaves
vinaigrette dressing
Wash and chop the lettuce and garlic mustard. Mix together with the sprouts, pour on the vinaigrette and toss.

Jack's cough syrup
Modern analysis of the plant also shows that the glycosides of the mustard oil have slight antibiotic properties. While not understanding why, country folk knew from experience that chewing the leaves could help heal mouth ulcers. The 17th-century herbalist William Salmon recommended that they be made into a syrup to keep colds at bay and to soothe a sore throat.

Handful of fresh garlic mustard leaves
1 clove of garlic
1 small jar of runny honey

Chop the leaves very finely and crush the garlic in a mortar with pestle. Place the leaves and garlic in a clean jam jar and allow to rest for 10 minutes. Fold in the honey, cover and leave overnight. Take 1 tsp as necessary.

Wildlife

If you would like your garden to offer a home to the orange-tip butterfly, then let garlic mustard flourish. You will be doing a good service towards conservation of this delicate species. Although widespread, numbers have been falling as agriculture has intensified and meadows have been lost. The green caterpillars are hard to spot, but they depend on garlic mustard for nourishment, along with one or two other Brassicaceae, such as lady's smock.

You may also see the caterpillars of the green-veined white butterfly on garlic mustard. These are shorter than those of the orange-tip, and a lighter green. This is a successful butterfly, probably benefitting from the warmer summers. It is distinguished from the small white by the dark 'veins' on the underside of the pale yellow hind wings.

Hawthorn (*Crataegus monogyna*)

Rose family (Rosaceae). Deciduous shrub/small tree. Pollinated by beetles and flies. Propagated by seed. Edible.

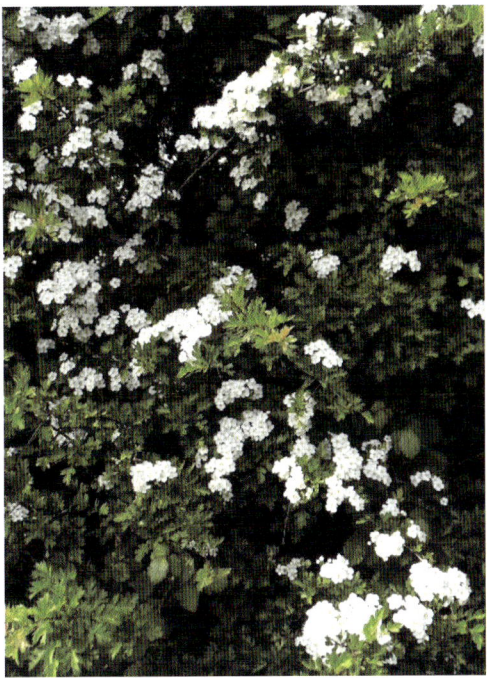

By allowing our hawthorn hedges to grow tall, we benefit from the beautiful clusters of white flowers in the spring.

THE LEAVES AND FLOWERS

My earliest memory of hawthorn as a country child is of picking the deeply lobed leaves and buds in spring and making a meal of them. We called them 'bread and cheese' and munched them eagerly. I have no recollection as to how they had earned this name as they bore no resemblance to a cheese sandwich in either taste, texture or appearance. In fact, they have rather a pleasant nutty flavour. It has been suggested that the peasants of Europe depended on hawthorn leaves for nourishment when food was scarce and so the shrub was given the name 'bread and cheese tree'. Indeed, they are very nutritious.

No other plant is so closely associated with a month of the year as hawthorn, the blossom being referred to as 'may'. It is unclear whether the old saying 'Ne'er cast a clout 'till may be out' alludes to the month or the blossom. My feeling is that it probably indicates the latter, although there can still be very cold spells during May as Shakespeare reminds us in a line of his famous sonnet (no. 18, 1609) – *Rough winds do shake the darling buds of May*. Certainly, it is wise not to be lured into putting away winter clothes by the warmth of early spring sunshine during March or April. Most British people do still take note of this old-fashioned dictum.

Hawthorn seeds itself very easily around our garden, mostly with the fortuitous assistance of birds, so, although a shrub or small tree, I do class it as a 'weed' in the sense that it is often a plant in the wrong place. It is sometimes given the name of 'whitethorn', perhaps on account of its beautiful sprays of blossom or the light greyish hue of the bark. Hard to spot in a large country garden such as ours, the pale slender stem that pushes up blends easily into the background. If it is not pulled up in the early stages, it quickly develops a long tap root and then becomes increasingly difficult to dig out. Cutting off the shoot is only a minor delaying tactic as hawthorn grows vigorously and will sprout energetically. You can recognise it by the alternate leaf buds up the new stem and slender sharp thorns, which are often produced at an early stage. If we find the seedlings growing in an inconvenient position, as we often do, we use them to fill the gaps in our hedges.

Folklore

Hawthorn seems to compete with blackthorn for the honour of being the tree from which Christ's crown of thorns was made. *Crataegus monogyna*, the common or one-seeded hawthorn, is native to Europe, but some relatives do grow in the Middle East. Tradition has it that Joseph of Arimathea, wealthy great uncle to Jesus and secret disciple, had a staff grown from the crown of thorns. He came to Britain after the crucifixion to establish Christianity here. On his arrival at Glastonbury, he thrust his staff into the ground and, fatigued after his long journey, promptly fell asleep. When he awoke, the staff had taken root and the tree subsequently became revered. To this day there is a sacred hawthorn at Glastonbury, which, unlike the British native species, flowers at Christmas as well as in late spring. It could indeed have originated from Palestine where winter-flowering hawthorns can be found.

Revered on the one hand, hawthorn is also associated with bad luck. On no account must one bring the blossoms into the house as this can be a portent of death. Perhaps it is the somewhat obnoxious aroma of the cut flowers that generated this belief because it is thought to resemble the stench of death. It is interesting that the chemical trimethylamine, which is produced during the process of decomposition, is also found in the flowers, so there is some substance to the old superstition. Despite this, Queen Elizabeth II was apparently glad to accept the winter hawthorn blossoms sent to her from Glastonbury and placed them on her breakfast table on Christmas morning.

Crataegus, with its sharp thorns and dense twigs, makes an excellent hedging plant, keeping stock secure. Perhaps on account of this practical reason it has earned the reputation for having protective qualities. It was therefore often planted outside a house to keep away evil spirits and also, incidentally, made a useful clothes horse. Believed to be the meeting place of fairies, it was traditionally inadvisable to harm a hawthorn tree, as they were likely to seek revenge. William Allingham (1824–89) records this succinctly in his poem 'The Fairies':

> If any man so daring
> As dig them up in spite,
> He shall find their sharpest thorns
> In his bed at night.

The month of May has for centuries been a period of transition between spring and summer, when herds would be driven out to pasture, a time of hope and a celebration of fertility and the harvests to come. There is no doubt that the sprays of pretty white blossom along the hedgerows anticipate summer, lift the spirits and remind one of the abundance of nature. The ancient Celtic festival of Beltane still takes place at this time, when purifying fires are lit. In some parts people decorate a maypole with hawthorn blossom and dance around it, and a pretty young woman dresses up as the May Queen. I remember holding one of the colourful maypole ribbons as a small child and being fascinated by the plaited patterns created as we wove in and out of each other.

Poets have sometimes associated the hawthorn with the sweet talk of lovers, as in Oliver Goldsmith's (1728–74) lines from the 'Deserted Village':

> The Hawthorn-bush, with seats beneath the shade,
> For talking age and whispering lovers made!

Indeed, not only did the aroma of the flowers remind people of death, they were also thought to arouse carnal desire. Medieval writers in particular considered both the month and the blossom to be 'lusty'. In the 15th century Sir Thomas Malory (1415–71) writes in *Le Morte d'Arthur*:

> For, like as herbs and trees bring forth fruit and flourish in May, in like wise every lusty heart that is in any manner a lover, springeth, and flourisheth in lusty deeds. For it giveth unto all lovers courage, that lusty month of May.

Uses

It seems surprising that John Gerard in his *Herball* of 1597 fails to list hawthorn, which grows so abundantly in the British countryside. As for Culpeper, he mentions it only briefly. It seems therefore that they had no knowledge of how it contributes to the healthy functioning of the heart muscle or how it improves circulation and lowers harmful cholesterol. Yet the physician Dioscorides from ancient Greece wrote about the virtues of hawthorn, and Chinese herbalists used it to treat high blood pressure, arteriosclerosis and angina in the 7th century. Although at least one French physician, Dr Leclerc, used hawthorn for heart conditions a millennium later, not until the end of the 19th century did this knowledge penetrate European herbals more generally, and only after the secret remedy of an

Irish physician, Dr Green, was revealed to the world by his daughter after his death in 1894.

By the 21st century, chemical constituents of the leaves, flowers and berries had largely been analysed and clinical studies carried out. Among the active ingredients discovered are flavonoids (including rutin and quercetin), which act to dilate blood vessels as well as being antioxidant, so providing protection from damage. It seems that the leaves and flowers may be richer in flavonoids than the berries, but all have therapeutic qualities. Also found are triterpene acids, which have been shown to normalise low blood pressure.

Hawthorn preparations can also act to inhibit certain enzymes which constrict the blood vessels. In a healthy person these 'ACES' (angiotensin converting enzymes) help to move the blood around the body efficiently, but if the vessels are already partly blocked with fatty deposits, then the opposite action is needed. The opening-up effect of *Crataegus* soothes angina and improves circulation to the extremities, keeping hands and feet warm, a blessing for the elderly.

One of the flavonoids, rutin, promotes the elasticity of the blood vessel walls, thus protecting against arteriosclerosis or hardening of the arteries. All the antioxidants together revitalise the components of the cardiovascular system and diminish deterioration through ageing.

In clinical trials hawthorn extract has been shown to improve the pumping action of the heart muscle and thereby increase a person's ability to exercise. It also has a stabilising effect and is therefore prescribed for arrhythmic or irregular heart beat or any kind of weakness of the heart. At the same time it acts to reduce the 'bad' cholesterol and remove any build-up of plaque in the arteries, cutting the risk of arteriosclerosis as a result.

Needless to say, heart conditions can be extremely serious and therefore none of the remedies suggested here should be taken without consulting your doctor.

Mayflower tincture

The tincture is prescribed to assist with regularising blood pressure and normalising the heart beat, to protect against hardening of the arteries, to ease mild angina and as a general heart tonic. Use the hawthorn tops when very fresh.

50 g/2 oz hawthorn flowers and tender leaves
570 ml/1 pint vodka

Chop the flowers and leaves and put into a jar. Pour the vodka over them, cover and leave in a cool place for a fortnight, giving the jar a shake each day. ♦ Arrange a cotton cloth over a sieve and strain off the liquid through this into a bowl. Squeeze the cloth to catch any remaining tincture and pour this into sterilised glass bottles. Store away from light. It will keep for at least a year. ♦ As a general heart tonic, take 1 tsp each day. Herbalists normally prescribe 1 tsp three times a day for the conditions listed above.

NB: Do not take hawthorn preparations together with beta-blockers or any other cardiovascular drug without consulting your medical practitioner.

Wildlife

We have two long hawthorn hedges bordering the road. Despite closeness to the traffic that passes through our village, small birds shelter here and build their nests, well protected by the sharp thorns from neighbouring cats, sparrowhawks and other predators.

Being a native shrub, it supports over 300 insect species. The leaves are an important food plant for the caterpillars of several moths, including the beautiful goldtail moth, which is on the wing in June and July. The golden hairs on the abdomen of this otherwise white insect are used to cover and protect the eggs which are laid on hawthorn leaves. You may spot the caterpillars in the spring with their black, red and white stripes along the length of the body. The larvae of the striking yellow brimstone moth also feeds on hawthorn and you may be lucky enough to see the adults when attracted to a lighted window in July. The hairy caterpillar of the grey dagger moth depends on hawthorn as a food plant, too. If these insects are plentiful, then not only will they take a role in the pollination of flowers, they will also provide a nutritious snack for the birds. Hawthorn therefore is well worth cultivating.

Herb-Robert (*Geranium robertianum*)

Crane's-bill family (Geraniaceae). Annual/biennial. Self-fertile. Propagated by seed. Medicinal.

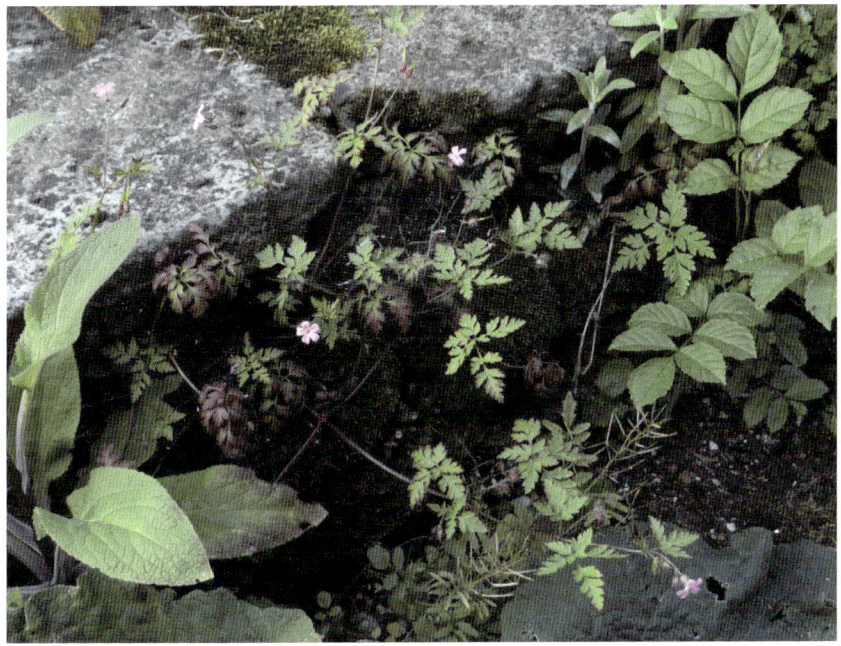

Herb-Robert grows anywhere in our garden, even in an old wall as here.

I have a particular affection for this plant, perhaps because it is the easiest to manage of the so-called 'weeds' and, with only a slim taproot, very quick to pull out. Despite its rather pungent smell, which has given it the unfortunate country name of 'stinking Roger', I deliberately leave any well-situated plants, the pink flowers adding warm, little dots to damp, shady corners. When the sun reaches the stalks, they turn a deep red as do the soft, feathery leaves.

After the flowers fade, a long, pointed 'beak' emerges which contains the seeds, each one in its own minute capsule. When disturbed, the seeds are thrown out explosively.

The abundance of herb-Robert around our house when we first arrived indicated to me that perhaps other members of the geranium family might find contentment here. This proved to be a useful clue. After planting just a couple of *Geranium endressii* in a sunny corner, this has since spread to cover the whole bed, its joyful pink flowers providing cheer for the entire summer.

Folklore

The name 'Robert' is thought to be derived from that of a medieval French saint who used herbs for healing, perhaps this one too. Another tradition connects the plant with the house goblin, Robin Goodfellow, who was reputed to have similar qualities, being red-featured and hairy, and generally carrying a candlestick. Yet, the name might simply have stemmed from the Latin *ruber*, meaning 'red'.

As for 'Geranium', this comes from the Greek geranos, or 'crane', a bird with a long beak, reflecting the shape of its seed pods.

Uses

As we have a very large pond, midges tend to proliferate after about 18.00 hours on a warm evening and can be very irritating. Having heard that Scottish people sometimes use the acrid juice of herb-Robert to deter them, I thought I would give it a try, with considerable success – another good reason to leave some of these 'weeds' in strategic places for immediate application.

To deter midges

Snap and crush the stalks in the fingers and dab the juice on to the forehead, back of the neck, wrists and any other area of exposed skin.

Remedy for a nosebleed

Herb-Robert has long been recommended for the healing of cuts and treatment of wounds. It can still occasionally be found in modern herbals for the stemming of nosebleeds.

Crush the leaves, then form into a ball. Use as a plug and, keeping the head back, insert gently into the nostril. This should help the blood to clot.

Wildlife

Despite its rather pungent aroma when the plant is crushed, the nectar of herb-Robert is evidently very appealing to many insects, including flies, butterflies and bees. Those with a long proboscis fare best as it is necessary to penetrate the narrow passage between petals down to their attachment points where the nectary is situated. Both hoverflies and the bristly empid flies will carry pollen on their backs, as will bees, notably the buff-tailed bumble bee. Empid flies are sometimes referred to as 'dance flies', as they will gather together in dancing swarms, generally above water.

Both the orange-tip and small white adult butterflies will feed on the nectar, while several species of beetle will devour the petals or leaves.

The larvae of plume moths may sometimes be found in the seed capsules or in the flower buds of herb-Robert. You can recognise the adults by their slim bodies and narrow wings.

Lady's Smock (*Cardamine pratensis*)

Cabbage family (Brassicaceae). Perennial. Pollinated by insects. Propagated by seed. Medicinal.

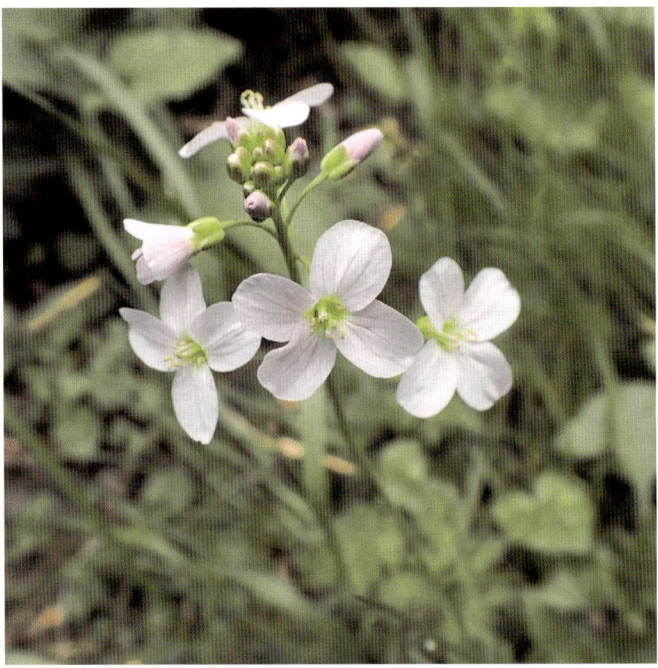

Lady's smock will only grow among grass that is reliably damp.

Some twenty-five years ago, the very first May after moving into this house, I was completely captivated by the delicate lilac flowers of lady's smock, or cuckoo flower, that appeared as if by magic on our somewhat neglected lower lawn. Our neighbours told us that there had been a dew pond in that position, but our predecessors had taken it upon themselves to put a drain in. Despite this the area was still damp, creating just the right conditions for this pretty plant. Eventually the seeds spread to the other damp part of our garden, the area around our pond.

In very warm parts of southern England, the flowers may open in April, just at the same time when a cuckoo can be heard – hence the other name. We are somewhat cooler here in the east, so need to wait a little longer for the buds to open.

Sadly, this beautiful plant is under threat in Europe due to extensive drainage and loss of valuable flood plain meadows. In the UK only 1,600 hectares of these wildlife-rich meadows remain, now needing special protection. The following quotation by the author Richard Mabey, from as recently as 1970, highlights the devastating effect that drainage can have: 'I always knew it by its other common name of Ladies Smock … I remember they grew in such abundance on my local common that I could pick armfuls every day. There are pictures of me with my arms full posing, ironically, beside the massive pipes which were soon to drain the common and denude it of its glorious pinky-mauve display.' Most of us will now never have the good fortune to see such a breath-taking show.

Like me, you may only be aware of this herbaceous perennial in May by which time the unmistakable pale lilac flowers have appeared. Each has four rounded petals with yellow anthers, several forming a cluster at the top of the upright stem. If you have a damp area, watch out for the rosette of spherical, toothed leaflets in the early spring. The main stem will push up from the centre. The upper leaves are quite different from the lower ones, being narrow and pointed.

Should you be lucky enough to have these dainty plants grace a moist patch, do not think of them as weeds! Rather tend them carefully and encourage them to multiply. They are in fact hermaphrodite, having both male and female reproductive parts, but are dependent upon insects for pollination. Established plants may develop stolons at the base which you can divide off and plant up. The seed pods are long and pointed and when ready will suddenly split open and propel the contents into the surrounding area. Obviously, you need to collect the pods just before this event. The seed is very fine but can be sown in a tray in April. Plant out in full sun or partial shade in the autumn or spring.

In May or June, if you place basal leaves flat on some compost, they will shortly produce fine white roots. After just two weeks, they should be big enough to put into a pot. Tend them carefully making sure that you keep them moist. Plant out when a strong root system has formed.

Folklore

During your investigations you may also notice some white, frothy blobs on the leaf axils of the cuckooflower. This is commonly called 'cuckoo spit' as it was thought that cuckoos spat on the eponymous plant while flying over! In fact, these are the homes of the larvae of the light-green insect, the meadow frog hopper.

It seems that the name of 'lady's smock' comes from Tudor times. Certainly, by Shakespeare's day, the plant had already acquired that name as we see from *Love's Labour's Lost*:

> When daisies pied and violets blue
> And lady-smocks all silver-white
> And cuckoo-buds of yellow hue
> Do paint the meadows with delight,
> The cuckoo then, on every tree,
> Mocks married men; for thus sings he:
> Cuckoo;
> Cuckoo, cuckoo! O, word of fear,
> Unpleasing to a married ear!

(Act V, scene II)

As with much of Shakespeare's work, subtle meanings lie beneath the words, 'cuckoo' being close to 'cuckold', the implication being that wives were being less than faithful, and their smocks, or undergarments, less than pure white. As for the other name of 'cuckoo flower', this seems to have been generally applied to any plant that flowered when the cuckoo was calling and here may refer to the cowslip.

Gerard's *The Herball* throws extra light on the possible origin of the name in describing the behaviour of the seed pods: '… though you put but your hand neere them, as profering to touch them, though you doe not, yet will they fly out upon you … and it may be called in English, Impatient Lady-smock …' Here we have the image of the smock suddenly flying open, a seductive invitation from an impetuous young woman!

It is easy to imagine why this pale, dainty, almost ethereal plant should have been thought to be sacred to fairies. At any rate, it was bad luck to remove it from its location and bring it into the home. Equally it would never be included in May Day garlands.

Uses

It seems surprising that there is so little mention of lady's smock or cuckooflower in traditional herbals, bearing in mind that it is in fact extremely rich in vitamin C, containing about 15 times more than lemons. Of course, most vitamins had not been identified until the mid-20th century, but nevertheless experience had shown that it helped to counteract the terrifying symptoms of the fatal disease scurvy, which wiped out many thousands of sailors on long sea voyages without access to fresh fruit and vegetables. Culpeper, however, astrologer-physician of more than 350 years ago, knew of its efficacy: 'They are good for the scurvy, provoke urine, break the stone, and effectually warm a cold and weak stomach, restore lost appetite, and help digestion.'

Wildlife

Lady's smock, along with various other Brassicaceae (flowers with four petals forming a cross), is important in the wildlife chain. It is the main food plant of the agile orange-tip butterfly and the attractive green-veined white. Thanks to our lady's smock, together with the hedge mustard and garlic mustard, we have the pleasure of seeing these attractive butterflies on the wing in summer. If you look carefully just under a bud, you may see the tiny egg of the orange-tip, first white then orange, which will develop into a pale-orange, later green, caterpillar. Evidently it relishes the sharp, peppery taste of this plant!

Lords-and-Ladies (*Arum maculatum*)

Lords-and-Ladies family (Araceae). Perennial. Pollinated by midges and small flies. Propagated by seed. Poisonous berries.

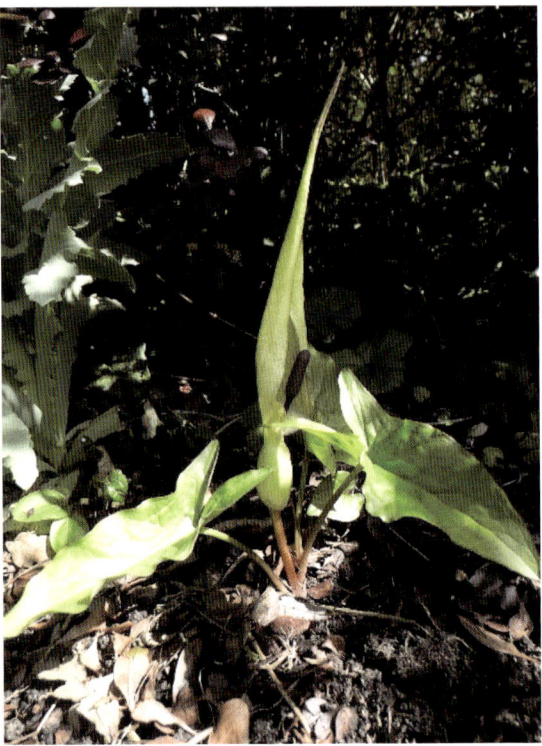

This is a very successful fly trap.

You may have noticed as early as March the large, pointed, shiny, green leaves, some purple spotted, that have pushed up through the ground from buried tubers. By May the strange purple spike, or 'spadix', will have appeared, hooded by a light-green 'spathe'. Gerard, writing in 1597, offers a lively description: 'Arum or Cockow pint hath great, large, smooth, shining, sharpe pointed leaves, bespotted here and there with blackish spots, mixed with some blewness… It beareth also a certaine long hose or hood, in proportion like the eare of an hare: in the middle of which

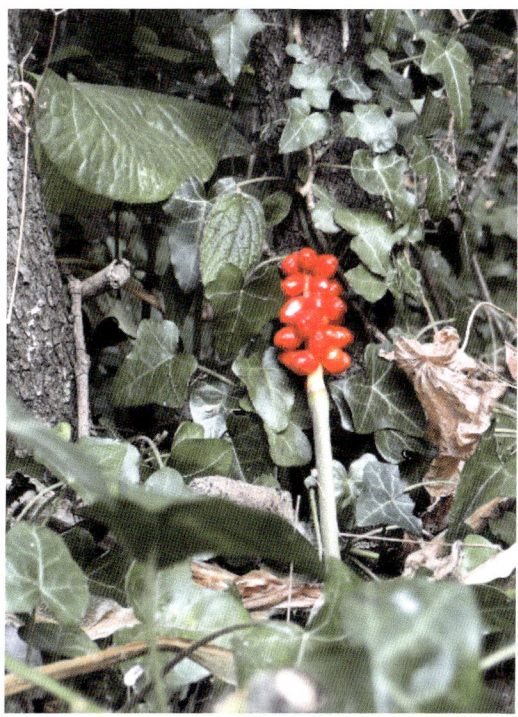

It is well worth allowing lords-and-ladies to develop, as the bright red berries complement the dark greenery. The plant is also known as 'cuckoo pint'.

hood commeth forth a pestle or clapper of a darke murry or pale purple colour.' Although this 'clapper' may look like the flower, these are in fact hidden from view in the bulge at the bottom of the spathe. Tiny carpels, the female part of the flower, encircle the base of the spadix with a ring of male stamens clustered above them.

This is a truly extraordinary plant, displaying nature at its most cunning because just above the male stamens are hairs which are hooked downwards to create a fly trap. Moreover, the spadix is able to raise its temperature and give off a foul, putrid odour, both of which happen to be extremely attractive to midges and small flies. Having already visited another cuckoo pint, the flies pollinate the female part of the flower. After a few days the pollen from the stamens becomes ripe and falls to the bottom of the spathe where the flies are trapped. The hairs then wither, allowing the pollen-covered insects to escape and be lured to another cuckoo pint to repeat the pollination cycle.

By the autumn, the spathe will have died away, but meanwhile the female flowers will have turned into bright orange-red berries, which can positively glow in a dark woodland corner.

Folklore

The phallic shape of the plant gave it lusty associations and it is thought that the word 'pint' from the popular name of cuckoo pint is actually a corruption of 'pintle', a long-forgotten word for penis. 'Cuckoo' may simply refer to the fact that the plant comes into flower when the cuckoo is calling. On the other hand, it could be a derivation of the Anglo Saxon *cucu* meaning quick or lively. This brings us to another innocent-sounding description with equally bawdy connotations: 'wake Robin', this name being derived from the French *robinet* for tap. The most amusing along these lines, and the least subtle, is 'Willy lily'!

I remember from my childhood that the plant was often referred to as 'jack-in-the-pulpit' or 'parson-in-the-pulpit'. Were these, along with 'lords-and-ladies', more decorous versions concocted by prudish Victorians to save the blushes of decent society? No one knows for sure. As far as lords-and-ladies is concerned, another possibility is that this refers to the powder and patches worn by the well-to-do in the 18th century. Indeed, the starch contained in the tubers was used in a French cosmetic known as 'cypress powder', which gave the face a fashionable pallid look. Patches first came to be worn to hide the scars of smallpox before becoming modish. Perhaps the purple spots on the leaves gave people this idea. All in all, from among the many common names, 'wild arum' can be counted as the most seemly!

The lustrous, orange-red berries that can so enliven a shady recess are in fact very poisonous. One folk tale is that the adder obtained its poison by eating cuckoo pint. They contain oxalates of saponins, its crystals causing irritation, burning and swelling to such a degree that anyone foolish enough to try them will not only suffer pain but will have great difficulty in breathing. If you have children, therefore, you may consider this plant should be dug up and removed from your garden. If, however, you value the unusual architectural shape and the gleaming colour of the berries, as we do, then you may decide to let it be.

Another curious attribute of cuckoo pint is that the pollen has a slight glow in the dark. When Irish folk came over to the Fens to look for work during their famine, they called them 'fairy lamps'. The local bargemen referred to them as 'shiners'.

Uses

At one time cuckoo pint was cultivated for its tubers which produce a starch that was used to stiffen the fine lawn of ruffs, collars and cuffs. Laundry women suffered greatly, however. Gerard points out in his *Herball* that it was 'most hurtfull to the hands of the Laundresse that hath the handling of it, for it choppeth, blistereth, and maketh the hands rough and rugged, and withall smarting'.

The root was also roasted and ground up to produce 'Portland sago', a popular drink among the common folk before the arrival of tea and coffee. Additionally, it was used like arrowroot for thickening.

Culpeper, in his herbal book, lists a number of possible remedies but acknowledges that these come from other sources and adds with some humour: 'for my part, I have neither spoken with Dr. Reason nor Dr. Experience about it.' Such remedies are no longer in use and one wonders whether they might have done more harm than good.

Wildlife

One of the flies that pollinate this plant is the owl-midge *Psychoda phalaenoides*. The insect gets trapped in the flower and is covered with pollen which is then carried to new plants. It is also known that *A. maculatum* is one of the food plants for the macro-moth *Noctua janthe*, the lesser broad-bordered yellow underwing. The larvae feed on the leaves until the adults become airborne in summer.

Common Sorrel (*Rumex acetosa*)

Knotweed family (Polygonaceae). Perennial. Pollinated by wind. Propagated by seed. Edible.

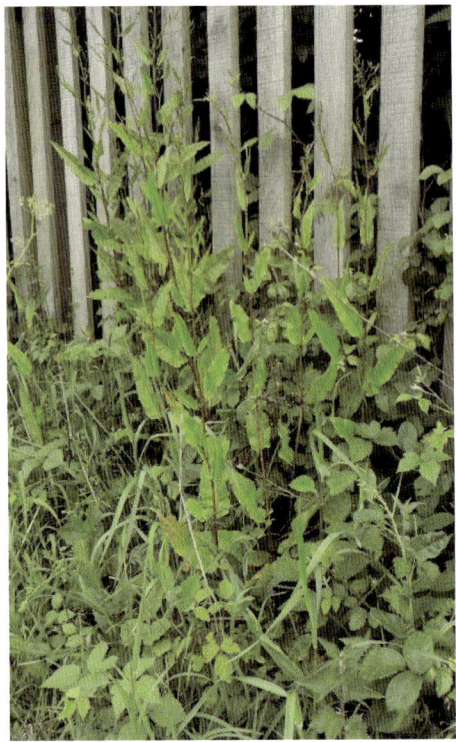

Sorrel may be plain in appearance, but its tangy leaves are praised by chefs.

Opinions vary significantly about this plant. Like dock, this hardy perennial is a tenacious weed, its long taproot making it extremely difficult to pull or dig out. Gardeners and farmers alike therefore generally curse its appearance. On the other hand, cooks and chefs with an interest in wild plants praise its culinary virtues. They even encourage its cultivation – at any rate the broad-leaved variety – for its lemony tang, which adds piquancy to the more delicately flavoured foods, such as fish and eggs or creamy cheeses. As for cattle and sheep, they will devour it greedily.

Common sorrel favours grassy places, so, luckily for us, ours grows harmlessly on our meadow, mingling with the unmown long grasses. In the early summer the reddish spikes of flowers, arranged in loose whorls up the stems, are easily spotted, later on deepening in shade to browny purple.

Folklore

There are very few records concerning the folklore surrounding sorrel. Mrs Grieve in her herbal book of 1931 does mention the old country name of 'cuckoo's-meate'. The underlying belief was that by pecking at sorrel the bird was then able to clear its throat before making its call!

Uses

If work in the garden leaves me hot and thirsty, I find that munching one of the arrow-shaped sorrel leaves is remarkably refreshing. Indeed, the poet John Clare describes how parched field workers used to chew the leaves. I will also pick a few young ones to add to a salad. If chopped fine and stirred into cottage cheese, they give a pleasantly sharp flavour. However, the plant does contain oxalic acid, so it is sensible to take it in moderation.

Although I have never tried it, the juice of common sorrel has been used to take rust spots out of linen. In Scotland and Wales it was reckoned to be very good as a dye for wool, the roots when boiled producing a rich red colour. Conveniently, the leaves could then be employed as the fixer. Without question, however, its main worth is as an ingredient in a sauce to accompany fish.

Sorrel sauce

Handful young sorrel leaves
1 oz/25 g butter
double cream

Simply pick a handful of young leaves, wash and shred finely. Melt the butter in a pan, then stir in the sorrel. Cook gently to allow the flavour to permeate, then add the cream to your preferred consistency. Heat through and serve with a white fish.

Wildlife

If you have *Rumex* growing under a hedge, have a look at the leaves in spring. If you see larval spinning this could belong to the moth light grey tortrix which feeds on sorrel. Indeed, the leaves are eaten by the larvae of several other species of moth.

Perhaps the prettiest of these is the blood-vein, which has pink fringing to its wings. When these are extended, you can see a red band running right across its fore- and hindwings. There are two generations, the first flying in May to July and the second in August to September. You are more likely to see it in the south rather than the north of England.

Often found in a suburban setting is the brown spot pinion, which has chestnut colouring and black markings on the edges of the forewing. This flies later in the year, September to October, and is attracted to light, so you may see it in the evening by a window.

During the 20th century numbers of the brightly burnished small copper butterfly declined dramatically, due largely to the intensification of agriculture. It would be very good to help it by letting *Rumex* flourish by your fence or hedge, especially if you live near unploughed grassland, heathland or woodland with open rides. Sorrel is its main food plant. The white eggs are laid singly on the upper side of a leaf, but the caterpillars, which are green, feed underneath, creating 'windows'. Brush autumn leaves into a pile nearby, because this is where the caterpillars will transform into pupae.

Star-of-Bethlehem (*Ornithogalum umbellatum* subsp. *angustifolium*)

Asparagus family (Asparagaceae). Perennial. Pollinated by insects. Propagated by seed and bulb offsets. Irritant. Toxic.

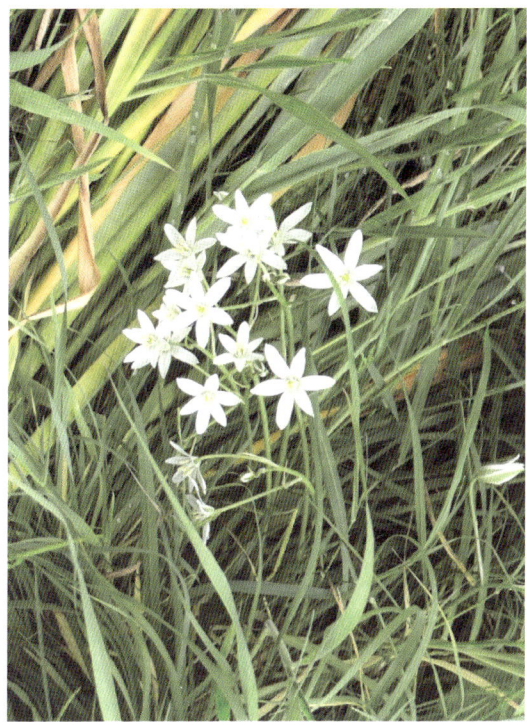

We were delighted to see star-of-Bethlehem appear spontaneously among the daffodil stalks.

There is an area of our front lawn which has been planted with spring bulbs – the crocuses, daffodils and anemones making a delightful show. When the flowers have finished, we allow them to die back naturally so that the goodness returns to the bulbs, leaving the patch unmown. Amid the remaining stalks we have been thrilled to see wild plants emerging. One year two bee orchids showed their faces, and now we have a little group of star-of-Bethlehem well established. This seems surprising because normally they prefer a sandy soil. However, they have been recorded in the wild in East Anglia since the 18th century.

Whether or not they were originally a garden escapee has not been definitively decided. My *Flora of Suffolk* tells me that *O. umbellatum* probably was formerly cultivated, but that a sub-species named *O. angustifolium*, which has fewer flowers per head, is most likely the one that is native to East Anglia – and the variety now in our garden.

The flowers are hermaphrodite, containing both male and female organs. There are six tepals (i.e. the petals cannot be distinguished from the sepals) each of which has a green stripe on the reverse. The slim, pointed leaves have a white band running down the centre on the upper side.

Folklore

When the sun shines, the pointed, white tepals open fully. One can see immediately why these charming flowers were named after the star associated with Jesus' birth: 'star of wonder, star of light' according to the well-known hymn. Indeed, they reflect the light beautifully.

Uses

There was a long tradition in the Middle East to dig up the onion-like bulbs, dry and store them, then use them as a source of nutrition on long journeys, especially when making pilgrimages to Mecca. The bulbs were commonly referred to as 'doves' dung'. As mentioned in the Second Book of Kings (vi, 25) in the *Bible,* there was a great famine in Samaria when under siege by the king of Syria, so much so that 'the fourth part of a cab of dove's dung' was sold for 'five pieces of silver' – a huge sum.

More recently, when star-of-Bethlehem was growing profusely in the woods near Bath, the cut plants, while still in bud, were sold as a vegetable and known as 'Bath asparagus'. Needless to say, this kind of commercial foraging is no longer acceptable.

One has to be careful before eating them as some varieties of the star-of-Bethlehem contain cardenolides, steroids which can be heart arresting and therefore toxic, so do **not** attempt to eat the bulbs. The sap can also irritate the skin. Despite this, the plant is used in a Bach™, Flower Remedy and is reputed to provide comfort in cases of shock or trauma.

Wildlife

The fully open flowers of the star-of-Bethlehem are extremely attractive to insects, so much so that the Royal Horticultural Society lists this plant as being especially beneficial for pollinators. Therefore, if you wish to see more bees in your garden, this would be a good choice.

Common Vetch (*Vicia sativa*)

Pea family (Fabaceae). Annual. Pollinated by bees. Propagated by seed. Mildly toxic.

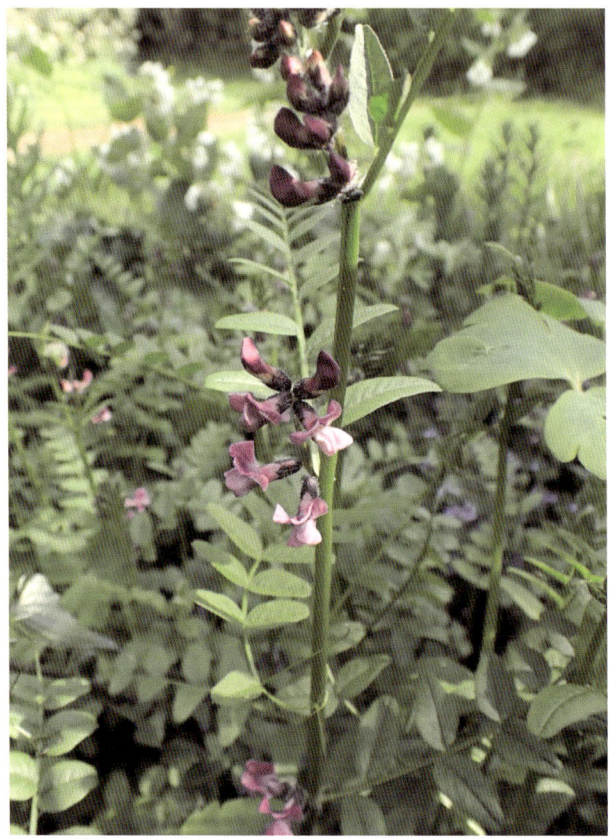

Vetch is easily recognised by its pea-like flowers and waving 'ladders' of leaflets.

Unless you leave some long grass in your garden, you are unlikely to see this plant as it favours meadowland. The common variety rambles happily in patches through our unmown grass, its pea-like petals providing little points of bluish purple among the green. The long stems also scramble over a sunny hedge, its curling tendrils twining themselves around the twigs to keep itself upright.

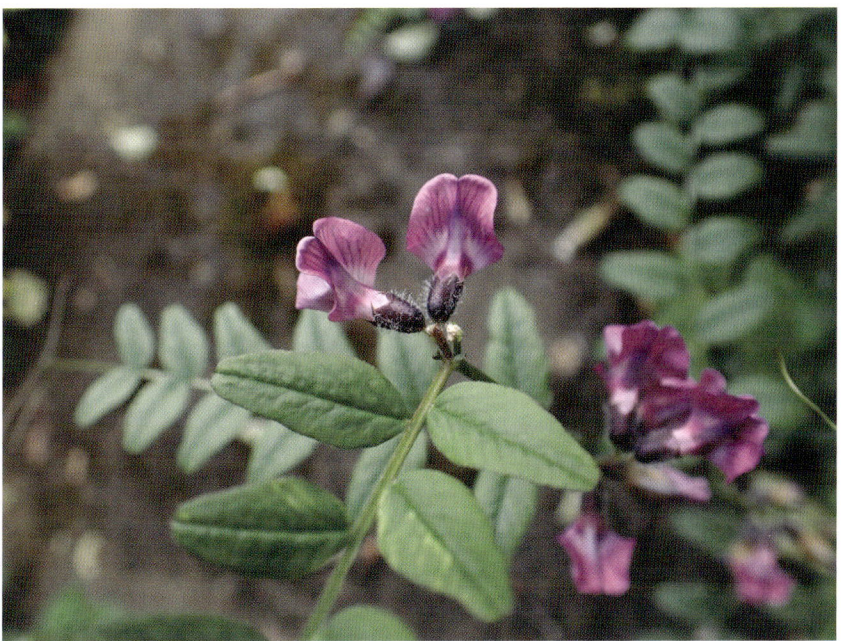

The pea-like flowers may appear singly or in pairs, as here.

There are five petals to each flower, the side pair overlapping the lowest two which are joined. The upper one is the largest. Just one or two of these flowers lie at the base of each petiole or small leaf stalk. Above is a waving 'ladder' of leaflets in opposite pairs, the grasping tendrils at the tips. They are spaced out and oval in shape.

In the autumn pods are produced, dark brown when ripe, each containing up to 12 seeds. These, if split, are somewhat like lentils and have even been illegally sold as such. Dispersal is mostly nearby, which explains the patches on our meadow.

Folklore

Other than the country description of 'poor man's pea', vetch has rarely been associated with plant lore. Its former common name was 'tare', especially when linked with animal fodder or an unwelcome corn weed. In the *Bible*, Matthew narrates Jesus' parable of the tares of the field in which they are the 'children of the wicked one' sown by the devil. This seems rather harsh, but crops were very precious with difficult growing conditions.

Uses

Although belonging to the pea family, vetches are no longer recommended for human consumption, being somewhat toxic if eaten in any quantity. No doubt this is the reason why the plant is not mentioned in herbals. Yet, in times of great hardship and starvation, meal has been made from the seeds. It has been recorded that Bernard of Clairvaux shared bread of vetch meal with his monks during the famine of 1124–26. Indeed, the meal was found in the meagre diet of the very poor until as recently as the 18th century, and it even occurred on the black market in France during World War II.

Common vetch is, however, nutritious for ruminant animals and it is often grown as fodder. Perhaps its most interesting attribute, like other plants of the pea family, is that it can make its own nitrogen from its cylindrical root nodules. It is therefore most useful as a soil fertiliser.

Wildlife

Bees are readily attracted to the sweet nectar and painstakingly crawl in and out of each flower, thereby pollinating the plant. It is very important to encourage bee-friendly wild flowers as these essential insects are increasingly under threat with loss of habitat, impaired immune systems and poisoning by certain pesticides. Vetches are sometimes deliberately grown for honey bees. Other insects also use vetch as a food source. If one should spontaneously appear in your garden, as ours did, do care for it and enjoy its visitors.

Wood Avens (*Geum urbanum*)

Rose family (Rosaceae). Perennial. Pollinated by bees and other insects. Propagated by rhizome and seed. Medicinal.

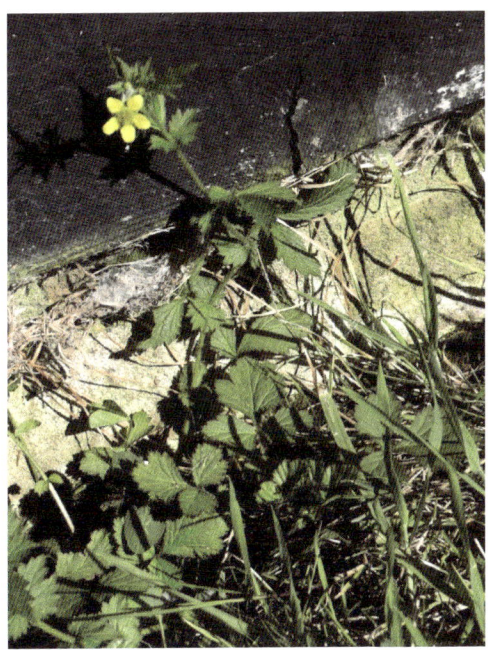

Wood avens are likely to pop up in your garden as they thrive in rich soil, unlike most wild flowers.

Despite its bright-yellow, cheerful flower, this plant has caused me some frustration. Each time I tried to pull it up, the stems broke leaving the tough roots intact. The only way to get it out was to lever it up with a fork dug well below the centre point of the spreading roots.

Much as I love our wild flowers, there were simply too many wood avens! They seemed to thrive in the moist corners around the house and places shaded by our tall trees. They also managed to thrust their roots down between paving slabs of paths, making it extremely difficult to get them out. Once established in a garden, they are likely to endure as they flourish in rich soil unlike many wild flowers. Not only are they perennials that persist each year, but their little, round, hooked burrs catch on the fur of animals or on the clothes of humans, unwittingly transporting the seeds to another area for germination. I have often found them entangled in my dog's hair or stuck to the back of my jeans.

One day I was expressing to my husband my inability to keep the wood avens under control only to discover, much to my astonishment, that he liked them! 'They're tough little things,' he said in some admiration. 'Let them be.' This encouraged me to take more interest in them. Looking closely at the flowers, I realised that the green, pointed sepals alternated with the yellow petals, giving each a somewhat startled appearance.

Folklore

Some country folk give the plant the descriptive name of 'gold star'. My mother, however, had always referred to it as 'herb bennet'. Wondering where this name came from, my researches pointed to the Latin *Herba benedicta* or 'blessed herb'. In medieval times the plant was considered to be blessed indeed as it was reputed to ward off evil spirits, even the devil, perhaps because of the spicy aroma of its roots. It was certainly popular with stone masons, and, if you look carefully when next in a centuries-old cathedral, you may see the flower carved as a motif.

Uses

In the early 17th century, Culpeper said of it: 'The root in the springtime, steeped in wine, doth give it a delicate flavor and taste, and being drunk fasting every morning, comforteth the heart, and is a good preservative against the plague or any other poison.' One cannot help surmising whether it was the wine on an empty stomach or indeed the herb itself that gave the patient such a soothing feeling! In fact, modern herbal medicine indicates that the root contains little in the way of active ingredients other than some tannins and essential oils. Nevertheless, it is still recommended for digestive complaints and poor appetite. The tea can also be used as a gargle to treat a sore throat or if applied to the skin can help to alleviate rashes, acne and eczema.

Herb bennet tea

2 tsp finely chopped fresh leaves
275 ml/½ pint boiling water
Pour the boiling water onto the leaves. Allow to infuse for 15 minutes. Strain and drink before meals to aid digestion, but not more than once a day. Makes 1-2 cups. ♦ Use as a gargle when lukewarm. For skin complaints, apply when cool.

Wood avens moth repellent

The Elizabethans trusted this herb, with its scent of cloves, to deter moths and other insects.
Roots of several wood avens plants
Wait until the plant starts to die back, then fork out the roots. Clean gently without soaking, then cut into small pieces. Dry in a very low oven, turning occasionally. Place in a muslin bag and hang in your wardrobe.

Culinary tip

If you run out of cloves, pieces of wood avens root can be used instead. It is very good in apple pie!

Wildlife

Wood avens is used by many insects as a food plant, including the larvae of flies, beetles and macro-moths. There is just one butterfly, the grizzled skipper, which favours the smaller members of the rose family and may well choose wood avens. If you live in the south of England or the Midlands, then you might spot this small brown and white butterfly on a warm day with its wings extended soaking up the sunshine. The little green caterpillar has a black head and brown stripes along its back. It will spin a silk 'tent' before feeding, leaving noticeable blotches on the leaves.

A macro-moth which visits gardens and is attracted to wood avens is the beautiful golden Y. This can be either amber coloured or even dark brown, with a velvety appearance. The adults are on the wing during June and July.

SUMMER

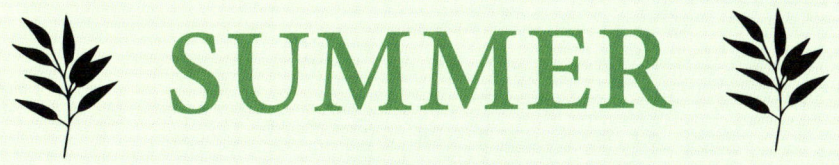

O Spirit of the Summer time!
Bring back the roses to the dells;
The swallows from her distant clime,
The honey-bee from drowsy cells.

Bring back the friendship of the sun;
The gilded evenings calm and late,
When weary children homeward run,
And peeping stars bid lovers wait.

Bring back the singing; and the scent
Of meadow-lands at dewy prime;
Oh, bring again my heart's content,
Thou Spirit of the Summer-time!

'Song: O Spirit of the Summer-Time' by William Allingham (1824–89).

JUNE

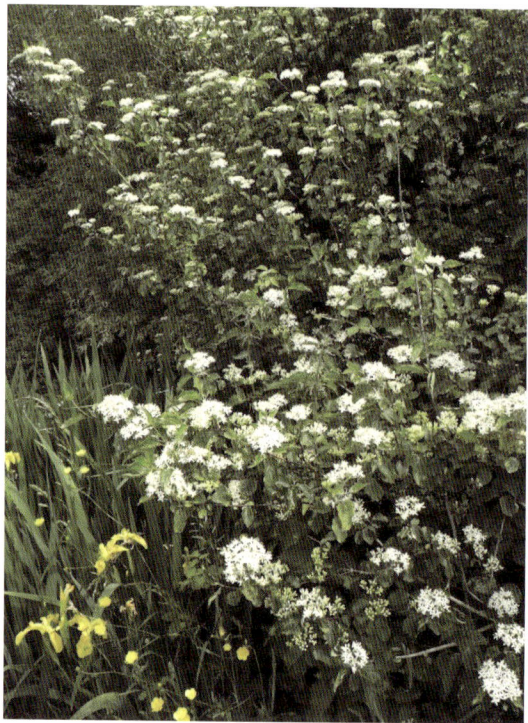

Although generally recommended for its attractive red stems in winter, dogwood also provides a summer show of creamy white blossoms.

This is a truly joyful month, with our garden full of colour. Our magnificent yellow flag irises bordering the pond are in full bloom and foxgloves have planted themselves in the cracks of paving stones. Along the side of the house, the wisteria is rich with drooping clusters of delicate lilac flowers and nearby the scent of the honeysuckle wafts through open windows. Our roses are putting on a good show, old-fashioned garden varieties mingled with the rambling stems and simple open petals of self-planted wild ones, which I have left to grow here and there. It always surprises me that the rather aggressively spiny pyracantha can produce such dainty, cup-shaped white flowers, which are well set off by the dark-green, glossy leaves.

I notice from Gilbert White's journal, written in 1784, that he, too, enjoyed mixing wild native plants with more exotic garden flowers, honeysuckle and vetch scrambling amidst the crown imperial fritillaries and fiery lilies. In that year the early summer weather was atrocious, with hailstorms so severe that several of White's windows and garden frames were smashed, costing him £2-5-10 for 'garden lights and hand glasses'. There seems to have been little let-up throughout the month as, day after day, he records rain, gales and deep fog. With global warming, our British summers seem to be more reliably sunny. We might consider this to be a good thing if it were not for the worry that our unremitting production of greenhouse gases will result in rising sea levels, unpredictable storms and catastrophic droughts.

Ambling through our small meadow is a real delight. The summer breeze ripples through the tall grasses, which are now displaying their delicate flowers, sending waves of nodding heads first one way then another. As the stems bend, the sunlight casts a silver sheen over them, creating a mesmerising dance. Each time I tread, dozens of tiny, buff-coloured grasshoppers spring out of the way, forming flying arches around each foot. Impossible to see until they move, these provide excellent nourishment for birds with sharp enough eyes and the speed to catch them. If we had mown the meadow, we would have had no grasshoppers and therefore fewer birds.

Around the other side of the house there is a different sort of activity. Here bees, in particular the white-tailed variety, are clustered around the cotoneaster that now emits a sweet perfume from the flowers. Underneath, white clover vies with the shrub for this buzzing attention. It is good to see so many healthy bees in our garden as these important pollinating insects have been having a hard time lately. Thirty of the 250 British bumblebee species are already extinct, and half of the rest are in perilous decline, with losses of up to 70 per cent since the 1970s. One theory is that pesticides are affecting bees' brains, blocking electrical signals between neurons, and preventing the insects from navigating to the best nectar sources and back home again. Here in East Anglia, which is intensively farmed, loss of wild flowers has been dramatic. Most bees need a varied nutritious diet which is impossible to find in a monocrop. Needless to say, malnourished bees are more susceptible to disease. Many beekeepers are reporting total colony collapse. Hence the crucial importance of providing nectar-rich flowers in our gardens, especially from native wild plants – or 'weeds'!

This month the bright pink flowers of common mallow are a particular favourite as these put on a show just when the spring plants are past their best.

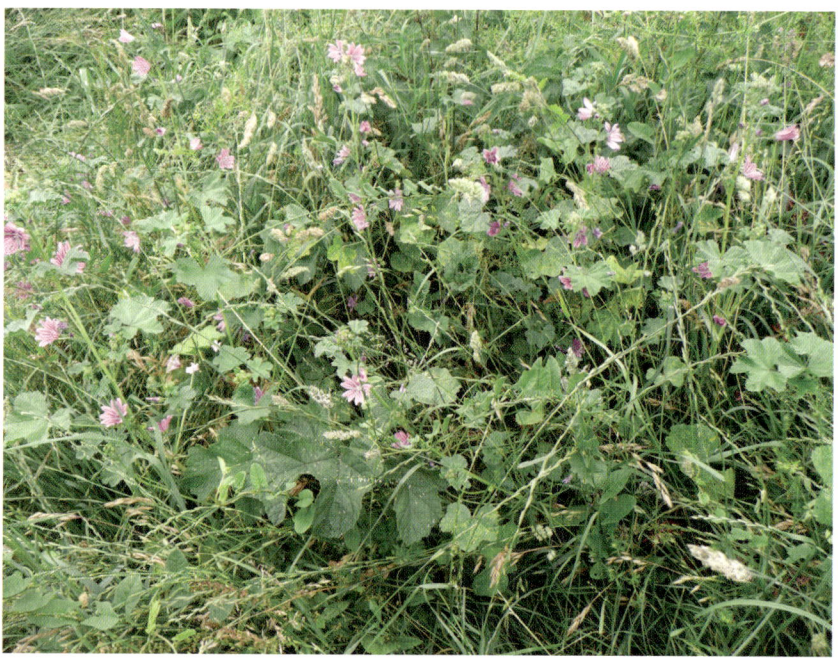

The flowers of common mallow provide a colourful display in the early summer.

Bittersweet (*Solanum dulcamara*)

Nightshade family (Solanaceae). Perennial. Pollinated by insects, especially bees. Propagated by seed. Poisonous.

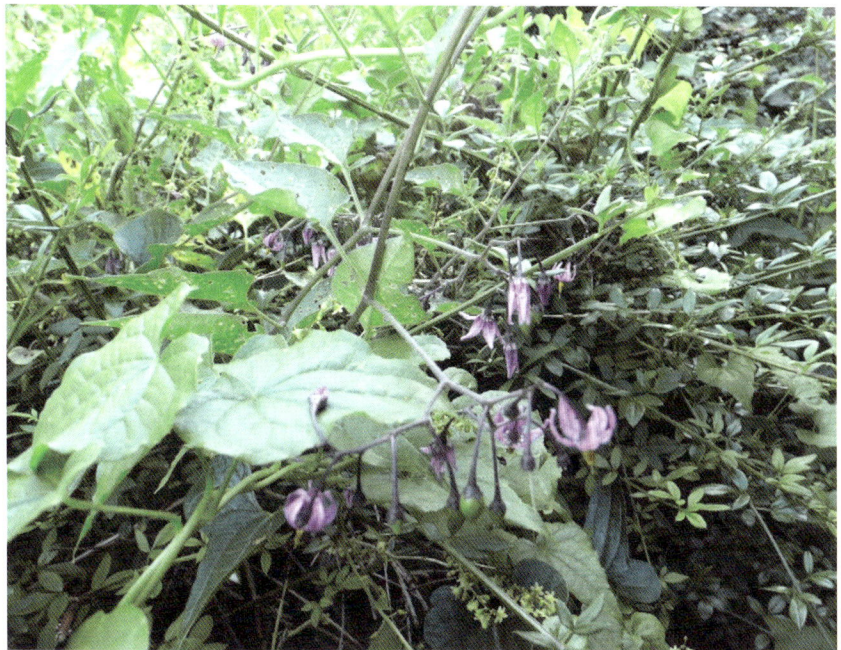

The purple petals of bittersweet are unusual in that they bend backwards.

We have a jasmine hedge planted along by our house, close to windows, which cheers us up in winter and early spring when the bright-yellow flowers finally burst into life, defying the wet and the cold. One year a somewhat straggly, slightly downy stalk appeared, rambling up and over the low hedge. This produced at first some lance-shaped, green leaves with a couple of rather odd lobes at the base of each, which Gerard, writing in 1597, likened rather charmingly 'unto two eares'.

Then, by the early summer, the most exotic-looking, purple flowers showed their faces, their five-pointed petals rolled back to exhibit a stunning yellow column of stamens. I counted as many as twenty flowers

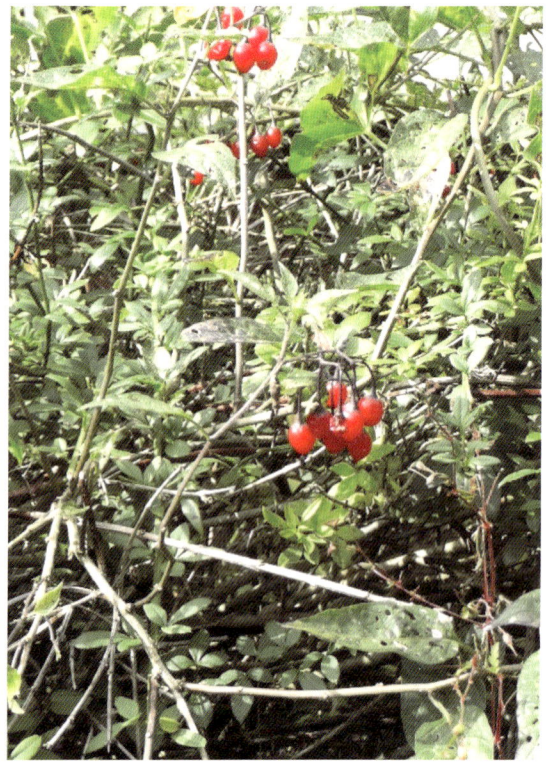

Tempting as these berries may look, do not try them, as they are both intensely sour and poisonous.

in one cluster alone. How could any busy bee not be tempted by such a striking display? Indeed, the nectar was clearly rather special as the plant was positively vibrating with their buzzing.

Folklore

Bittersweet, also called woody nightshade, is somewhat poisonous, although not as pernicious as deadly nightshade. I was particularly curious to know how this plant had been given its name of 'bittersweet'. Evidently, anyone so bold as to try eating the glossy, red berries in the autumn will have a nasty surprise as they are intensely sour. Having survived this unpleasant experience, there is reputed to be a sweet aftertaste, but it is definitely not recommended that you try it. Mrs Grieve, in her herbal book of 1931, notes that it is the chewing of the root and stem that tastes first bitter then sweet. Personally, I feel disinclined to test this out! Be that as it may, the Latin botanical name derived from *dulcis* (sweet) and *amarus* (bitter) is therefore erroneous; rather than *dulcamara* it should really be the other way round. Shakespeare's Isabella had the right idea:

> I should not think it strange, for 'tis a physic
> That's bitter to sweet end.

(Measure for Measure. Act IV, vi)

As you see, Shakespeare thought of the plant as therapeutic which seems somewhat astonishing bearing in mind its poisonous nature. Nevertheless, it was a known narcotic. Salmon, writing in 1693, says that an extract of the plant is 'soporiferous and operates much like Opium'. He comments, however, that it should be administered 'by a wise hand' – no doubt good advice.

Rather than taking the juice internally, there seems to have been an ancient custom of threading the berries to make necklaces or wreaths, either to ward off some kind of harm or to offer protection. It is interesting to note that when Tutankhamun's coffin was discovered a wreath of bittersweet berries was found on top of it. Perhaps it was thought to aid with a safe journey into the afterlife.

Culpeper believed that if the threaded berries were tied around the neck they would alleviate 'the vertigo or dizziness of the head'. In Germany, cattle wore bittersweet to avert evil or danger. Gabrielle Hatfield in her *Herbal* of 2007 reported that, until quite recently here in East Anglia necklaces of the berries were reputed to help infants with their teething.

Uses

Some herbalists recommended external application of the plant's juice for various skin conditions. Gerard suggested that it would heal bruising of 'them that hath fallen from high places', while Peachey later thought that the leaves administered externally would relieve inflammations and swellings.

Experience of bittersweet must have indicated to former physicians that it contained properties capable of alleviating certain skin conditions. Science now proves them right as alkaloids in the plant have been shown to have antidermatophytic activity. The stems have been officially approved in Germany for external use in cases of chronic eczema. The plant's narcotic ability is also now officially attributed to solanine, an alkaloid glycoside, which, unfortunately, has the debilitating side effects of vomiting and convulsions.

Wildlife

Being poisonous to humans and livestock, I wonder what part bittersweet plays in natural systems. The red berries clearly provide a special delicacy for certain birds in the autumn as they seek them out and quickly strip the plant, leaving the whitish stem (compared with 'the colour of ashes' by Gerard) looking rather forlorn. Thrushes, in particular, seem to thrive on them and are evidently immune to the poison. This plant not only ensures survival through pollination by bees but also disseminates its seeds via hungry birds.

Black Bryony (*Tamus communis*)

Black Bryony family (Dioscoreaceae). Perennial. Pollinated by insects. Propagated by seed and tuberous shoots. Poisonous. Irritant.

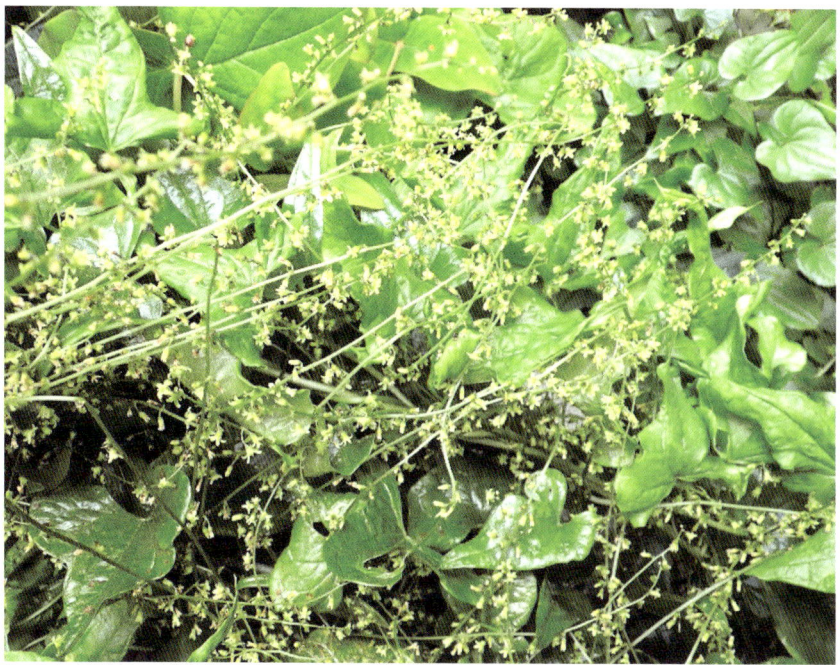

The glossy leaves of bryony are more noticeable than the tiny flowers.

I first noticed the long stems of black bryony when pruning some mature shrubs. Able to climb a considerable height, these seemed to be hanging on very effectively without tendrils, each twining itself in a clockwise direction around the supporting branches. The leaves, being a dark, shiny green and heart-shaped, were particularly attractive. Wondering how this weed might develop, I decided to leave it for a while. By the early summer, it had produced pale, yellowish-green flowers, each with six pointed petals, some in long racemes (male) and the others in small clusters (female).

While the flowers of black bryony are unremarkable, the garlands of glossy, bright-red berries make a spectacular show in the autumn, just at

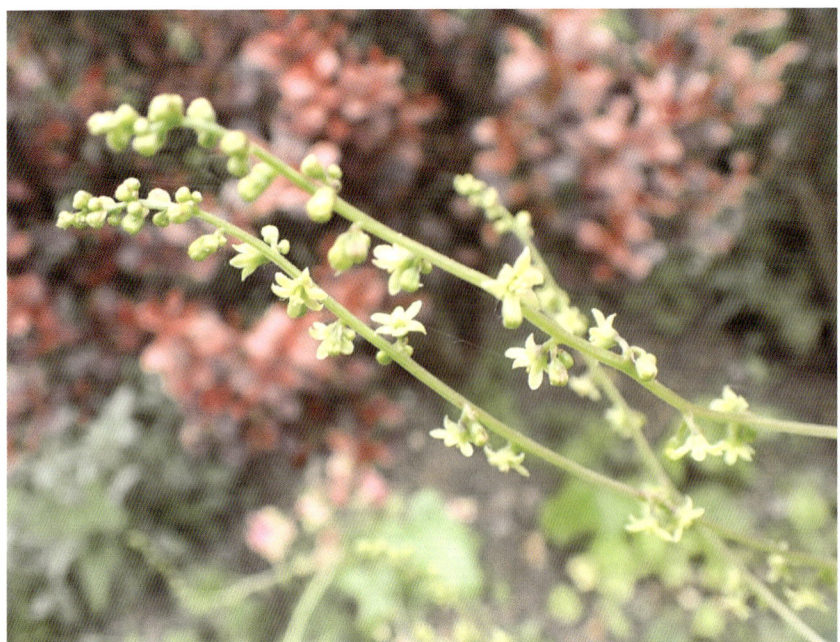

Close-up of black bryony flowers

the time when visual interest in the garden is waning. Although these look very tempting, they are in fact poisonous, so this is not a weed to encourage where children might be playing.

Folklore

As a relative of the yam, the root is a tuber, but, unlike its cousin, it is not edible, being acidic and an irritant. Despite this, farmers here in East Anglia would shred it and mix it in with horses' feed in the belief that it would enhance the shine of their coats. Perhaps they simply took this idea from the gloss of the leaves and berries.

Being a sufferer of chilblains as a child, I recall all too well the difficulty of pulling on shoes over swollen, itchy toes, then the agony of walking to school. As ours was a religious household, my mother would not have suggested the folk remedy in which the berries and roots were thoroughly soaked in gin before applying to the painful red swellings! Indeed, black

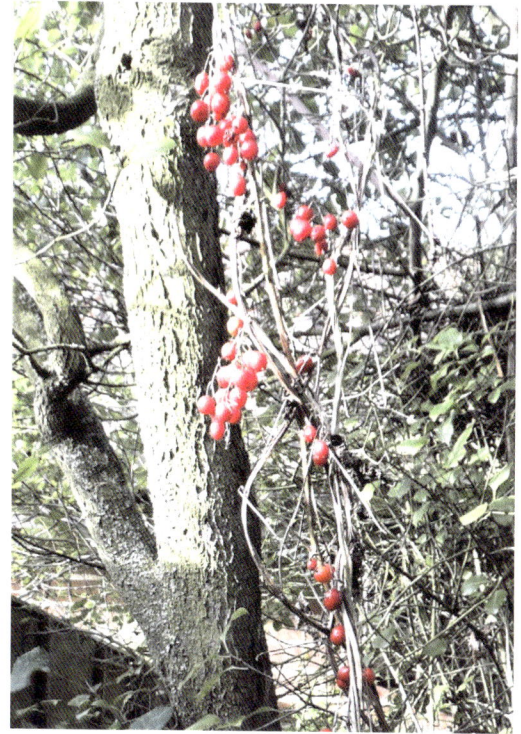

It can also be found hanging gracefully from small trees. We leave the plant here and there to benefit wildlife from the strings of bright red berries and to enliven dark days later in the year.

bryony had earned the name of 'chilblain-berry'. Whether it was the plant or the gin that was efficacious is hard to determine.

The French had an altogether different name for it: *Herbe aux femmes battues* – herb for beaten wives. Gerard seemed to agree, stating that the roots 'do very quickly … consume away blacke and blew marks that come of bruises and dry-beatings'. Perhaps the irritation caused by the remedy simply disguised the sting of the beatings.

Uses

While there are no known uses for black bryony growing in Britain, scientists have discovered that a Mexican relative of this plant, *Dioscorea composita*, contains the chemical compound sapogenin. They found a way of converting this into progesterone, which was subsequently used in the birth control pill.

Wildlife

I have noticed how black bryony grows from beneath a shrub or hedge or by a fence, scrambling upwards as it develops. Doubtless this is because a bird has perched above and dispersed the seeds after eating them. Although poisonous to humans, these apparently have no ill effects on the birds.

Two minute flies, the gall midge and a thrips will somewhat surprisingly use black bryony as the food plant of their larvae. Gall midges are attracted to light, so you may well find them in your kitchen if you have a window open. You will recognise them from their orange bodies. A thrips is generally black or brown with two pairs of feathery wings, although it is hard to see these without a microscope. Thrips are those annoying little insects that are evident during warm and humid weather and are therefore sometimes referred to as 'thunder flies'. Nevertheless, both the midges and the thrips are good pollinators despite their small size.

Red Clover (*Trifolium pratense*)
White Clover (*T. repens*)

Pea family (Fabaceae). Perennials. Pollinated by bees, butterflies and moths. Propagated by seed; *L. repens* also by stolon. Edible. Medicinal.

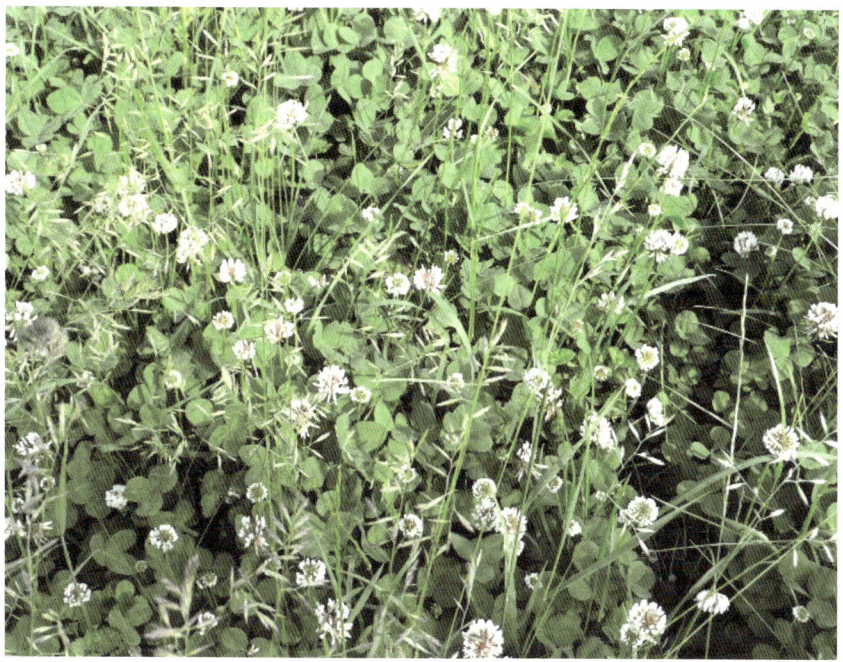

We have to be careful where to tread as this clover patch is often humming with bees.

Lucky enough to have a country childhood, I clearly recall picking clovers in nearby meadows and sucking the sweet nectar from the flower heads. Delicious! Each head is composed of a number of individual florets which cluster together into a ball-like shape. There are five slim petals to every floret, the two on the sides hiding the lower two which are joined, while the upper one is the broadest and most conspicuous.

Both clovers are perennials, but the white variety has creeping stems that root themselves at the nodes. Each bears the familiar three leaflets on a short stalk, yet there are differences: those of white clovers are rounded, whereas red clovers have oval leaflets, often with a light-coloured, V-shaped mark. As rain threatens or as night descends, the leaves will fold up protectively.

Clovers are well known for their ability to fix nitrogen in the soil and are therefore often deliberately planted for this reason. Do not root them out of your lawn as they compete with other weeds and will survive mowing. They also offer natural protection against plant diseases.

Folklore

Should you find a four-leaved clover, you will be lucky indeed – or so we are told. How I used to search in the hope of finding this charm, but it remained stubbornly elusive! Today, sadly, they are genetically engineered in America and sold to the unwary. However, if you happen to dream that you are lying in a meadow of clover, then it means you will be brought both happiness and good health. The expression 'to live in clover' signifies a life that is comfortable and carefree. Perhaps this comes from its use as a nutritious cattle feed.

The shamrock is of course the emblem of Ireland. Saint Patrick offered it as a metaphor for the Trinity, the Three in One, and on his commemoration day white clover was traditionally worn in hats. It was believed to have protective powers, especially against the spells of witches, and could even cure madness if brought indoors, or so it was said.

Uses

Red clover in particular has been traditionally used in plant medicine, and native American Indians knew of its efficacy in alleviating fevers. The dried heads would be kept to make a tisane that could treat coughs as well as skin conditions, including eczema and psoriasis. It is interesting that the active ingredients of tannins, glycosides and phenols are found in the plants. There are reports from the north of England as well as from Ireland of such a tea being used to treat bowel cancer and to thin the blood. Indeed, research carried out more recently has shown a certain anti-tumour capacity and also an anti-coagulant effect.

The proteins and sugars in clover mean that it can be foraged as a survival food. The flower heads will sweeten salads, and the leaves, if harvested when very young and tender, can be added to soups. Whole red clover plants can be picked and boiled for five or ten minutes to be eaten as a vegetable. The deep roots can also be dug up and are edible when cooked.

Red clover cough medicine

5 flower heads of red clover, fresh or dried
275 ml/½ pint boiling water
½ tsp honey

Put the flowers in a tea pot and pour on the boiling water. Allow to stand for 10 minutes. Strain as you pour into a cup and stir in the honey. ♦ For a bad cough, drink up to 3 cups a day.

Wildlife

The sweet nectar of red clover is particularly appealing to butterflies. We have seen the normally secretive small skipper feeding on the flower heads in our garden. In very warm sunny weather, a little later in the year, you may be fortunate enough to see the beautiful clouded yellow butterfly, whose caterpillars use clovers as their main food source. White clover attracts a micro-moth known as metallic coleophora due to its silvery sheen. It flies in the summer, then the larvae feed on the seeds in the early autumn.

Bees, of course, relish clover nectar, as do a variety of other insects. Not only are clovers very pretty when mingled with grasses, they provide sustenance for our pollinators. Do allow them to flourish in your garden.

Dog-rose (*Rosa canina*)

Rose family (Rosaceae). Deciduous shrub. Pollinated by insects. Propagated by seed or cutting. Edible. Medicinal.

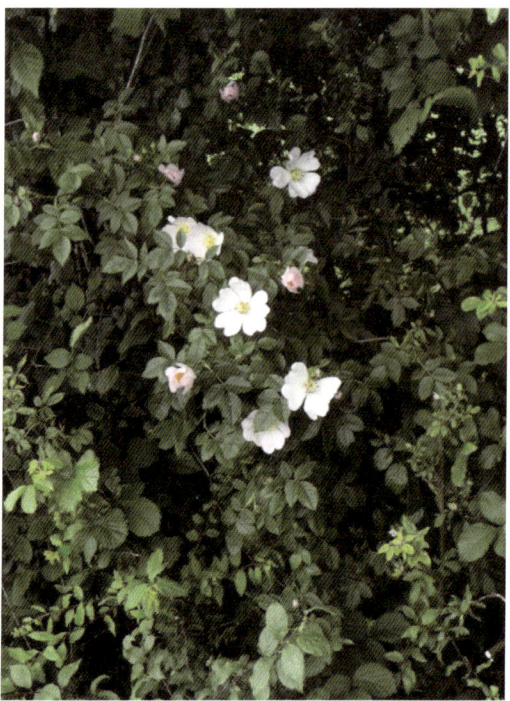

We welcome the wild beauty of dog-rose and are delighted when it turns up in a hedge, its tender petals peeping out shyly.

THE LEAVES AND FLOWERS

I am always struck by the contrast between the delicacy of the wild rose petals and the savagery of the thorny stems. Each of the five petals is almost heart shaped, often white near the yellow centre but blushed pink towards the edge. No wonder the flower is often used as a symbol for love! In the well-known poem by Christopher Marlowe, 'The Passionate Shepherd to his Love', the young man invites his love to live with him and declares:

> There will I make thee beds of roses
> And a thousand fragrant posies.

As for Thomas Lodge's 'Rosaline':

> Her lips are like two budded roses …
> Heigh-ho, would she were mine!

The plant certainly thrives in our heavy clay soil, often springing up in borders and around shrubs and trees. Much as I adore the beauty and simplicity of the flower and appreciate the usefulness of the hips, it is necessary to be discriminating about whether to leave, prune or dig up. One planted itself directly under a willow tree, sending up long, arching stems and attaching itself to the trunk and branches with its sharp thorns. After the flowers appeared, it looked such a picture that we decided to leave it *in situ*. Others we have had to remove as they were in quite the wrong place and crowding out valued garden plants.

The petals are not only extremely pretty, the pink coloration tells us that flavonoids, or vitamin P, are present. In nature, these pigments are designed to attract pollinating insects. Equally, the red hips invite the birds for a feast, which subsequently disperse the seeds.

Folklore

It is unclear where the term 'dog' comes from. There are two possibilities. Pliny the Elder, according to his *Natural History*, believed that by making a decoction of the root, the bite of a mad dog could be cured. Alternatively, the word might simply be a corruption of 'dag', short for dagger, descriptive of the long, sharp thorns.

Uses

Laboratory research has shown that flavonoids have several therapeutic actions, including anti-inflammatory, anti-microbial and anti-cancer. The petals also contain tannins, which have a mildly astringent effect. In the

Middle Ages they were commonly used to treat diarrhoea, while modern herbalists recommend them for care of the skin. It is therefore worthwhile to make an oil from the petals, which can be massaged in to help alleviate dryness and even reduce wrinkles. It is also reputed to calm tattered nerves. Salves can be made, too, to heal sore or chapped hands and lips.

Rose oil

Collect the petals just before they are about to fall, allowing insects to make maximum use of the nectar. Mix the wild ones with the cultivated, just as you wish, selecting those with a sweet perfume. Almond oil is best for this recipe, but good sunflower or olive oils are also effective. Addition of the wheat germ oil, at about 5 per cent, will help to prevent the infusion from becoming rancid.

Several handfuls of rose petals
almond oil
wheat germ oil

Place the petals in a wide-necked transparent glass jar. Cover with the almond oil and seal with a lid. Place in direct sunlight and allow to infuse. When the petals turn brown, replace with new ones. Repeat until the oil is pink-tinged. ♦ Strain when ready and stir in some wheat germ oil. Transfer to a dark jar with stopper. ♦ Massage into the skin as necessary.

Rose salve

Have ready several small, clean jars with lids.
275 ml/½ pint rose oil (as recipe above)
25 g/1 oz beeswax, grated
boiling water

Pour the oil into a heat-proof jug or jar and stir in the beeswax. Place this in a large pan and surround with the water to the level of the mixture. Return gently to the boil and simmer until the beeswax has dissolved, stirring from time to time. ♦ Remove from the bain-marie and, after a little cooling, pour into the small jars and allow to set before replacing the lids.

Wildlife

The leaves of our native wild rose provide useful sustenance to no less than 20 species of moth. If you notice a long 'mine' that winds round a leaf, turning back on itself, that will almost certainly indicate the presence of the larvae of the rose leaf miner moth. It is tiny, with a wing span of up to just 6 mm/¼ inch. It has bronze-coloured wings with a green-red sheen.

Another moth with a metallic lustre, but much larger, is the green brindled crescent. This seems to be quite happy in a suburban setting and is on the wing in the autumn. You may notice the dark-grey caterpillars on rose leaves earlier in the year. Do leave them alone! They could become a tasty snack for a local song bird.

You can also find the grey caterpillars of the feathered thorn moth, so called because of the feathering on the antennae of the male adults. These are reddish brown with a dark-brown, narrow band across the forewings, which stretch to 45 mm/1¾ inches. Similarly, this flies in the autumn.

These and the many other invertebrates that use dog-rose leaves as a food supply are all part of the wildlife in your garden. Finding out what they are can become a fascinating study.

Elder (*Sambucus nigra*)

Moschatel family (Adoxaceae). Deciduous shrub. Pollinated by insects. Propagated by seed. Flowers and cooked berries edible. Medicinal.

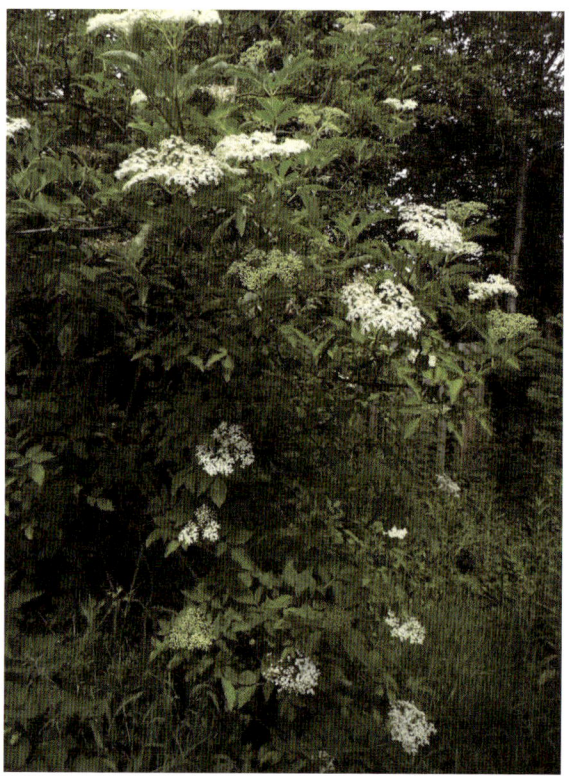

Many superstitions surround the elder, being associated with black magic as well as supposedly having protective powers.

THE LEAVES AND FLOWERS

Despite its unprepossessing, rather straggly appearance, elder is a most useful wild shrub to encourage in the garden. The creamy-white flowers, which form in June and July, are sweetly scented and extremely pretty, forming a 'corymb' or cluster with a flattish top, made possible by some of

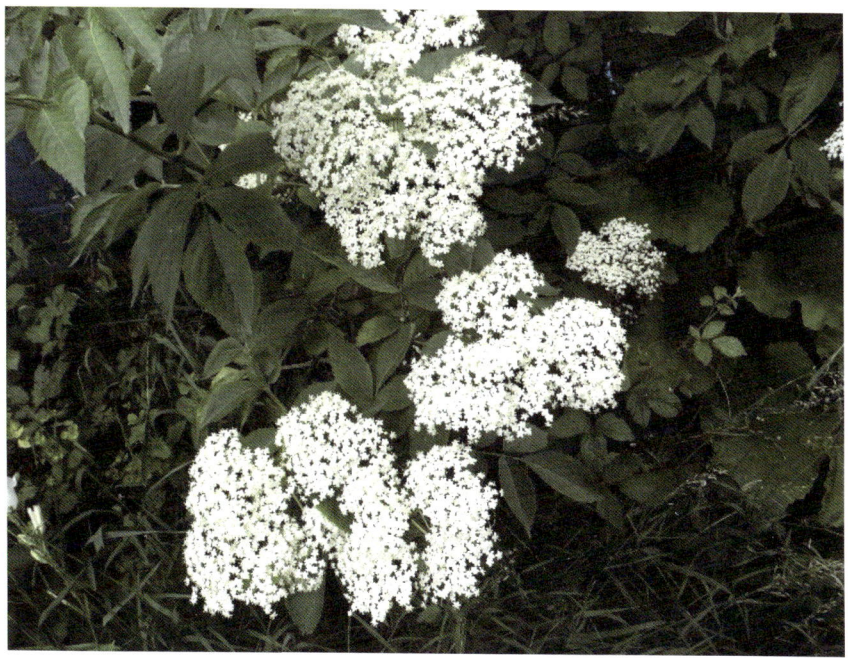

Close-up of elder flowers

the lower flowers having longer stems. They make a refreshing snack eaten straight off the tree or delicious fritters when dipped in batter and fried, and the cordial is, of course, sold commercially and widely available. As for elderflower 'champagne', this is without doubt the best sparkling country wine. The flowers form the basis of many remedies, being particularly helpful in easing skin conditions. Indeed, every part of the plant has had a use in folk medicine.

Unfortunately, elder tends to spring up in the most inconvenient places. The trick is to watch out for a young one, then move it to a better location before it becomes too big. You will recognise the oval, pointed leaves, with sharply toothed edges, set opposite each other with several on each stalk. The main stem is greyish-brown in colour.

It seems a shame that elder is currently regarded as a weed. In the 18th century it was deliberately planted as a fast-growing hedge, sometimes in double rows, each plant being staggered so that the blossoms formed attractive arching patterns in the summer. As a minor part of a hedge, however, it can quickly overshadow its neighbouring plants due to its rapid growth. Therefore, it is better to let it flourish somewhere on its own and allow it to achieve its full height.

Folklore

Despite its many nutritional benefits to us, the elder has been associated with black magic, witches and the devil, and bad-tempered fairies at various times in history. A great many superstitions have surrounded the plant which can be traced even into the middle of the 20th century. For some long-lost reason, it was believed during the Middle Ages to be the tree to which Christ was nailed, though I have yet to see one which could bear the weight of a person, many of its branches being largely hollow with soft pith. That said, the heartwood is very tough. The following Scottish rhyme implies that the tree took on its unprepossessing appearance because Jesus was nailed to it:

> Bour-tree, bour-tree, crookit rung,
> Never straight, and never strong,
> Ever bush, and never tree,
> Since our Lord was nailed t'ye.

No doubt, this Christian association gave rise to the superstition that it was very unlucky to cut elder down or destroy it. Here in East Anglia to burn the green branches brought dire consequences: 'you'll die with aching bones' was the threat. At the same time the religious connection seems to have endowed the bush with protective powers, so that if you stood under it in a storm the belief was that the lightning would not strike you. Elder was often planted next to the house to keep away bad spirits or fixed to doors and windows, as in the Isle of Man. There were, however, pragmatic reasons for this custom as the odious smell from the leaves deterred the flies. Equally, bunches of leaves would be hung on a horse's harness or on the door of a cowshed to give relief to the animals.

Yet Jesus' betrayer, Judas, was said to have hanged himself on the elder, summoning up ominous associations. The dramatist Ben Jonson used this idea in his comedy of 1598 *Every Man out of his Humour*, in which each character represented a vice, two such described thus: 'He shall be your Judas, and you shall be his elder-tree to hang on.' Records from medieval assizes show that witches had used the elder in black magic, and there was a long-held conviction that fairies resided in the hollow stems, who would wail each night if the branches were cut.

There were so many good uses for the elder that I'm left wondering how people found a way around these superstitions. One seems to have been to ask permission of the druids, or fairies as the case may be, before taking anything from the shrub. You may like to invent your own incantation!

Uses

Elder has been comparatively well researched, and it has been discovered that the main biologically active ingredients are the flavonoids and triterpenes (see Glossary). Laboratory studies have shown that remedies made from various parts of the elder display in particular anti-viral, anti-inflammatory and diuretic actions. Both the flowers and the berries offer good support to the immune system (see also under September). Yet, generations before such scientific studies were carried out people knew from practical experience how valuable the different parts of this shrub could be – roots, bark, leaves, flowers and berries. Gabrielle Hatfield in her *Herbal* lists many folk remedies, including the use of the bark as a painkiller and emetic, the buds as a gentle laxative, the root for rheumatism and the pith against ringworm.

An infusion made from the flowers is a classic remedy for the promotion of a fair complexion. Mrs Grieve in her *Modern Herbal* of 1931 says: 'Elderflower water in our great-grandmother's day was a household word for clearing the complexion of freckles and sunburn and keeping it in a good condition.' The anti-viral actions of the flowers help to hasten recovery from colds and 'flu if either the cordial or tisane is drunk hot and taken regularly. The decongestant effect also helps to loosen up catarrh and clear sinuses. Some people have discovered that it can be a helpful remedy for hay fever. Besides tea, soothing ointments and creams can be made from the flowers, which have been used to encourage healing of both eczema and dry, chapped hands.

The leaves have therapeutic properties too and are said to ease the symptoms of insect bites if rubbed directly onto the affected area. However, be aware that the leaves, along with the bark, seeds and raw, unripe fruit contain the cyanogenic glycoside sambunigrin, which is potentially toxic in significant doses. Such remedies are best used externally therefore and are not recommended if pregnant or breastfeeding.

The leaves can also be boiled up in water and used as a spray against mildew and aphids. This is well worth a try. It seems that the caterpillars that strip a gooseberry bush bare dislike elder leaves, so lay some elder branches underneath for protection.

Drying the flowers

On a sunny day, cut off the corymbs whole. Gently remove any insects. Hang each separately upside down from the main stem. Choose a dry place where there is a movement of air. This discourages mould from developing. Leave them for several weeks until the flowers are crisp to the touch. They can be stored in a darkened glass jar until the following year.

Elderflower infusion

Three teaspoons of dried flowers infused in a pint of boiling water will help to alleviate colds and 'flu when drunk hot, or freshen and tone the skin when patted on cold. It also soothes sore and tired eyes if a clean cloth is soaked in the cooled infusion and placed over the closed lids. Any remaining infusion can be poured into the bathwater.

Soothing elderflower ointment

This ointment is made by infusing the oil with the flowers, then mixing with beeswax to thicken which has its own healing properties, being naturally anti-bacterial. The ointment is excellent for rough, chapped hands and will help to heal minor cuts. Have ready some sterilised, wide-mouthed jars with lids.

Several elderflower heads, freshly picked
275 ml/½ pint almond oil
25 g/1 oz yellow beeswax, grated

First fill a 275 ml/½ pint jar with the flowers cut from the stalks. Cover the flowers completely with the oil. Seal the jar and leave in a warm place for at least two weeks, allowing it to infuse. Check it from time to time. It is ready when it has taken on the colour of the flowers. Strain thoroughly. ♦ Pour the oil into a pan and stir in the beeswax. Heat very gently until it melts, then transfer to the jars and leave to set. Screw on the lids.

Wildlife

Wildlife profits from elder, the nectar attracting many insects in summer, while the berries provide nutritious food for birds in the autumn (see under September). Indeed, it is the birds that help to propagate the shrub. If you have elder in your garden, you will notice the many hoverflies that visit the flowers, along with numerous small beetles. It is quite easy for the tiniest of insects to acquire the nectar as it is shallow and readily available. Small solitary bees will come along for the same reason. All of these insects will of course pollinate at the same time.

There is a grey moth with small, white dots that seeks out elder on which to lay its eggs. Its name is the white-spotted pug. There are in fact two generations of this moth, the first flying in May to June and the second in July to August. It so happens that by the time the larvae have hatched from the spring generation the elderflowers are in full bloom, offering a rich food source. You may see them feeding. They are pale green with dark, green-brown patches.

Another particularly pretty moth that favours elder is the V-pug, so called because of the two distinctive V-shaped marks on the green wings. When resting, it forms a characteristic triangular shape making it easy to identify. There are also two generations of this moth, each flying at the same time as the white-spotted pug, although in northern parts of Britain there may only be the earlier one.

Foxglove (*Digitalis purpurea*)

Speedwell family (Veronicaceae). Biennial. Pollinated by bees. Also self-fertile. Propagated by seed. Poisonous.

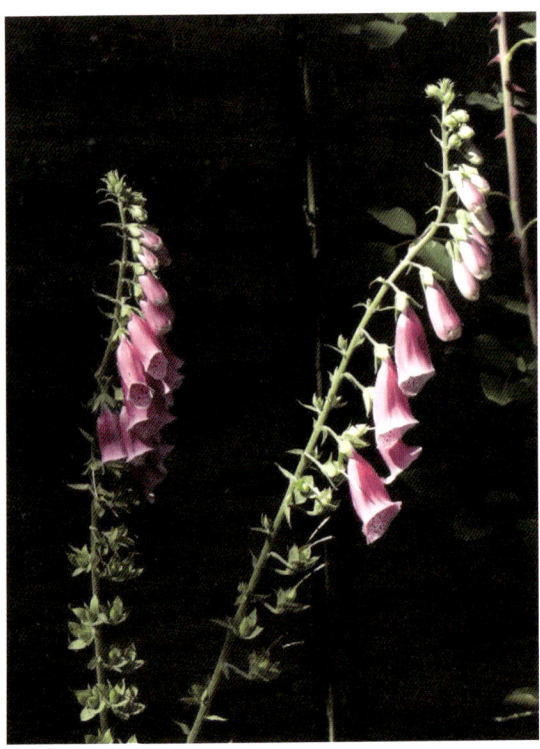

Foxgloves self-seed freely around our garden.

I always look forward to the moment when our foxgloves push up beyond the height of a certain window ledge. Our computer sits right next to this window and it is such a joy to be able to glance sideways at these majestic plants now and then while working. Their tubular, pinky-purple flowers, spotted inside and arranged so elegantly on just one side of the tall stem, have the effect of lifting the spirits. I was astonished to read that a single plant can produce up to 80 flowers.

Our foxgloves appeared 'out of the blue', probably transported by wind or rain, and have re-seeded themselves ever since. Somehow, they manage to survive just in a crack of the path, perhaps enjoying the cool, shady place by the house, a human-made substitute for the woodland glade which would be their natural setting.

The spear-shaped leaves with their downy hairs are beautifully soft to the touch, spiralling up the stem from a basal rosette, each with its own short stalk. In fact, being biennials, you will see only the rosette of leaves in the first year, the flower spike appearing in the second. If I notice one that has started to put down roots in an inconvenient place, I dig it up and carefully replant it in a more suitable location. Foxgloves are reputed to prefer acid soil, but ours seem to be perfectly content with our clay. Gardeners say that they are excellent companions to other plants as they encourage their growth and help to protect them from diseases.

Folklore

The scientific name comes from the Latin *digitus*, meaning finger. Since time immemorial children have fitted the flowers over their fingers and chased each other, purple 'claws' at the ready: hence the association with gloves. Yet no one seems to be sure why they should be connected with foxes. Could it be that the velvety hairs on the stem and leaves have reminded people of a soft, furry animal? Or is it that the plants grow in shady places most likely to be frequented by foxes? Whatever it is, the origin of the popular name is now lost in the mists of time. The association is not always with gloves, however, as fairies are often reputed to use the flowers as thimbles or hats.

As recently as 1948, Lewis Spence reported of the more sinister aspects of Irish superstition, whereby the juice of foxglove would be used to test whether or not an infant was a changeling. It involved giving three drops of the juice on the tongue and three in each ear, then putting the baby on a shovel and swinging it out of the front door three times while chanting, 'If you're a fairy, away with you.' If the child died that night, then that proved it was a fairy; if not, then the infant was no changeling and would recover.

Bearing in mind that digitalis is a poison, one wonders how many were 'proved' to be not entirely human and allowed to die.

People in southern England believed, for some unknown reason, that if a foxglove appears one spring in your garden, as ours did, then that is a sign of good luck and you should tend it lovingly. If, however, you transplant it, then your good luck will turn bad. Since I have been responsible for both actions, I can't say I have been aware of any significant changes in my fortune!

Uses

The history of the foxglove being employed as a herbal remedy is extremely interesting. Culpeper listed various uses, including the healing of sores, wounds, phlegm and falling sickness. Above all, he was 'confident that an ointment thereof is one of the best remedies for a scabby head'. It was also used in folk medicine as a diuretic, but the patient often failed to survive. Knowing of its toxicity, Gerard wisely agreed with 'the Ancients' that it had no place in medicine. How wrong he was proved to be!

Serious scientific work on the plant was eventually carried out by Dr William Withering (1741–99), a physician and botanist. It so happened that the young lady he was in love with was a keen amateur artist, especially of painting wild flowers, and it was this that prompted him to investigate their properties. It is generally considered that his book *An Account of the Foxglove and Some of its Medical Uses* was pivotal in initiating a break between time-honoured herbalism and the modern approach to the development of drugs. The book records in detail the benefits on the heart of the right dose of digitalis, slowing its beat and at the same time fortifying the muscle. An 18th-century rhyme captures this precisely:

> The Foxglove's leaves, with caution giv'n,
> Another proof of favouring Heav'n,
> Will happily display:
> The rapid pulse it can abate;
> The hectic flush can moderate;
> And, blest by Him whose will is fate,
> May give a lengthen'd day.

Experience of treating patients suffering from 'dropsy', or fluid retention, also showed that the diuretic action could help to alleviate this condition. Here again, exact dosage was vital to avoid doing more harm than good.

Finally, the active ingredients of the plant, digitoxin and digoxin, were isolated and the heart drug thereby derived came into general use. The naturalist Richard Mabey reminds readers in his *Flora Britannica* that during World War II foxglove leaves were gathered from limestone areas as they were particularly rich in digitalis. The European foxglove *Digitalis lanata* is now usually preferred for the making of the heart drug.

Wildlife

Here again we have a wild plant, all parts of which are poisonous, yet the purple flowers are highly attractive to bumble bees and seem almost to have been made for them. They can conveniently alight on the protruding lower petal, then make their way inside the tubular flower, where they can reach the nectar undisturbed. At the same time, of course, the plant is pollinated. Wild bees are in dramatic decline and desperately need gardeners' help. Honey bees, too, are suffering from pesticide poisoning and disease.

The foxglove pug moth is both common and widespread and, during May to July, it will find its way to its special food plant to lay its eggs. It is not very large with a wingspan of up to just 22 mm/¾ inch, but you may see it if you have an outside light. Its wings have broad bands of grey and brown. After the larvae hatch out from the eggs they will feed inside the flowers, consuming both the stamens and then the seeds. They have a greenish brown body, dark on top but quite pale beneath.

As you see, foxglove plays an important role in wildlife ecology. Do therefore consider growing this beautiful native plant, particularly if you have some shady places, and preserve those that arrive by accident. Watch out for that rosette of downy leaves.

Goat's-beard (*Tragopogon pratensis*)

Daisy family (Asteraceae). Annual/perennial. Pollinated by insects. Also self-fertile. Propagated by seed. Edible.

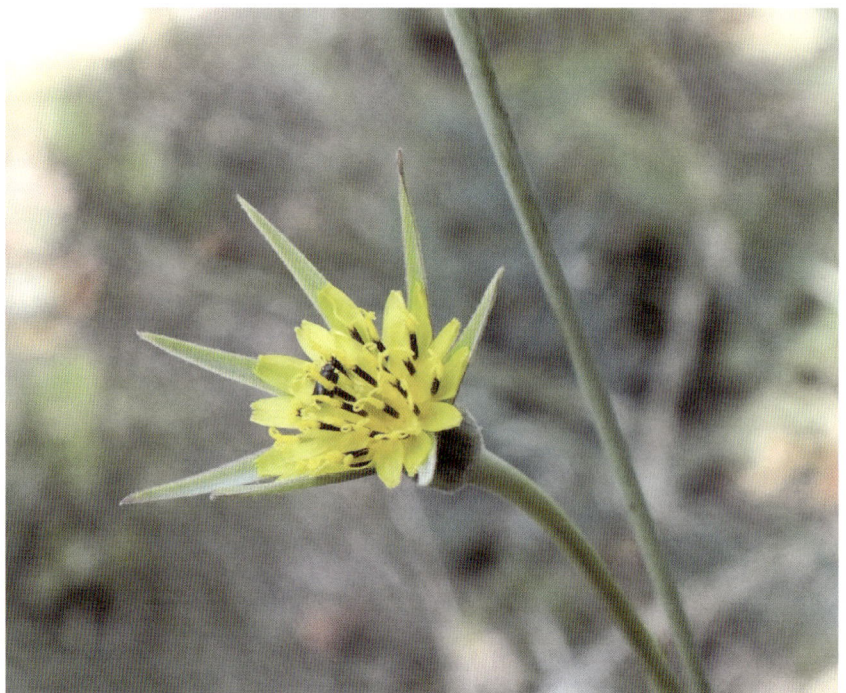

The long bracts are a particularly notable feature.

I find this so-called 'weed' truly beautiful. The many bright, yellow florets, so carefully cradled by long, pointed bracts, make it one of my favourites. The flower head gently sways on the slender stem, surrounded by sprays of narrow leaves, each with a white vein running along the centre of the blade. If you break a stem, milky sap will ooze forth. Not only is it beautiful in flower but the following seed head is truly spectacular, creating a 'clock' considerably bigger than a dandelion. If you look very closely, you will see that each 'parachute' is formed like an inside-out umbrella, with many

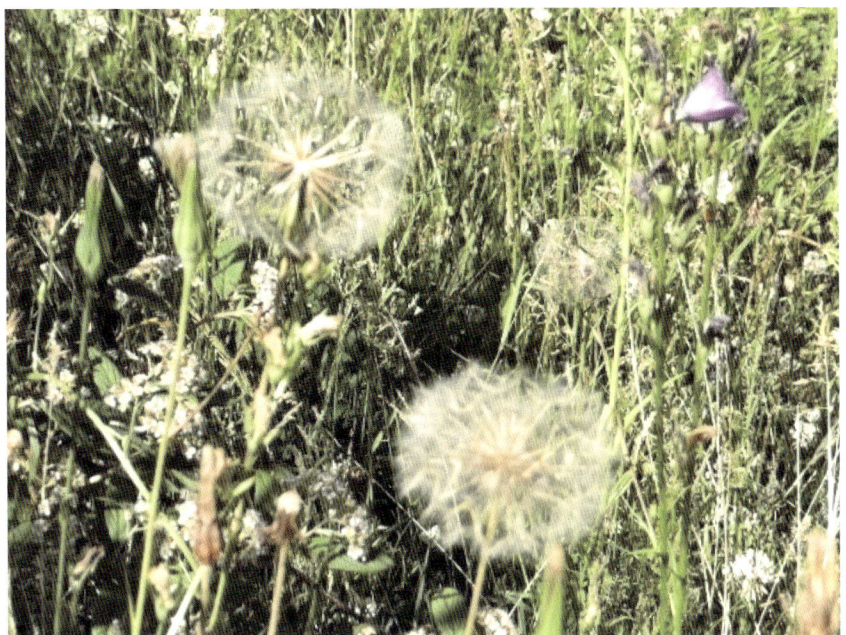

The seed heads of goat's-beard form even more impressive 'clocks' than dandelions.

spokes, each supporting a multitude of fine hairs, perfect for wafting the precious seed long distances on the wind.

It plants itself frequently in the paving cracks outside our greenhouse, although its normal habitat is grassland or waste land. Depending on conditions, it can grow to 60 cm/2 ft or more. It is certainly a successful species, being both self-pollinating and also pollinated by insects.

Folklore

It is really only possible to appreciate the charm of goat's-beard in the mornings as, come noon, it hides its face. This is what Gerard says about it in *The Herball* (1597):

> … it shutteth it selfe at twelve of the clock, and sheweth not his face open untill the next daies Sunne doth make it floure anew, whereupon it was called Go to bed at noone.

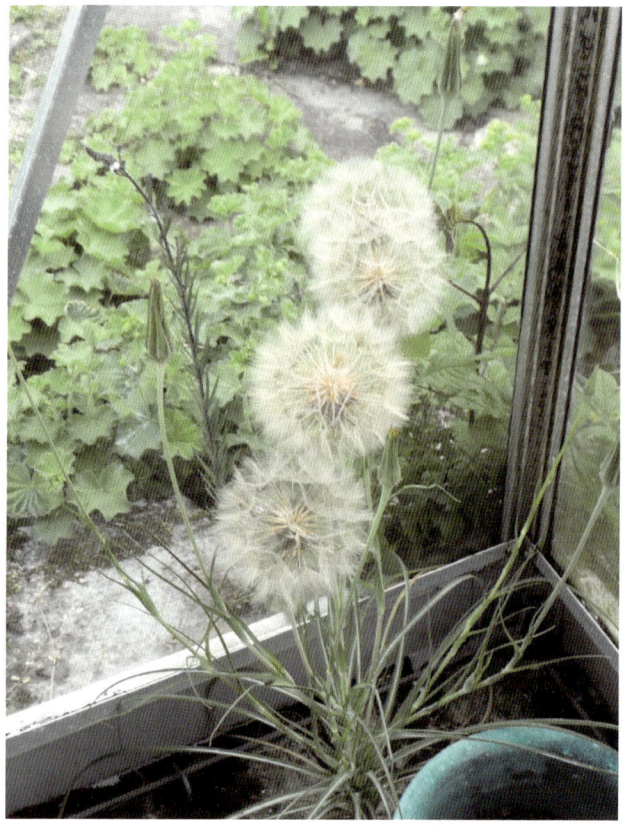

Here you can see that it managed to put its roots down in the greenhouse.

Another common name was 'noon tide' or even 'Jack-go-to-bed-at-noon'. The flower head will also close with impending rain. Perhaps it is this elusiveness that makes it even more attractive. I have to say I have found it tricky to do it justice in a photograph as the slightest breath of wind causes it to move and blurs the picture.

Uses

Being related to salsify, the long taproot can either be eaten raw in a salad or cooked like parsnip. Gerard is impressed with its qualities when boiled and buttered:

> … A most pleasant and wholesome meate, in delicate taste far surpassing either Parsenep or Carrot: which meate procures appetite, and strengthneth those that hath been sicke of a long lingring disease.

Some decades later, Culpeper was in agreement, particularly recommending it for 'cold watery stomachs'. Recent research shows that the root contains inulin, causing it to be broken down in the body as fructose rather than glucose. The suggestion, therefore, is that it could provide useful nutrition for diabetics. Gerard has more to say about its therapeutic benefits:

> The roots of goat's-beard boiled in wine and drunk, asswageth the pain and pricking stitches of the sides.

If only I had known about such a remedy in my youth when doubled over in pain on the sports field! However, perhaps Culpeper's treatment with the distilled water rather than the wine would have been more appropriate.

Wildlife

The micro-moth grey tortrix may select goat's-beard as the preferred food plant for its larvae, although it may use many other plants. The adult is greyish brown with patchy markings and a wing span of up to 22 mm/1 inch. It flies in July to August from dusk onwards. To begin with, the smoky-grey larvae will mine a leaf, then roll it into a tube. This family of micro-moths may also spin the flower petals together with silk.

Honeysuckle (*Lonicera periclymenum*)

Honeysuckle family (Caprifoliaceae). Deciduous climber. Pollinated by moths and bees. Propagated by seed, cutting and layering. Medicinal. Seeds mildly toxic.

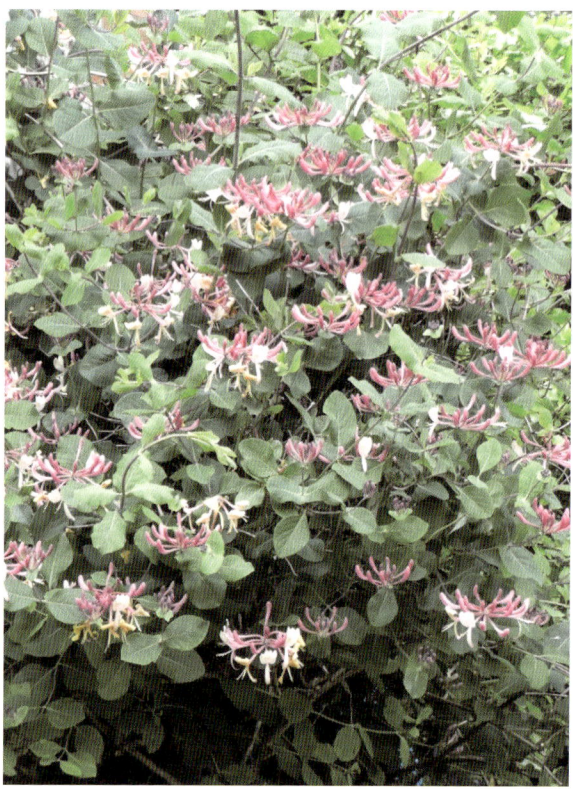

We cultivated this self-planted honeysuckle to benefit from its alluring perfume.

What could be more glorious than the sweet, intoxicating perfume of honeysuckle flowers wafting through an open bedroom window on a warm summer's evening! There is good reason for this night-time scent as many species of moth are attracted to the nectar and thereby pollinate the flowers. These small creatures are able to sense it as far away as half a kilometre/¼ mile.

JUNE

In our garden the pinky-orange and cream flowers are well and truly open in early June. Their delicate, tubular shape is most unusual, described by William Bulleyn in 1562, most aptly, as being like ladies' fingers:

> … how frendly doe this herbe … imbrace the bodies, armes and branches of trees, with his long windyng stalkes, and tender leaues, openyng or spreding forthe his swete Lillis, like ladies fingers, emong the thornes or bushes.

These are formed by the joining of the five petals, the lower one curling back at the tip, allowing the five stamens to protrude visibly from the tube. There can be anything between four and 30 flowers in a single cluster. Being a strong climber, honeysuckle will quickly take to a trellis on a sunny wall and can grow up to 10 m/34 ft. As the shrub naturally twists itself in a clockwise direction, other supports can also work very well, such as poles or canes, or a dead tree or bush.

Once you have one honeysuckle, more will surely arrive. If you are passionate about native wild plants, as we are, then you will be hunting for new locations into which to transplant the seedlings. Even though honeysuckle is supposed to thrive best in dryish loamy soils, ours seems to like to put its roots well down into our clay, usually in the most inconvenient places. A favourite is to wrap itself around a rose bush, weighing down the slender branches and obscuring the flowers. If there has been no more space under a bedroom window, then we have replanted it in our roadside hedge where it can scramble at will through the hawthorn, giving any passer-by a treat with its heady perfume.

Being semi-evergreen, some leaves will last through the winter. You will see that they are paired, growing opposite each other and are of a simple oval shape, slightly pointed. Underneath, their colouring has a bluish tinge. Each has a very short stalk or none at all.

In the autumn the flamboyant flowers are transformed into attractive crimson berries, each with several seeds. Tempting as they look, it is not recommended that you eat them as they are somewhat poisonous. There are some 180 species of honeysuckle worldwide, but only 20 native to

Europe and just two to Britain. The other is fly honeysuckle (*L. xylosteum*), a stockier shrub, whose flowers are smaller and less showy.

Folklore

The name *Lonicera* was given to the species in memory of Adam Lonicer, a well-known botanist of the Renaissance period. As for the common name, this surely comes from country children's habit of picking off the trumpet-shaped flowers and sucking out the sweet nectar.

In earlier times, honeysuckle was often referred to as 'woodbine', descriptive of its binding and twining nature, and how it is often found in a woodland setting, using trunks and branches as supports. Chaucer believed 'woodbyne' to be symbolic of steadfastness in love, and it was therefore a popular plant to have entwined around a bower. Most famous of all quotations are those from Shakespeare's *A Midsummer Night's Dream* in which Oberon, king of the fairies, describes the bank where Titania sometimes sleeps as being 'quite over-canopied with luscious woodbine'. Later in the play, Titania, while drugged with a love potion, declares to Bottom:

> Sleep thou, and I will wind thee in my arms …
> So doth the woodbine the sweet honeysuckle
> Gently entwist.

What could be more conducive to feelings of love than the luxuriant pleasure of the perfume, combined with the sight of the plant entwining itself around the bower, just like embracing arms!

The sensuous nature of honeysuckle was considered to be so evocative that it was believed by the people of the Fenland district to have a corrupting influence on young girls. It should not therefore be taken into any house where they were residing as it would cause them to have erotic dreams!

Uses

Being strong and flexible, the long stems have been used as rope since time immemorial. Evidence of this was found just a few years ago when 'woodhenge', dating to the Bronze Age, was excavated in north Norfolk. It was the ideal material for binding together pieces of wood to make shelters or in this case a temple.

As far as remedies are concerned, Gerard notes that 'the floures steeped in oile, and set in the Sun, are good to anoint the body that is benumbed, and growne very cold'. This would seem to be a most pleasant and efficacious preparation, highly likely to encourage any patient to feel better, even if not much warmer. More usually, however, an infusion of the flowers was made to alleviate the discomfort of asthma. In 1694 the physician Pechey declares that 'Tis chiefly used in an Asthma, and for a Cough. It helps Difficulty of Breathing'. The tea was also taken for nervous headaches and applied to the skin for the healing of spots and pimples. In the mid-18th century, a sweet conserve made from the flowers was kept in the store cupboard as a guard against asthma attacks in the family. Extra honey might well be stirred into it and a tablespoon taken night and morning.

Modern herbalists still prescribe honeysuckle for respiratory problems. One helpful constituent of the flowers is salicylic acid, which has a natural pain-relief effect. Drinking an infusion can alleviate a headache, while gargling with it should ease a sore throat. However, there is nothing to beat honeysuckle infused in its namesake. The honey enhances the antiseptic properties of the flowers.

Soothing honeysuckle honey

Honeysuckle flowers
clear honey

Pick both the buds and the open flowers, remove any insects, then fill a jar almost to the top with the petals. Pour in clear honey to cover them. Put the top on, then leave in a warm place for a couple of weeks, making sure that none of the petals are exposed to air. Strain and store in a sterilised jar. ♦ Take 2 tsp night and morning as required. Alternatively, pour hot water onto a spoonful of the honeysuckle honey to make a soothing drink.

Wildlife

During the day, bumble bees will be buzzing busily around this attractive food source, pollinating it at the same time. Then, in the evening, when the aroma from honeysuckle flowers is particularly fragrant, a wide variety of Lepidoptera may be found feeding on the sugars, including some of our most striking moths, such as the garden tiger, mottled beauty and swallow-tailed. More recently, with the warming of the climate, I have even seen hummingbird hawk moths hovering by the flowers and using the long proboscis to push into the delicate petal tubes and suck up the nectar.

Honeysuckle is also an important caterpillar food plant of the beautiful white admiral butterfly. If you live in southern districts within a woodland setting, then you may be fortunate enough to see this gorgeous insect with its distinctive white markings. You will search for its chrysalis in vain, however, as it is perfectly camouflaged, looking just like a dead honeysuckle leaf!

The Royal Society for the Protection of Birds (RSPB) has a good tip: if you prune the plant hard, the twisting stems will bush out, providing ideal roosting cover and nesting sites for small song birds. In the autumn, finches, warblers and thrushes will feed on the red berries voraciously. Despite slight toxicity to humans, they clearly have no ill effects on the birds.

Common Mallow (*Malva sylvestris*)

Mallow family (Malvaceae). Perennial. Pollinated by insects, especially bees. Propagated by seed. Edible. Medicinal.

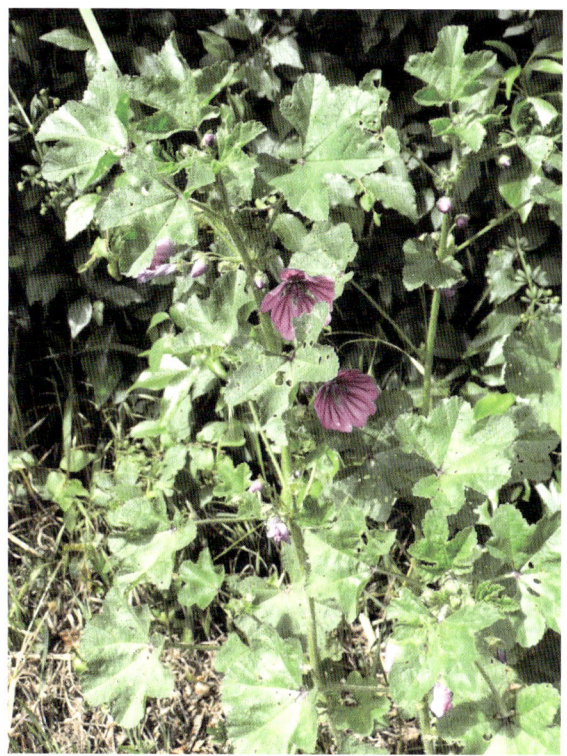

Common mallow, with its appealing, purple-veined petals, is an agreeable arrival beneath the hedgerow.

There is a particular steep roadside bank not far from our house, too awkward to mow, which is ablaze with vivid red poppies in the late spring. When common mallow begins to appear in early June, the poppies are still putting on a show. The two together, the deep pinky-purple of the mallow along with the scarlet of the poppy petals, make an eye-catching colour clash.

This attractive plant may well stray into your garden, indicating that some of the cultivated varieties could also do very well there. Musk mallow (*Malva moschata*), for example, is a very pretty perennial, with saucer-shaped, rose-pink flowers on tall spikes in the early summer. It is well worth seeking out. The self-seeding hollyhock, so popular in cottage gardens, is closely related, as is the more delicate hibiscus.

If it were not for the fact that common mallow tends to become rather untidy as it passes its best flowering period, then it would most certainly be a welcome addition to any garden. The five notched petals have several deep mauve stripes running from the centre. The flowers are so striking, they have been compared to clematis. The stalked, downy leaves have a roundish shape overall, with three to seven lobes. As for the main stem, it is thick, strong and hairy and can be either erect or spreading. The common mallow that occasionally finds its way from the hedgerows into our garden is of the low and spreading type.

Folklore

The fruits of mallow are round and somewhat flattened, so that when dried they could make interesting necklaces. Alternatively, they would be strung up and kept for medicinal use. In Norfolk they were called 'cheeses' and children would nibble at them. This was encouraged by the adults as they have a mildly laxative effect. As a result, the whole plant is still called 'pick-cheese'.

It is sad indeed that wild marsh mallows are now so scarce, not only for the loss of a beautiful plant but also because country folk used to believe that they would only flourish close to a home that is happy.

Uses

Everyone has heard of marshmallows, the soft, rather gooey sweets that are a favourite present at Christmas. Traditionally these were made from *Althea officinalis*, the once common marsh mallow. It is now scarce in the wild, and the modern marshmallow confectionery no longer contains the plant. However, it is not difficult to cultivate as long as you can provide it with dampish soil and a sunny place. Not only is it very beautiful with velvety leaves and soft, lilac-pink flowers arranged up its tall stem but it is also extraordinarily rich in healing properties, most especially mucilage, also tannins, anthocyanins and flavonoids. Common mallow has similar properties, although in smaller quantities. Nevertheless, it is still worthwhile as a medicinal plant, and both the flowers and leaves are edible.

In addition to being a useful soluble fibre, mucilage has soothing, anti-inflammatory properties. Mallow is safe to take and is therefore often recommended as a remedy for dry coughs and colds, stomach upsets and ulcers, as well as for urinary tract infections. Chewing the flowers and rubbing into the gum can alleviate toothache. When applied externally it can also help to ease the pain of stings, small wounds and bruises. A bath made from the leaves and flowers can lessen the inflammation that tends to surround fractures. Adding the flowers to salads not only makes them look more appetising, but they will also assist with digestion.

Drying the flowers

Pick on a dry, sunny day, then simply spread them out on paper in a cool and airy position. You will see that the flowers change colour, becoming blue as they dry.

Soothing mallow tisane

You can use either fresh or dried flowers and buds. If these are unavailable, then pick a couple of young leaves instead.

2 tsp mallow flowers
275 ml/½ pint boiling water

Pour the water over the flowers and leave for 5 minutes to infuse. Strain. ♦ Take one mugful three times a day to alleviate a cough or sore throat, ease digestion or the pain of cystitis.

Mallow poultice

This is a quick remedy for swellings, such as insect bites, stings, boils or abscesses.

Take several mallow leaves and mince up. Lay on the affected area and keep in place with a plaster so that the juice soaks well in. Repeat as necessary until the inflammation subsides.

Melokhia

This is a viscous, health-giving soup, especially popular in Egypt, which is made from the leaves of a plant very similar to mallow. It is reputed to boost the immune system and ward off all kinds of diseases. Pick the leaves when they are young and tender and use them fresh.

225 g/½ lb mallow leaves, chopped fine

1 tbsp butter

2 tbsp garlic, chopped fine

1 tbsp ground coriander

570 ml/1 pint stock

pitta bread

First you make the taqliya from the spices. You do this by melting the butter, then adding 1 tbs of the garlic and all the coriander. Turn up the heat and stir for about three minutes until the colour is golden all through. ♦ Put the rest of the garlic into a large pan with the stock. Add the leaves. When it is hot (not boiling) mix in the taqliya and simmer gently until well done, stirring from time to time. ♦ Serve with the pitta bread.

Wildlife

The larvae of various beetles, aphids and moths will feed on mallow. Among moths, the most likely visitor if your garden is in the southern half of England is the least yellow underwing. This flies during the summer and is best recognised by the reddish colour of its upper wings.

Common mallow may also bring the beautiful painted lady butterfly to your garden. Although its favourite food plants are thistles or nettles, it will also lay its eggs on mallow. As a migrant from north Africa, its arrival in Britain depends largely on prevailing winds.

Greater Plantain (*Plantago major*)
Ribwort Plantain (*P. lanceolata*)

Plantain family (Plantaginaceae). Perennials. Pollinated by wind. Propagated by seed. Medicinal.

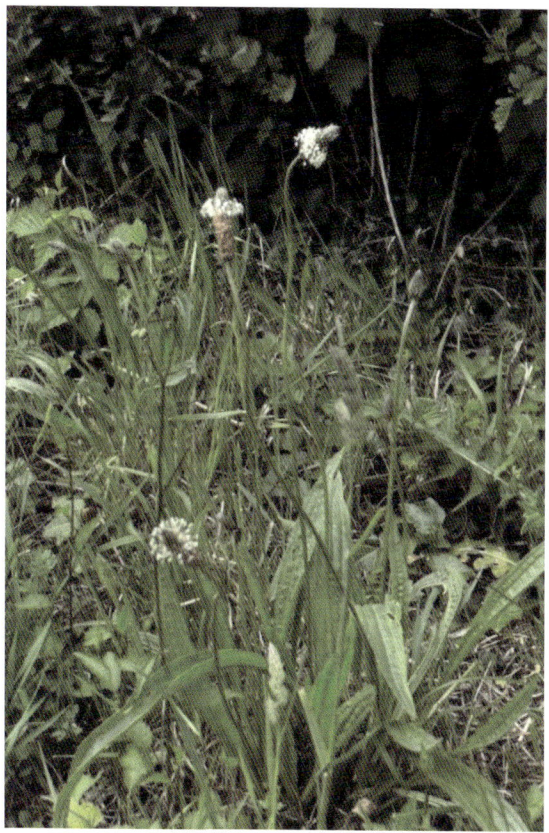

Ribwort, like greater plantain, is a valuable medicinal herb.

Who would imagine that such an insignificant, down-trodden little 'weed' as plantain would have such extraordinary properties? That rosette of leaves inhabiting our lawns is a familiar sight and most gardeners curse at it and dig it out or, worse, treat it with herbicide to get rid of it. Yet the

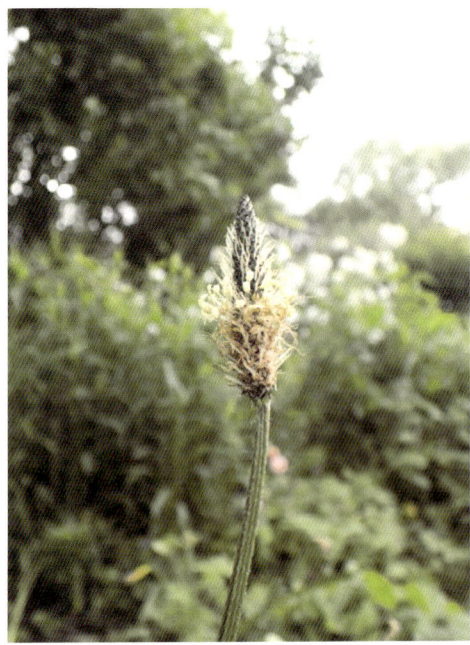

The flower head of ribwort plantain is edible and tastes a little like mushroom.

Anglo Saxons knew better. To them it was the 'mother of herbs' and one of nine most sacred plants, as described in the *Lacnunga*, a 10th-century collection of medical texts and incantations.

There are many species of plantain, but the two that grow most commonly in our garden are greater plantain and ribwort plantain. The first has broad oval leaves with more or less smooth margins and five or more prominent veins. The multitude of tiny, yellowish-green flowers grow on the slender spikes that push up from the centre of the rosettes. The prominent anthers are lilac to mauve in colour. Although the spikes generally reach to only about 15 cm/ 6 in, an astonishing number of seeds may be produced, on average about 14,000.

You can easily distinguish ribwort from greater plantain as it has narrow, lance-shaped leaves with prominent veins, as its name suggests. The flower heads at the top of long stems are much smaller and are brown with protruding, white stamens. A single plant can produce 2,500 seeds or more, but fewer on poor soils.

Plantain has an extraordinary ability to survive compression, either being walked over or mown. The rosettes of leaves simply flatten themselves out to avoid damage, and for this reason plantain survives very well in lawns. You may believe this plant to be a nuisance, but before throwing these valuable herbs away, please do consider their benefits.

Folklore

Since time immemorial this herb has been associated with the feet, either for comforting them when tired or swollen, or relieving blisters and other sores. Hence the name *Plantago*, which is derived from the Latin *planta*, sole of the foot. Moreover, the seeds seem to have been carried by foot from country to country as it is now found worldwide. The American Indians referred to it as 'white man's foot', as it arrived on that continent along with white settlers and then seemed to spring up wherever they went. An early English name for plantain is 'Waybroed' or 'Waybread' as it was so often found alongside roads and tracks:

> And you, Waybread, mother of worts,
> Open from eastward, powerful within,
> Over you chariots rolled, over you queens rode,
> Over you brides cried, over you bulls belled;
> All these you withstood, and these you confounded,
> So withstand now the venom that flies through the air,
> And the loathed thing which through the land roves.
>
> From 'Lay of the Nine Healing Herbs' in the *Lacnunga*

The flower heads of ribwort have been used for centuries by children as 'ammunition' in a game of soldiers. The stem of the plant is wound around itself, just below the head, to form a noose. By pulling sharply, the head will fly off towards the opponent. Another game is to strike your opponent's flower head with yours in the attempt to knock it off. In Scotland this was known as 'Carl and Doddie', referring to Bonnie Prince Charlie and George III, each trying to decapitate the other. Any ribwort surviving such attacks was greatly prized.

Uses

Long before the Anglo-Saxon texts, plantain was valued as a healing herb by the Ancient Persians and Arabians, who used it to cure dysentery and many other conditions affecting the digestive tract. Centuries ago in India it was noticed that a mongoose would instinctively eat plantain if bitten by a cobra. It was presumed that the herb had some kind of neutralising effect on the venom. The Roman Pliny recommended plantain to help someone bitten by a rabid dog. At later dates others believed it to be the best antidote for various stings, bites and poisons. Even the famous classical scholar Desiderius Erasmus (1466–1536) stated that plantain was the herb of choice to combat the poisons of spiders.

The headaches suffered by Alexander the Great (356–323 BC) were alleviated by plantain. Some 270 years later the Greek physician Dioscorides prescribed the herb for its soothing and cooling effects. Herbalism was one of King Henry VIII's (1491–1547) many interests and his personal collection of recipes is held by the British Museum. One of his prized and most-used herbs was plantain. Shakespeare, too, mentions its virtues in several of his plays. Romeo says to his friend:

> 'Your plantain leaf is excellent for that, Benvolio.'
> 'For what, I pray thee, Romeo?'
> 'For your broken skin.'

(Act I, ii)

It seems curious, therefore, that although Gerard admits in *The Herball* that juice of plantain is helpful for eye conditions, he dismisses the advice of 'antient writers' as 'ridiculous toyes'. Culpeper, on the other hand, extols its blessings to the extent that it seems to heal practically every common disorder, both internal and external, including all kinds of swellings, itchings and bleedings, as well as ridding the body of worms.

Plantain is still recommended as an instant remedy for nettle stings and insect bites. Ribwort leaves are the best if available, because they are juicier than greater plantain and can be quickly crushed and applied.

It has been demonstrated that plantain has antihistamine properties; a tea made from the leaves can help to soothe hay fever. As the leaves can be rather bitter, add a little honey. This is also effective as a gargle or mouthwash to soothe a sore throat or gums, or as a temporary relief for toothache. Ribwort tea is very good for the treatment of coughs.

Poultices made from the plant are used to diminish varicose veins as well as to alleviate skin rashes and cuts. They are also ideal for grazed knees. Plantain is still used to help draw out splinters, thorns, or any sort of ulcers, boils, or poisonous infections.

As for the seeds, these are rich in vitamin B1 and can be ground up to make a flour. The husks are fibrous and absorbent, swelling up when wet, and are therefore excellent for the relief of constipation.

A review of studies into *P. major*, reported in 2000, showed that extract of the plant had considerable biological effects, with 'wound healing activity, anti-inflammatory, analgesic, antioxidant, weak antibiotic, immuno-modulating and anti-ulcerogenic activity'. For a single herb, this list is truly astonishing. How right the Anglo Saxons were to think of it as the most sacred of herbs! Scientific analyses show why poultices of the leaves can heal wounds and ulcers and relieve sores, bites and stings so effectively. The anti-microbial compound is aucubin, while the cell-growth promoter is allantoin; the mucilaginous sap has a soothing effect and the flavonoids have healing properties. Moreover, the salicylic acid is a natural source of pain relief.

While the seeds will act as a laxative, a tea of the leaves will have the opposite effect, the astringency of the tannins being good for the treatment of diarrhoea, dysentery or incontinence, and even excessive menstrual flow. Also, many of the nutrients lost will be replenished by those in the herb, including potassium, iron and calcium and vitamins C, A and K.

Drying the leaves

The leaves are available most of the year, but it is advisable to pick and dry some in the summer in case of snow during winter – just at the time when you may need them to help cure a bad cough. You can also freeze them successfully. To dry them, lay them flat on sheets of brown paper in a warm place but out of direct sunlight. Each day turn the leaves over until they are dry and brittle (at least 2 weeks). Store in an airtight jar in a dark place.

Plantain oil

Plantain leaves, chopped
cold-pressed olive oil

You will need a lidded jar for the infusion. Fill the jar with the chopped plantain leaves, then pour in the oil to cover completely. Put on the lid and leave in a warm place for up to two weeks. By this time the oil should have absorbed the essential compounds from the leaves, changing the colour. Check that this is so; if not, leave a little longer. When ready, strain through a fine sieve and store the oil in a well-sealed dark jar. ♦ This will be usable for up to a year and is very soothing for insect bites and stings.

Plantain salve

275 ml/½ pint plantain oil (see above)
25 g/1 oz beeswax, grated

Put the ingredients into a heat-proof jug. Stand the jug in a larger pan and pour water around it until the level is just below the level of the oil. Simmer gently until the beeswax is melted, stirring from time to time. ♦ Pour into small, clean jars and leave to set. Screw on the lids. ♦ Usable for up to two years. An excellent remedy for rashes and itchy skin. Also safe for animal use.

Anglo Saxon foot remedy

'If a man's feet in a journey swell, take then waybread the wort, pound in vinegar, bathe the feet therewith, and smear them.' As vinegar is well known for bringing out bruises and reducing swelling, this, combined with greater plantain, is a potent remedy for tired, sore and swollen feet.

2 handfuls fresh leaves of greater plantain
vinegar to cover

First bruise the leaves by applying pressure with a rolling pin. Put in a small pan, add the vinegar and simmer very gently, without boiling, for about 5 minutes, until the leaves are soft. ♦ Apply the leaves to the feet and bathe the affected area with the vinegar. ♦ Alternatively, make a poultice by laying the leaves while still hot on a cloth. Fold the cloth over to make a pocket, then lay this on the feet until they feel soothed. This poultice is also useful to draw out thorns and splinters, and to hasten the healing of ulcers, bites, stings and rashes.

The Scots, being forever practical, down-to-earth people, have a simpler version of the foot remedy. Just lay some leaves of greater plantain inside your socks underneath and around the feet, and allow the juice to soak into the skin as you walk about.

Ribwort throat and chest mixture
By using the ribwort raw, you are preserving the vitamins.
Ribwort leaves
½ small pot clear honey
Put several handfuls of ribwort leaves into a juicer. Simply stir the resulting juice into the honey to fill the pot. ♦ Take 2 tsp as needed to help relieve sore throats, chest infections and colds. It will also soothe stomach ulcers. Stir before use.

Wildlife

It is well worth including plantain, a perennial, in a wildflower meadow as the leaves, seeds and flowers are of great benefit to wildlife. Many insects feed on this plant, hoverflies in particular enjoying the nectar. It is one of a range of food plants of certain moth caterpillars, such as the small fan-footed wave moth and the heart and dart.

The seed heads last for a long time into winter and provide nutritious food for several bird species, especially goldfinches. If you want to delight in seeing these colourful little birds in your garden, with their striking red faces and yellow-barred wings, then cherish your greater plantain.

Petty Spurge (*Euphorbia peplus*)

Spurge family (Euphorbiaceae). Annual. Pollinated by insects. Propagated by seed. Irritant. Toxic. Medicinal potential.

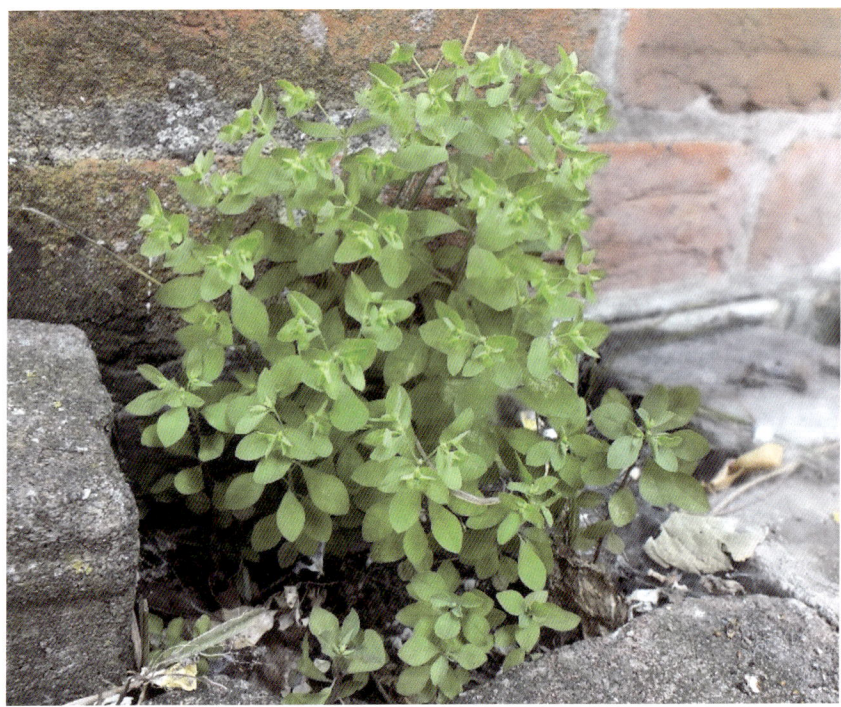

Researchers have been excited to discover that the sap of petty spurge has anti-cancer properties.

The botanical name of this small, rather unusual plant has an ancient history, going way back to the time of Anthony and Cleopatra's daughter Selene, whose husband, King Juba II of Numidia and later Mauretania on the north African coast, had a physician named Euphorbus. He discovered the laxative qualities of spurge. One hopes that he administered it with care as its effects, when taken internally, can be dire. Indeed, the common name of spurge comes from the Latin *purgare*, to purge, a process so extreme in this case, depending on quantities given, that the patient might not survive its effects. At any rate, the king named the plant after his physician, so one assumes it was put to good use. Much later, in the 18th century, Euphorbus was again honoured when the Swedish botanist Carl Linnaeus gave his name to the whole genus of plants.

As for the term 'peplus', this is ascribed to a Greek botanist and physician, Dioscorides, who saw the similarity between the shape of the upper and lower bracts and the folding over of the *peplos*, or loose-flowing garment worn by the women.

I first noticed a tiny specimen, no more than 10 cm/4 inches in height, in one of our tubs set against a south-facing wall. Here I generally plant annual climbers, such as morning glory or rambling nasturtium, to cling to the trellis and decorate an otherwise rather dull space. Realising that there were oval bracts rather than petals, I guessed at once that it must be some sort of *Euphorbia*. The petty spurge description fitted exactly, with its slim stem topped by the flowering upper branches. Looking very carefully, I noticed how each yellowish 'flower' nestled between two green, leaf-like bracts. Four minute long-horned, crescent-shaped lobes surrounded the flower, which I later discovered was the male. It had just a single stamen. Out of interest, I allowed the plant to flourish, and later saw how the seed pod emerged from the centre of each flower and, evidently weighed down by its contents, leaned over to be cradled by the adjacent leaves. This was so charming! When ready, the three-lobed pod will burst open and scatter the seeds with an explosive action. Bearing in mind the small size of the plant, each can produce up to a staggering 1,200 seeds.

Folklore

As this is a poisonous plant, it seems odd that the Gaelic name for it is *lus leighis* meaning 'healing herb'. Nevertheless, it is an indication that folk remedies were made from it. Other common names such as 'wartwort', 'wartgrass' or from Cornwall 'wartweed', suggest that the juice was widely applied to burn off these skin blemishes. Indeed, this seems to have been common practice here in East Anglia.

Uses

Culpeper was well aware of petty spurge's extreme laxative effect:

> It is a strong cathartic, working violently by vomit and stool, but is very offensive to the stomach and bowels by reason of its sharp corrosive quality and therefore ought to be used with caution.

His words of warning need to be taken seriously. Moreover, it is wise to wear gloves when handling spurge as the milky sap is a severe irritant. In particular never allow the juice to come near the eyes which can be permanently damaged from its burning effects.

The hazards apart, *Euphorbia peplus* has important therapeutic properties. Recent research has generated considerable excitement in relation to skin lesions and cancerous conditions. In 2011 the *British Journal of Dermatology* reported significant success with this plant in the treatment of non-melanoma skin cancers. The sap was applied to the tumours once a day for just three days. After one month, 41 of the 48 cases had shown no signs of malignancy. After 15 months, 30 of the 48 were still completely clear.

The active ingredient in the sap is called ingenol mebutate, which kills the cancerous cells and at the same time encourages the neutrophils (white blood cells of the immune system) to repair the damage. Trials are under way for the treatment of leukaemia as these malignant cells are known to be especially sensitive to petty spurge sap. The extract used works by activating an enzyme called protein kinase C which sets into motion controlled cell suicide.

Wildlife

Being basically a harmful irritant and toxic to domestic animals, I wondered what role petty spurge could have in the garden, if any. I was intrigued to discover that it has the ability to deplete boron in the surrounding soil. It is therefore probably a good idea to put any unwanted spurges onto the compost heap as borate minerals are not helpful here. These are somewhat toxic to some of the wriggly creatures such as centipedes, which are so important to the health of the heap.

Spurges have the capacity to raise the soil's temperature. They could, therefore, be good companion plants to others that are sensitive to the cold. It is said that moles dislike spurge! There is, of course, a great deal of advice about how to discourage these little creatures where they are a nuisance, some of which is effective and some not at all. However, you could try transplanting any spurges that you find to a disturbed border. I would be glad to learn of any successes.

White Stonecrop (*Sedum album*)

Stonecrop family (Crassulaceae). Perennial evergreen succulent. Pollinated by insects. Propagated by seed or cutting. Irritant.

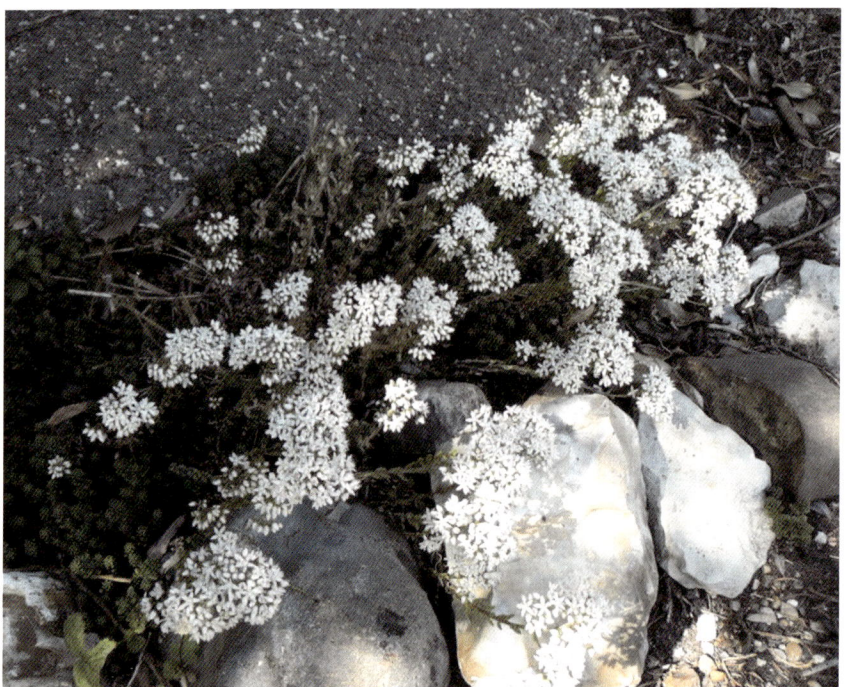

White stonecrop turned up in a dry stony area of our garden, indicating that cultivated succulents might thrive in similar conditions.

The people who owned our house before us had spread gravel over the driveway, much of which had subsequently become overgrown. We cleared and restored the part nearest the gate but decided to leave the rest as it was beyond the garage and rarely used for parking. Not realising it at the time, this well-drained shingle area later proved to be an ideal habitat for several new arrivals to our garden, one of which was white stonecrop.

    This small plant has distinctive succulent leaves, placed alternately on the stem, which are shiny green, occasionally red-tinged depending on

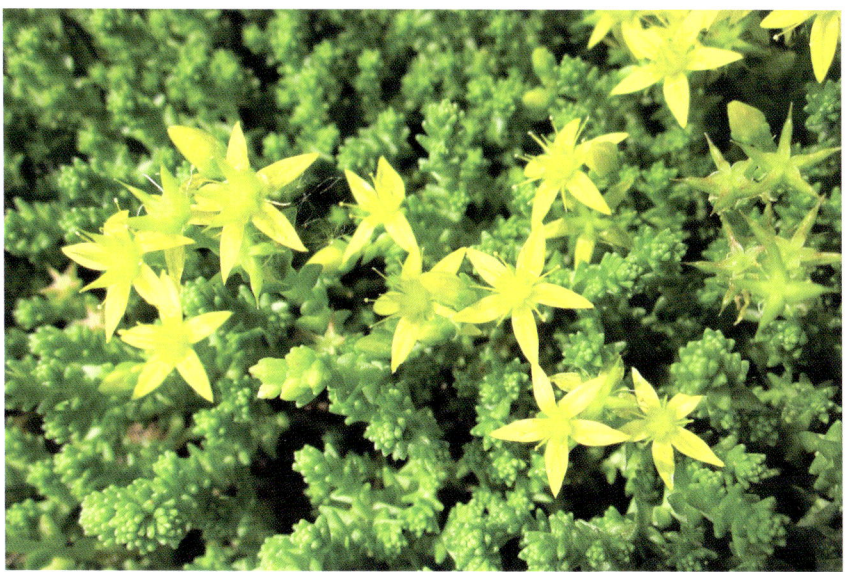

Golden or biting stonecrop is often sold as an attractive plant suitable for rockeries or gravel gardens. *Photo © Wikipedia Images*

the available amount of nutrients. This method of storing water allows the stonecrop to thrive in a dry environment with minimal soil and even through long-term drought. It conserves water very cleverly by opening its stomata to let in carbon dioxide only during the night when the temperature is cool and evaporation low. Indeed, it spreads itself happily across our gravel, forming a dense mat from which the flower stems arise. In the summer an otherwise dull patch of stones is transformed into a pretty spectacle as the white starry flowers open up. Each has five tiny, pointed petals, and several flowers are clustered together at the top of every stem to form a flattish cyme.

Folklore

Stonecrop was believed to have protective qualities and was traditionally planted on thatches. This may well have had a practical application as the succulent leaves perhaps provided some safeguard against fire caused by lightning strikes or sparks from the chimney.

Uses

Its main use in horticulture nowadays, apart from rockeries, is in cities for the creation of 'green roofs', as a way of introducing nature into an otherwise concrete landscape.

As for remedies, these have been restricted to the yellow-flowered relative golden or 'biting' stonecrop (*Sedum acre*), so called because of the peppery taste of the leaves. Its other, somewhat extraordinary, common name is 'welcome-me-husband-though-never-so-drunk'! One wonders whether the wife was simply being generous hearted or whether the welcome was in the form of a blisteringly hot-tasting remedy to bring the man to his senses. Today it is not used by herbalists as the sap can provoke rashes.

Wildlife

An occasional migrant from continental Europe is the beautiful Apollo butterfly, which uses stonecrop as its food plant. The adult is white with five black patches on each forewing and two prominent red and black 'eyes' on each of the hindwings. Although it used to be quite common on the Isle of Wight, it is now critically endangered due to loss of habitat. Its caterpillar is velvety black with two rows of orange spots. As it remains at this stage for two years, it is especially vulnerable to predation, despite the fact that it emits a foul odour as a defensive mechanism. If you have large lawns along with its food plant, then you might just have the good fortune to catch a fleeting glimpse of the Apollo as it likes wide open spaces.

JULY

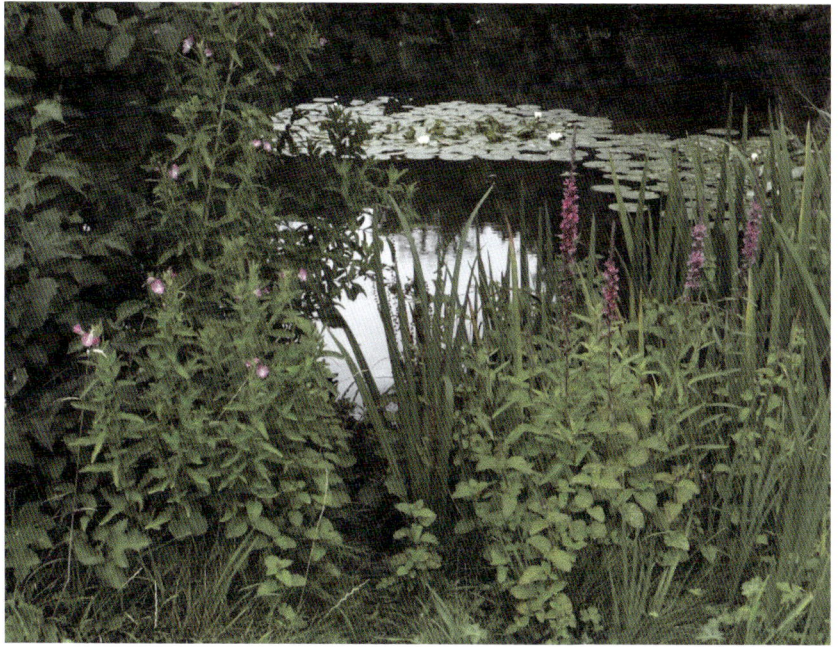

Our pond is a joy in July. Here great willowherb and purple loosestrife frame the picture, liking the damp pondside.

It is early in the month and the height of summer, with hot, humid days. Yesterday afternoon I was sitting under the awning of our front porch reading when a movement caught my eye. Looking up, I realized it was a snake idly sliding by in graceful wave-like motion, apparently unaware of my presence. I felt awe-struck. The two golden half-moons on its head indicated that it was a grass snake. It was fairly short, 45 cm/18 inches perhaps, so I surmised that it was last year's male. I watched for a while as it lazily crossed the lawn and disappeared into the undergrowth of some shrubs. What a privilege to be able to witness this shy creature! We had known for some time that grass snakes were breeding in one of our nice warm compost heaps as John, my husband, had found the remains of their rubbery eggs one day when turning the heap over to let in some air.

There is much activity in the garden. Our resident pair of moorhens have shooed away their first brood of four chicks, now that the second brood is fending for itself, no longer in need of the extra feeding help provided by the older siblings. The new generation will no doubt have to make do with damp ditches as so many of our local ponds have been filled in.

Our waterlilies have opened their pearly white petals and brilliant turquoise damsel flies rest on some reeds. High above, a fat-bodied chaser patrols to and fro. It is so good to have a break from the weeding every now and then to observe the wildlife. Indeed, if it were not for the weeds I would spend far less time in the garden!

The jackdaws, which nest each year in a hole high up in an ash tree, have been especially talkative recently. It seems that they were planning a journey! Several families have gathered together and flown off towards the south-west, amidst great chattering. I will miss their conversations. However, they will be back soon enough as most jackdaws pair for life and re-use the same nesting place each year.

Amidst this activity, many of our garden plants have paused for a rest and some are looking a little sorry for themselves. The roses have had their first flush and I have been doing much dead-heading so that the bushes will not waste energy on producing fat hips. This way we can expect many more blooms late into the autumn. The wild rose hips, however, I will leave for the birds.

Our meadow grass is beginning to look brownish, but we will avoid wasting water on it as it will soon spring up again with the next shower. It has done good work in providing a habitat for many small invertebrates which our songbirds depend on. Spiders, in particular, thrive here along with the lively grasshoppers. Grass-eating caterpillars have now turned into meadow brown butterflies, their chocolate-coloured wings fluttering close to the ground. This month the spring flowers will be seeding, producing more important food for our birds.

The task of weeding has now become urgent as plants that I would rather not have quite so much of in the garden grow apace. Rosebay willowherb is now taller than myself and some of it will have to go. However, the removed plants will not be wasted as I will dry the leaves for later use and make syrup from the flower spikes. The remaining clump will offer nectar to many insects.

We always leave a good patch of nettles in an inconspicuous place because it is a favourite food plant of several butterfly caterpillars, including the beautiful red admiral. Close inspection of the leaves reveals many tiny holes where these small creatures have been nibbling. Apparently, they do not suffer from stinging! What nettles lack in beauty, they make up for in wholesomeness, for they contain a wealth of health-giving vitamins and minerals, nourishment for both the garden and people – as you will see. Several nettle plants have strayed into other parts of the garden, however, and need to be dug up quickly, especially now that they are flowering. This is hard work as the ground is dry this year, after so little spring rain. The discarded plants will make an excellent liquid feed (see entry for common nettle, p.216).

I was just about to pull out the remains of the cow parsley along by our front hedge but then remembered the advice of the British Trust for Ornithology that we should leave them for the seed-eating birds that depend on tall plants. So, these must stay where they are for now. Perhaps they will attract our local finches.

There are many 'weeds' in flower this month which I treasure, in particular the bird's-foot-trefoil. This has taken hold along the footpath to our front door, its orange-tipped, yellow petals offering a warm welcome to our visitors.

Hedge Bindweed (*Calystegia sepium*)

Bindweed family (Convolvulaceae). Perennial. Pollinated by insects. Propagated by seed and rhizome. Medicinal.

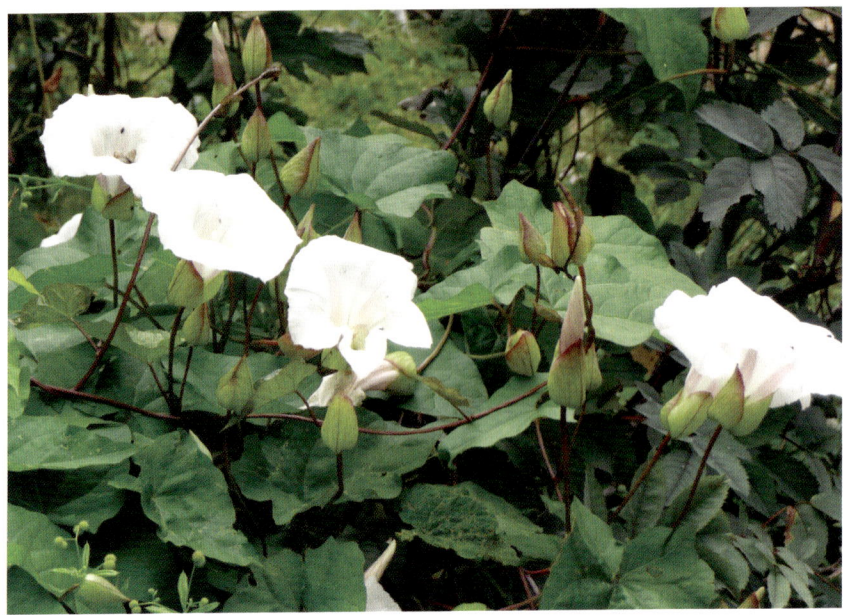

Hedge bindweed has a gorgeous flower, but the plant is very tricky to keep under control.

I have to admit that I was quite entranced by the beautiful white, trumpet-shaped flowers when they appeared unexpectedly one summer, ornamenting a rather dull green shrub at the bottom of the garden. Little did I realise how invasive this plant would prove to be! By next summer it had embellished the uninspiring wire fence and managed to entangle itself among our perennials in a nearby border. This was bad news as the long, creeping underground stems had invaded the roots of our garden plants, throwing up yet more bindweed which then began to strangle the perennials by winding itself up their stalks. Hours were then spent attempting to unwind the weed to give our flowers a chance!

Early the following spring I attempted to dig out the long roots but found it an impossible task because such a dense network had already been formed. I was then advised to give up on this and to pull off all the new leaves as soon as they appeared so that the plant was unable to photosynthesise. This was more successful. Even so, much of the vine escaped.

It seemed such a shame to cut off the appealing flowers, but when I learnt that the seeds could last for up to 30 years in the soil, I realised that I must not give in to sentimentality if the perennials were to survive. At least there was a practical use for the long stems which became an excellent substitute for twine, almost invisible among the plants it was supporting.

The large, white flowers are a delight, and the leaves are most attractive, spirally positioned and heart or arrow shaped. Yet, they have the effect of shielding light from the host plant and thereby weakening it.

Folklore

Country children will pick a flower and pinch the green calyx at its base which causes the white corolla to fly out. Meanwhile they chant 'Grandmother, grandmother, pop out of bed!' Perhaps the flimsy, funnel-shaped bloom floating away brings to mind a white cotton nightdress.

Uses

Most gardeners will not wish to allow bindweed to grow, despite its visual allure. That said, it contains the active ingredients of glycosides and tannins, and the sap is known to be an effective cure for constipation. The roots brewed into a tea have been taken as a laxative.

Wildlife

Although not originally a native of Britain, the soft fragrance of bindweed will attract tiny, black thunderflies which will suck the sap from the plant cells. Bindweed also provides food for the yellow and green caterpillar of the white plume moth, so called on account of its delicate feathery wings. Although small, you may sometimes see it by a lighted window.

Common Bird's-foot-trefoil (*Lotus corniculatus*)

Pea family (Fabaceae). Perennial. Pollinated by bees. Also self-fertile. Propagated by seed. Mildly poisonous.

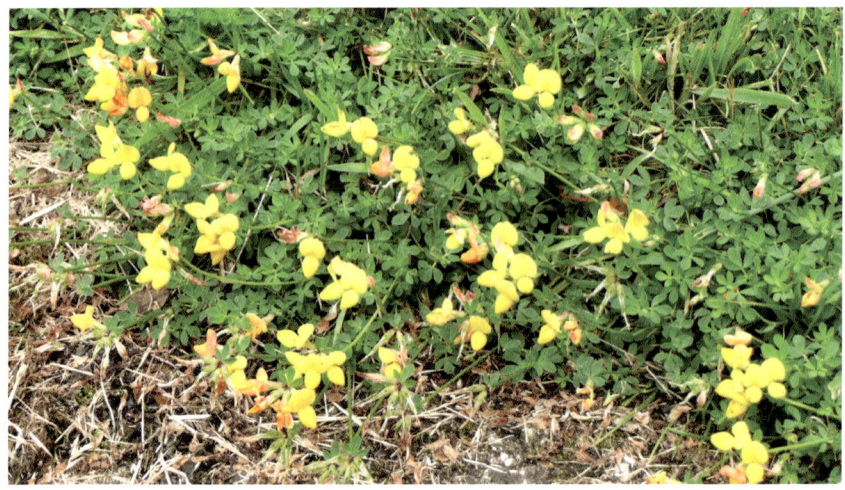

Alongside our front path, bird's-foot-trefoil gives our visitors a warm welcome.

This charming plant with its colourful pea-like flowers may well make an appearance on a sunny edge of your lawn. If it does, do leave it there as it will provide weeks of enjoyment through to early September. I had to rescue ours from my husband's spade as he is less tolerant of 'weeds' than I am. Now he agrees that it is as beautiful as any cultivated plant.

The clusters of flowers are deep yellow, often orange-red tipped or streaked, while the green of the leaves has a slightly bluish hue. There are five petals, with the upper one the largest, the lower two joined and the side two overlapping. The five sepals are the same length and joined, creating a tube into which the petals fit. The 'trefoil' is formed from three clover-like leaflets on a short stalk, the base of which carries two further leaflets or stipules. They are arranged on alternate sides of the main stem.

It is a perennial and will continue to bloom each summer. Self-fertile, the flowers are hermaphrodite, in other words with both male and female organs. It is readily pollinated by bees and other insects.

Folklore

The other common name of 'eggs and bacon' is perhaps more obviously descriptive of the plant than 'bird's foot' as the yellow and red coloration is often its most striking characteristic. The shape of the flowers with the large upper lip has inspired the sobriquets of 'lady's slipper' and 'Dutchman's clogs', reminders of old-fashioned footwear. However, from August the clusters of black seed pods will appear, and these can look distinctly claw-like. Perhaps they had something to do with the plant's darker associations, being indicative of revenge in the Victorian language of flowers. The other name of 'granny's toe-nails' is touched with a wry sense of humour.

Uses

The plant seems to have been used therapeutically in the 16th and 17th centuries for the treatment of wounds. At any rate, both Culpeper and Salmon mention it. Yet, it is no longer prescribed as it is somewhat toxic.

Wildlife

Bird's-foot-trefoil belongs to the pea family and therefore can fix nitrogen from the atmosphere. Not only does this benefit the plant itself but also those nearby.

This is a perfect plant for a wildflower meadow. It is very pretty and provides abundant nectar for many insects. The caterpillar of the silver-studded blue butterfly considers the leaves and buds a tasty treat as does that of the six-spot burnet moth.

All parts of bird's-foot-trefoil are mildly poisonous to humans, containing cyanogenic glycosides. When dried, however, these become innocuous, so it is acceptable in hay and often fed to cattle.

Bristly Oxtongue (*Picris echioides*)

Daisy family (Asteraceae). Annual/biennial. Pollinated by insects. Propagated by seed. Mildly irritant.

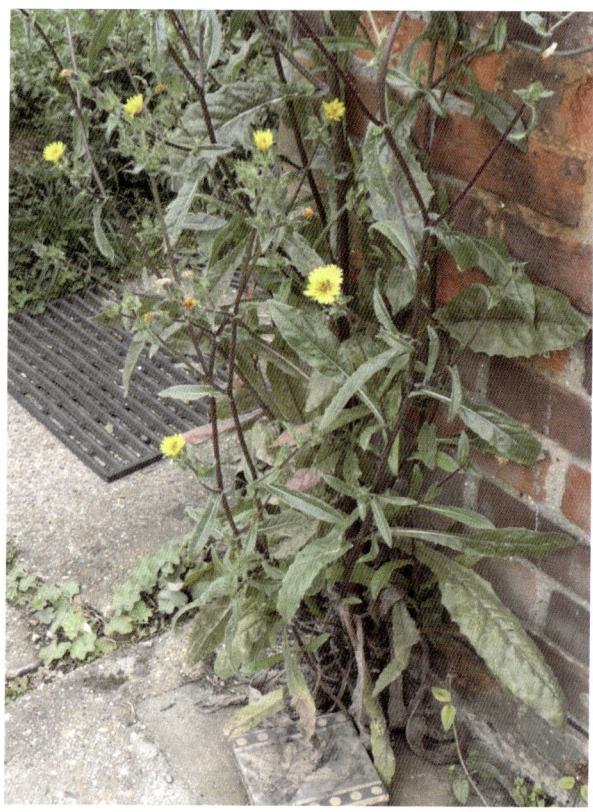

Bristly oxtongue is another 'weed' which can plant itself in the smallest of cracks.

When first the bristly rosettes of oxtongue leaves appeared on our meadow, I was puzzled as to their identification. Coming from the north of England, I had never seen them before. Originally a native of the Mediterranean, bristly oxtongue subsequently spread to much of the rest of Europe, including the south and east of England. My husband, being a local East Anglian, recognised the plant instantly.

I was fascinated by its development and watched it grow into a tall branching specimen, almost 1 m/3 ft high, with a sturdy, furrowed main stem. Its relationship to the dandelion was obvious when the yellow flowers finally appeared, each head of petals flattening out into a circle when mature. Most distinctive are the broad, heart-shaped bracts, also roughly prickly. Noticeable on the wavy lanceolate leaves are the whitish pimples at the base of each hair. A magnifying glass reveals the hooks at the tip of the hairs, compared to miniature grappling irons. Like the dandelion, it has a milky sap. The seeds are also blown away on feathery 'parachutes'.

The plant grew in my affections, perhaps because it seemed so strange to me, and so I have allowed it to flourish among tall grasses on our roadside verge.

Folklore

If you attempt to handle the plant without wearing gloves, you will surely suffer from numerous prickles. According to folk tradition the best way of curing these is as follows: cut off a flower head and throw it behind you, but be careful not to look round!

Uses

Little has been written about the plant as a beneficial remedy or for other uses. Perhaps people have found the bristles unappealing. Nevertheless, the leaves are edible but best when cooked. There is some evidence that they were used as a pot herb in the medieval period. They were also thought to help get rid of parasitic worms.

Wildlife

Bristly oxtongue is the food plant of the larvae of a small moth, *Cochylis hybridella,* which seek out nutrition within the seed heads. The adult has a white thorax with brown and black markings and a wing span of no more than 15 mm/½ inch. It can be seen flying from dusk onwards during the months of July and August. As it prefers the chalky habitats of southern

England and Wales, you are only likely to spot it if your garden is within such an area.

More widespread are the fruit flies which are attracted to the flowers. These flies are recognisable from their 'pictured' wings in the form of black shapes that adorn them. Some of these flies may cause galls to appear by injecting the plant tissues with a chemical at a time of rapid growth when cells are dividing quickly. Here the larvae will live and feed and find protection from predators.

It is worth examining the stem of a mature bristly oxtongue plant in search of tiny holes. These might well indicate that the larvae of a gall wasp, *Phanacis caulicola,* have been feeding on the pith. If you break the stem open, you may see the galls inside. The adult has a shiny black body and venation in the wings.

Lesser Burdock (*Arctium minus*)

Daisy family (Asteraceae). Biennial. Pollinated by insects. Propagated by seed. Medicinal.

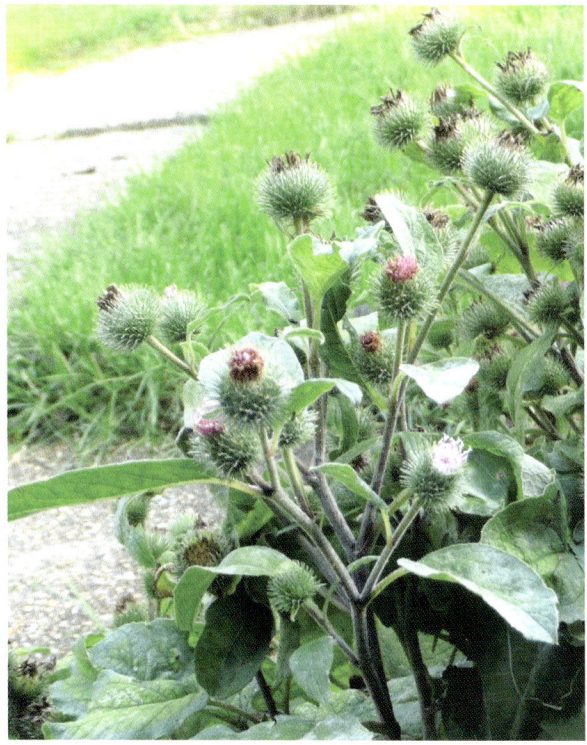

Once the flowers are over, the bristly seed heads of lesser burdock stick readily to clothing, as well as to our dog's fur!

One of the most difficult aspects of grooming my dog is trying to disentangle the burrs of burdock from his fur. The tiny hooks on the numerous bracts cling on persistently and are extraordinarily tricky to comb out without pulling unnecessarily on the hair. This is a remarkably effective way of dispersing seeds as the animal is likely to walk a fair distance before they drop out. Indeed, it was the fastening power of burdock's miniature hooks that inspired the Swiss inventor Georges de Mestral to develop Velcro.

Even lesser burdock can grow to quite a height, up to 1.30 m/4 ft 3 in, its large, lower, heart-shaped leaves forming a considerable spread. These have hollow stalks. The smaller, upper leaves are oval in shape. All are toothed.

Burdock is a biennial, so the reddish-purple, thistle-like flowers do not appear until the second year. These rather modest florets are made up of many small flowers; the five petals are joined to form a tube. In our garden we first notice the downy, pointed leaves of the plants which seem to establish themselves in the most inconvenient places, such as a crack in our front path. These we have to pull up. Others, however, choose a more suitable location, for example on waste ground next to our septic tank. Here they can stay.

Folklore

Over the centuries, country children have delighted in throwing the burrs at each other, their stickiness causing much hilarity.

In Scotland these games seem to have led to the tradition of the 'Burry Man' whose coat is entirely covered in burdock burrs. On a particular day in August he visits his neighbours in the town of Queensferry to collect donations. Afterwards his coat is removed and ritually burnt.

Uses

One of my favourite childhood drinks was dandelion and burdock. Only much later I learned how healthy it was as an effective cleanser and blood purifier. Burdock encourages the discharge of waste products from the body's cells, while dandelion, as a natural diuretic, flushes them out of the system. When in London recently, I was surprised to see this on sale in a café. Yet, some of these commercial drinks no longer contain the genuine ingredients, so it is wise to read the small print.

Along with essential oils and tannins, the root contains both mucilage and inulin. These are soluble fibres that help to lower the 'bad' blood fats, including LDL cholesterol. As such they can reduce the risk of heart disease and type 2 diabetes. They can ease constipation while at the same time increasing the abundance of the beneficial bacteria in the intestines.

Inulin is known to enhance immune function. If burdock appears in your garden, therefore, don't throw this valuable root away!

As for the large leaves, these make ideal poultices to relieve sore muscles or joints, skin eruptions such as acne or boils, and the pain of burns. They are naturally antiseptic and will accelerate healing. They can be applied hot (as described below) or cold according to the condition. For a quick remedy, for example to soothe a minor burn or the itchiness of eczema or psoriasis, simply crush a leaf and place over the problem area.

Health-giving gobo

In Japan, the root of burdock is used as a vegetable, known as gobo, tasting similar to artichoke. It is best to dig it up either the first autumn or the second spring. It can grow to a considerable length.

2½ tbsp sunflower oil
450 g/1 lb burdock root, peeled and cut into short, thin strips
1 tbsp soya sauce
1 tsp honey

Put the oil in a pan or wok and turn up the heat. When sizzling add the burdock strips and stir and toss for about 3 minutes. Reduce the heat and add the soya sauce and honey. Continue to stir-fry for a further 3 or 4 minutes until tender. **NB: Do not eat if pregnant or gluten intolerant.**

Burdock hot poultice

Pick a large leaf and put in a steamer for a few minutes until soft. Apply it immediately to the condition needing treatment and keep it warm by putting a hot water bottle over it. Leave the poultice in position for at least half an hour. Healing will take place as the therapeutic properties soak into the skin and blood is drawn to the area.

Wildlife

If you love butterflies as much as I do, then you will want to keep some burdock in a quiet corner, despite the annoyance of burrs sticking to clothing. It provides perfect nourishment for the larvae of the painted lady.

Cut-leaved Crane's-bill (*Geranium dissectum*)

Crane's-bill family (Geraniaceae). Annual/biennial. Self-fertile. Propagated by seed. Formerly medicinal.

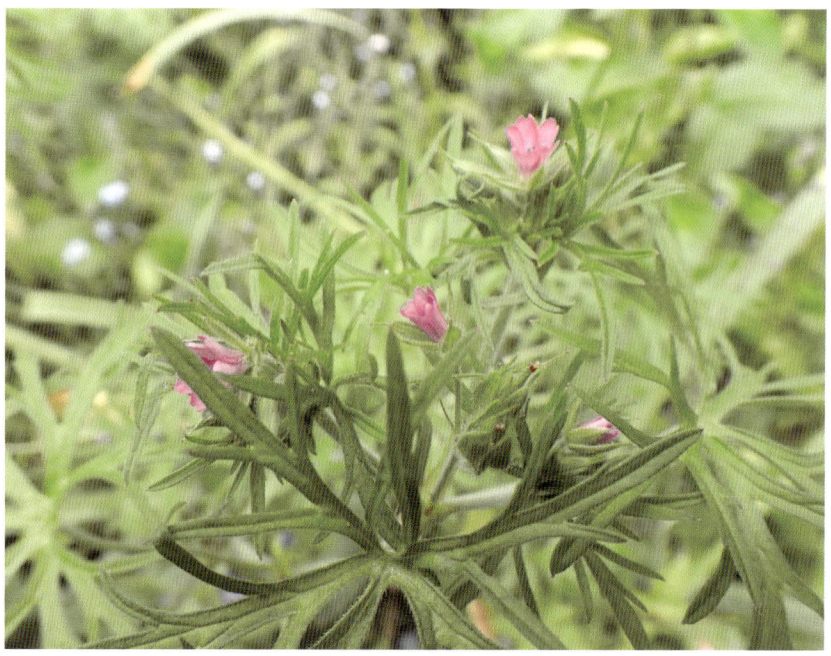

The pink flowers of cut-leaved crane's-bill are tiny and the deeply cut leaves are typical of this plant.

It seems odd that there is remarkably little information available about this native annual plant, especially as it is so common. Perhaps the reason is that it is very similar to herb-Robert (*Geranium robertianum*) and therefore undeserving of individual entries. However, there are essential differences. Although the shade of pink is comparable, the tiny flowers have notched rather than rounded petals. As indicated by its name, the leaves are deeply lobed, being divided nearly to the base.

The overall appearance can only be described as rather straggly. Like many weeds, it favours poor waste ground, yet it seems to have no difficulty

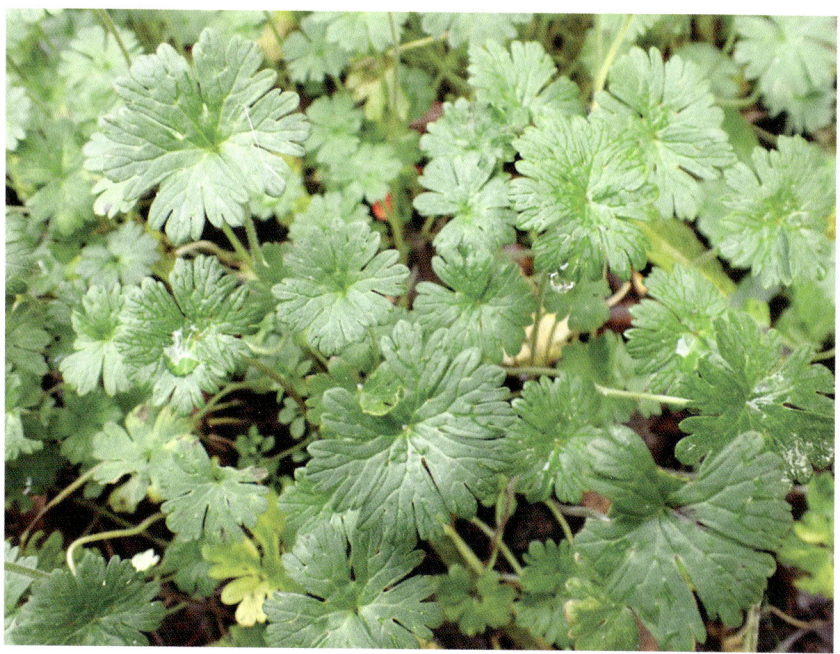

The leaves of the seedlings are already deeply divided, as its name implies.

flourishing on our clay. It is never a problem in our borders as it is very easily removed.

Perhaps the most interesting feature of the plant is its mode of seed dispersal. The seeds form in a long, beaked capsule, each in its own segment. When the pod is ripe, a thin strip of the beak coils suddenly upwards, flicking the seeds out. It never fails to astonish me how clever nature is!

Folklore

The common name of 'crane's-bill' is descriptive of the long beak-like seed pod before its seeds are explosively dispersed. Centuries ago cranes would have been a regular sight in the English countryside before losing their habitat to development and being shot to extinction. There would have been an obvious analogy between the striking bill of the bird and the seed pod of the plant.

The derivation of *Geranium* is from the Greek *geranos* meaning 'crane'.

Uses

In Norfolk and the area of the Fens, species of geranium were thought to aid in the healing of cuts. In an emergency, leaves would be crushed and placed on the wound, allowing the juice to penetrate.

Mrs Grieve would have agreed with this, as she lists 'styptic' as one of its properties in her *Modern Herbal*, especially if the plant is used before flowering when its constituents are most active. She also suggests that an infusion of 1 oz of herb to 1 pint of water can help to relieve diarrhoea. However, crane's-bill is rarely used in current herbal practice.

Wildlife

Around August to September time the brown argus butterfly lays its eggs on crane's-bill, especially in limestone districts of the south and east of England. If you live in such an area, then you might just spot this small butterfly flitting close to the ground, stopping often for nectar or to bask in the sun. Although mostly brown, the edges of the wings are adorned with a line of orange crescents and white fringes.

You will find it hard to spot the caterpillars, being leaf green with just a fine pink line. However, some excited ants might give the game away. Brown argus is related to the 'blue' butterflies, which have a symbiotic relationship with ants. Their caterpillars secrete a sweet, nectar-like substance which the ants consume. In return, the ants protect and care for the caterpillars. What an extraordinary association!

Common Figwort (*Scrophularia nodosa*)

Figwort family (Scrophulariaceae). Perennial. Pollinated by insects, especially wasps. Propagated by seed. Medicinal. Mildly poisonous.

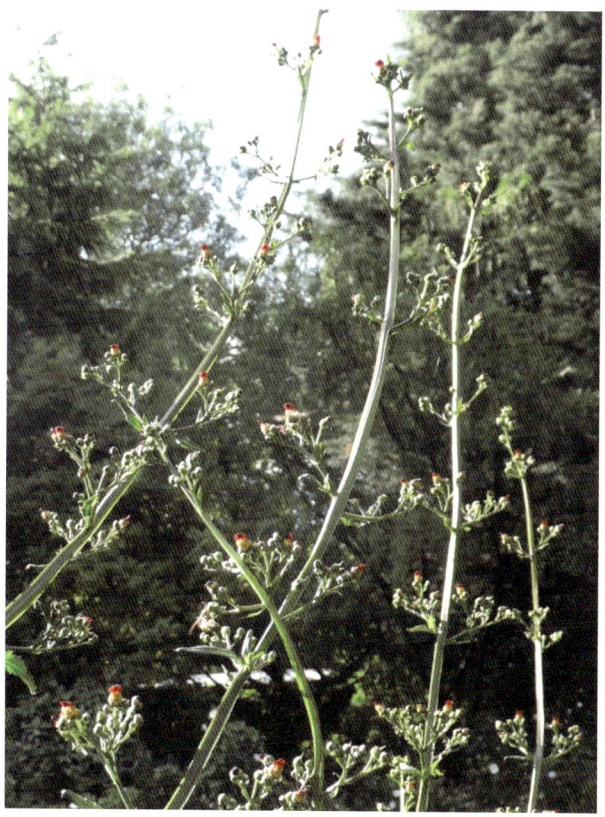

Despite its rather odd scent, figwort nevertheless appeals to wasps and other insects, which pollinate the plant.

Although described as 'common', this was another plant I had never previously seen, so I was baffled when a tall square stem began producing rather peculiar brownish-purple flowers on side shoots. These seemed too small and out of scale with the rest of the plant, which was statuesque in character. The large, pointed, dark-green leaves placed opposite each other

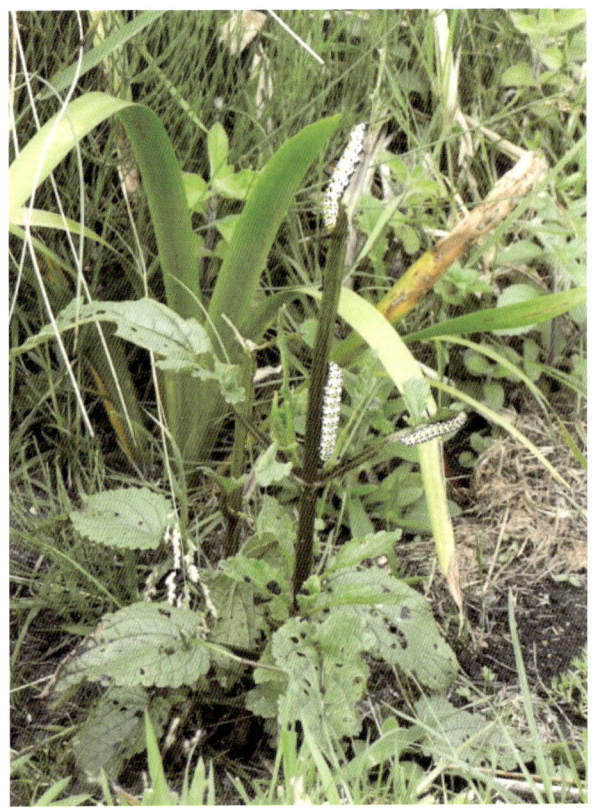

We were fascinated to see the caterpillars of the mullein moth eat their way through this figwort, their other food plant.

and toothed along the edges added to this impression. The first that arrived in our garden grew under a willow tree, followed by several that turned up by the pond. Clearly this damp position was favoured as they have grown here ever since, whereas the willow location was a one-off.

Looking closely at the flowers, I could see that the upper two petals were the longest, overshadowing the three lower ones, all joined towards the base to form a globular shape and here becoming greenish in colour. The five sepals are also green. Taking a sniff to test for a perfume, it struck me as being expressive of its looks – rather odd and not particularly attractive. Yet, evidently it does appeal to wasps which are its main pollinators.

Folklore

Scottish folk in the Hebrides believed in the protective qualities of figwort. When placed in the byre the cows would thrive, so they thought, and produce plenty of milk.

Uses

The Latin name is as unlovely as the plant – *Scrophularia* – referring to its apparent ability to cure the disease known as scrofula, a tuberculosis of the lymph nodes in the neck. No doubt this belief derives from the Doctrine of Signatures in which the plant is supposed to portray the 'signature' of the disease it is able to cure. The globular tube formed by the joined petals and the gaping 'mouth' of the flower, along with the swellings on the tubers beneath the soil, must have collectively pointed to the swollen glands of scrofula. Otherwise known as the 'king's evil', Culpeper thought that there was no better remedy than figwort, or 'throatwort' as he called it. He also recommended it for 'any other knobs, kernels, bunches or wens growing in the flesh wheresoever; and for the haemorrhoids, or piles', to which bruised leaves would be applied. Indeed, the name 'fig' is the old word for piles.

Research has shown that there are useful active ingredients in the plant. Most particularly it is an anodyne with considerable pain-relieving properties. Gabrielle Hatfield in her *Herbal* reports that mothers used to gather and dry the stems, cutting them into small pieces and threading them into necklaces for their infants. The child would chew on the 'beads' which eased the pain of teething. However, as figwort is somewhat poisonous, no such remedy should be attempted.

At Kew, laboratory tests have shown that the plant contains iridoids that have anti-bacterial activity and that stimulate fibroblasts, the cells in connective tissues that synthesise collagen. In theory, therefore, figwort could turn out to be an important treatment for leg ulcers.

Wildlife

The figwort sawfly deserves mention here. This looks just like a wasp with black body and fine yellow bands. However, the difference is that it lacks the 'waste' of a true wasp. Flying from May to August, the front edges of its forewings have an orange hue. The larvae are surprisingly large at twice the size of the adult, reaching 30 mm/1¼ inches. They have an off-white, black-spotted body and a dark head. In the autumn they feed on the leaves of figwort and then hibernate, emerging the following year in the late spring.

In addition to the mullein moth (see p. 210), the frosted orange may also feed on figwort. It flies at night from August to October, with a wing span of up to 43 mm/1¾ inches. The resting adult moth is virtually invisible, as the orange and brown speckled wings blend perfectly with the autumn leaves. The larvae, also autumn coloured, but with the addition of black dots, are scarcely ever seen as they feed internally inside the stems and roots of the host plant.

Ground-elder (*Aegopodium podagraria*)

Carrot family (Apiaceae). Perennial. Pollinated by flies and beetles. Propagated by rhizome and seed. Edible. Medicinal.

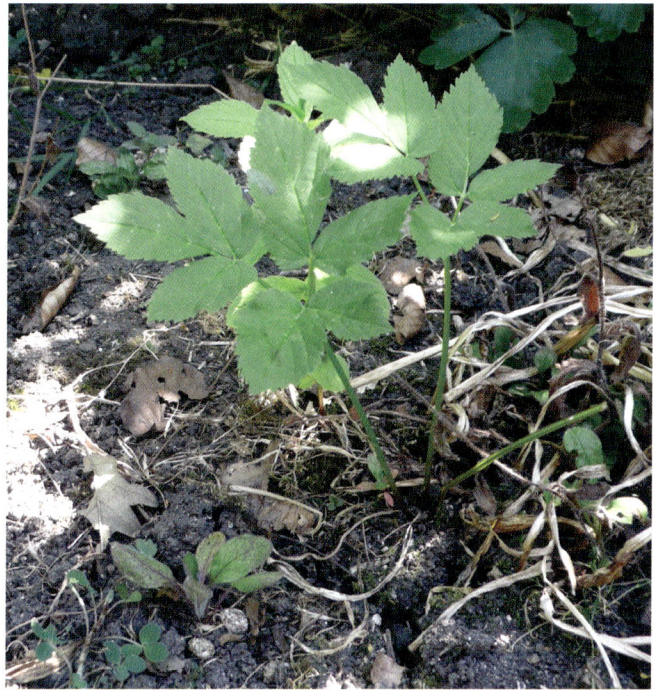

If seedlings of ground-elder appear in your borders, you may want to dig them out quickly!

Pretty as the umbrella-shaped, white flower heads are, this is definitely not my favourite 'weed'. If only it could be easily contained, then I would welcome it gladly into our garden on account of its therapeutic properties. The underground stems, however, creep along and throw up new plants everywhere among our border perennials and, try as I might, there is no way of getting on top of it. Even digging up the whole bed, carefully pulling out the long runners and replanting everything, failed to succeed in abolishing it. If even a tiny piece of root is left behind this will produce a

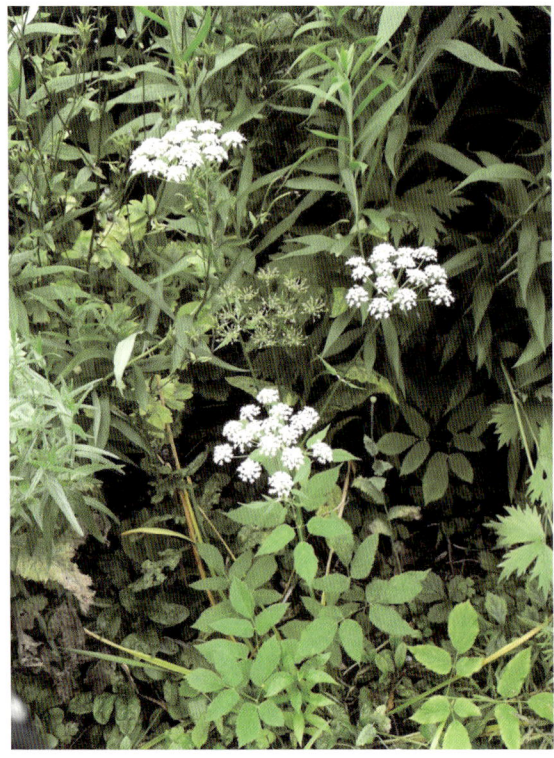

Ground-elder is one of the few real problem weeds, as even a fragment of root left in the soil will result in another plant.

new plant. Mrs Grieve in her *Modern Herbal* of 1931 thinks that buckwheat could drive away ground-elder, but I haven't tried it.

The best piece of advice for organic gardeners is to hoe off the leaves below ground level as soon as they appear, and thereafter each week. The plant will then be unable to photosynthesise and will eventually give up and die. Our problem is the large size of our garden. By the time I get round to them again, a week has long since passed and new ground-elder is already well established. The 16th-century apothecary John Gerard puts it well:

> It is so fruitfull in his increase, that where it hath once taken root, it will hardly be gotten out againe, spoiling and getting every yeere more ground, to the annoying of better herbes.

However, the tender young leaves are not wasted, as they can perk up a salad, being 'of a resonable good savour' as Gerard admits.

You will recognise the plant by its serrated, pointed, oval leaves, which are in threes on each stalk. The main stem is hollow and grooved, branching out at the top. If you pull it up, you will see how it is attached to the long underground runner. Be careful not to leave any behind! These rhizomes can grow up to 90 cm/3 ft in a year. Each flower has five minute, white petals with the tips curved inwards. The flower head is a collection of up to 25 small umbels to form one large compound umbel.

Folklore

The first part of the botanical name is rather odd as, literally translated, it means 'goat and little foot', *aigos* being the Greek for 'goat' and *podos* for 'foot'. Apparently, this was inspired by the shape of the leaves. *Podagraria*, however, makes better sense as this is derived from *podagra*, or gout. A particularly appealing and descriptive common name is 'Jack-jump-about', due to the seed pods which, when they are ripe, become detached and are whipped away by the wind.

Uses

In the Middle Ages, it was well known as an effective treatment for gout. Indeed, it was recommended in texts of the period, such as Hildegard von Bingen's *Physica*. It is often referred to as 'herb Gerard' as the saint of this name was believed to relieve the pain of gout sufferers. Alcoholic beers were drunk in large quantities at this time as the water was unsafe, so no doubt gout was extremely common. It is hardly surprising, therefore, that 'goutweed' became another popular name. It seems that ground-elder was taken to northern Europe by the Romans as an appetising green vegetable. From there monks brought it to Britain as a pot-herb and remedy, and, like it or not, here it has stayed.

A tisane made from ground-elder is still recommended by some herbalists as a good cleanser of the kidneys as it is a natural diuretic. Poultices from the boiled-up roots and leaves, if laid on swollen joints, can offer relief as the essential oils will permeate through the skin. Homoeopaths still use minute quantities of the plant to treat rheumatism and gout.

A cleansing tea

Handful of fresh young leaves and roots of ground-elder
275 ml/½ pint boiling water
1 tsp lemon juice
1 tsp honey

Chop and crush the herb and place in a pot. Pour on the boiling water, then stir in the lemon juice and honey. Cover and allow to infuse for 10 minutes. ♦ Take in small doses throughout the day.

Goutweed poultice

You will need a piece of muslin or thin cloth to make the poultice. Amounts of ingredients will depend on the size of the area to be treated. Plain white flour can be substituted, but barley is best. You can make this yourself by grinding up pot barley in a coffee grinder.

Fresh young leaves and roots of ground-elder
barley flour
boiling water

Chop the ground-elder into small pieces and crush. Mix with equal amounts of flour. Pour on boiling water, just sufficient to make a paste and stir well. With a spatula lay the mixture on to the muslin and fold over the corners. Apply hot to the affected area and secure with clingfilm or a bandage. Repeat as necessary.

Gerard's 'spinach'

Be sure to pick the leaves well before the plant has flowered when they are still pleasantly piquant. You will need plenty as they boil down.

25 g/1 oz butter
fresh young ground-elder leaves
2 tbsp water

Melt the butter in a large pan then add the leaves and the water. Cover. Cook very gently, stirring from time to time to avoid sticking.

Wildlife

Ground-elder is most commonly found among ancient ruins, particularly those with ecclesiastical associations. Indeed, our garden is composed of former glebe land belonging to the local church. Perhaps this explains why ground-elder so thrives here! It also follows that the caterpillar of a moth, the grey dagger, which has a special liking for old walls, should have developed a taste for ground-elder. While the hairy caterpillar has colourful red and white stripes, the sombre tones of the adult moth blend so perfectly with stone ruins that it is virtually impossible to detect, except perhaps by the sharp eyes of a passing bird.

Another caterpillar which relishes ground-elder, amongst a wide host range, is that of the dot moth, so called on account of the two white spots on its wings.

Hogweed (*Heracleum sphondylium*)

Carrot family (Apiaceae). Biennial/perennial. Pollinated by insects, especially hoverflies. Propagated by seed. Irritant.

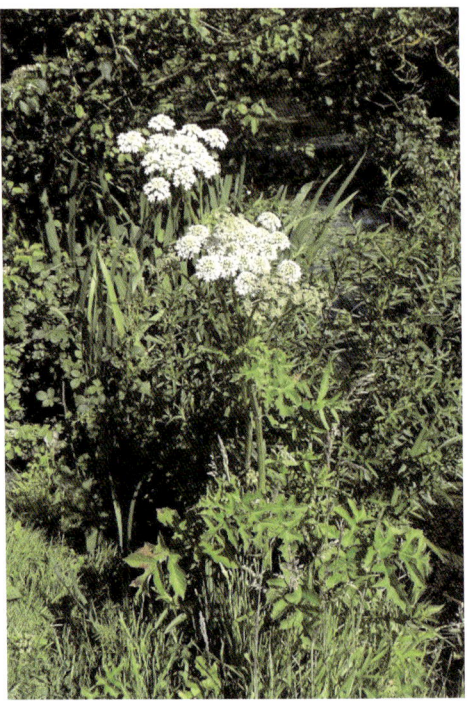

The petals of hogweed are its most distinguishing feature. If you look closely, you will see that those on the outside of the inflorescence are longer than those on the inside.

When a plant with dark, rather coarse, green leaves pushed itself up to a statuesque height near our pond, I observed it with considerable caution. Was it simply our native common hogweed, or could it be the non-native invasive and highly toxic giant hogweed? When it eventually stopped growing at a little taller than myself, I was reassured, as the giant variety will reach more than double that. Even so, it is wise to wear gloves when touching even common hogweed as some plants can produce the same

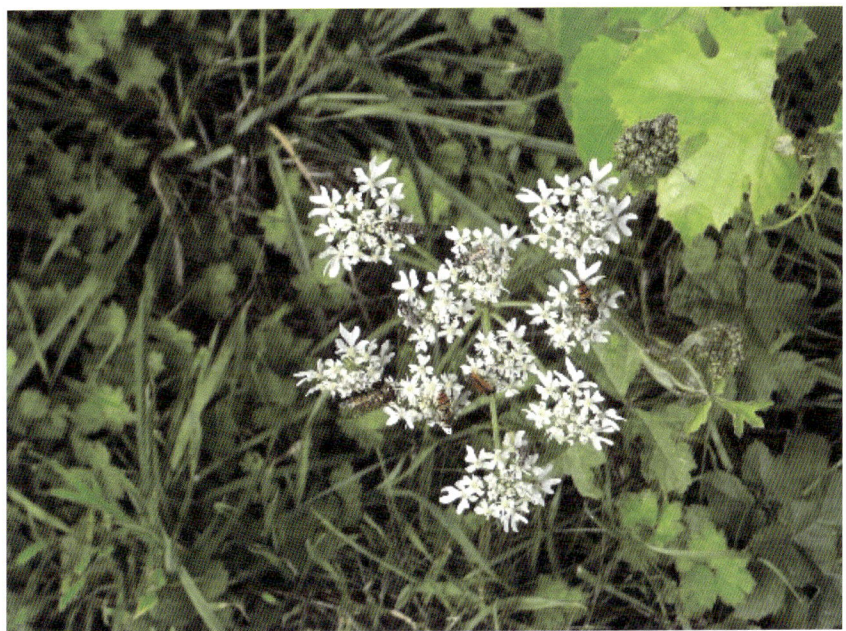

The flowers are very attractive to hoverflies.

toxic chemicals in their sap, the furanocoumarins, that cause the skin sensitivity especially in sunlight known as phyto-photodermatitis.

The flower heads were beautiful, large flattish umbels, made up of as many as 30 rays, each with a great many buds shaped like tiny 'parcels'. I was fascinated by the way they opened, by unfurling their notched petals. These are generally white, although sometimes with a pink tinge. I noticed that the flowers on the edges of the umbels had unequal petals, the longest and more deeply notched of the five being the outermost.

The seed pods, when they appeared, were flat and more or less round in shape, with a seed in each half. Because the plant is so tall, wind dispersal is effective as it sways to and fro.

Folklore

It is not entirely clear where the common name came from. There are reports of the plant being fed to livestock, but these generally allude to cattle rather than pigs. Indeed, its other common name is cow parsnip. However, the flowers do have a slightly pig-like odour, so perhaps it was this that prompted the name.

The tall stem is hollow inside, so country children have favoured it either as a sword for playing at soldiers or else as a pea-shooter. When dry, it is ideal for making a bee 'hotel', simply by cutting it to short lengths and placing these inside some sort of tube and hanging this in a warm, dry place. Wild bees will nest here.

Uses

Although not prescribed by modern herbalists, common hogweed has long been a favourite plant of foragers. It belongs to the carrot family and is edible. The young shoots in particular have an asparagus-like flavour and are very good when steamed. The flower buds can be added to stir-fries. Later in the year, the seeds provide a piquant snack. However, you must be one hundred per cent sure of identification before consuming any part of this plant on account of its similarity to the poisonous giant hogweed. Apart from its size, the main difference is that this Asian species has purple blotches on its stem.

Wildlife

In addition to the fact that our hogweed looked rather splendid beside our pond, I decided to allow it to flourish when I noticed how attractive the flowers were to insects. My researches indicated that as many as 118 different species will visit hogweed, particularly hoverflies and sawflies. Apparently, they find the smell of pigs most alluring! The grey and orange soldier beetle will soon turn up to feed on the numerous smaller insects.

Great Mullein (*Verbascum thapsus*)

Figwort family (Scrophulariaceae). Biennial. Pollinated by insects, especially hoverflies. Propagated by seed. Medicinal.

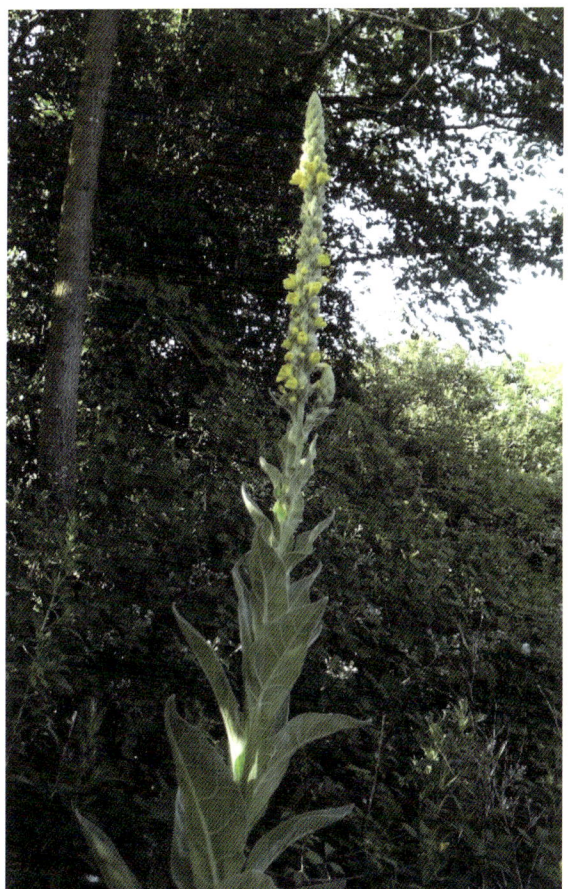

We were amazed when mullein arrived in our garden as this plant generally prefers quite dry conditions rather than our damp clay.

About five years ago, a tall, majestic spike of great mullein appeared under one of our willow trees. Ever since I have watched out for its grey-green, woolly leaves, but year after year it has failed to reappear. This is hardly

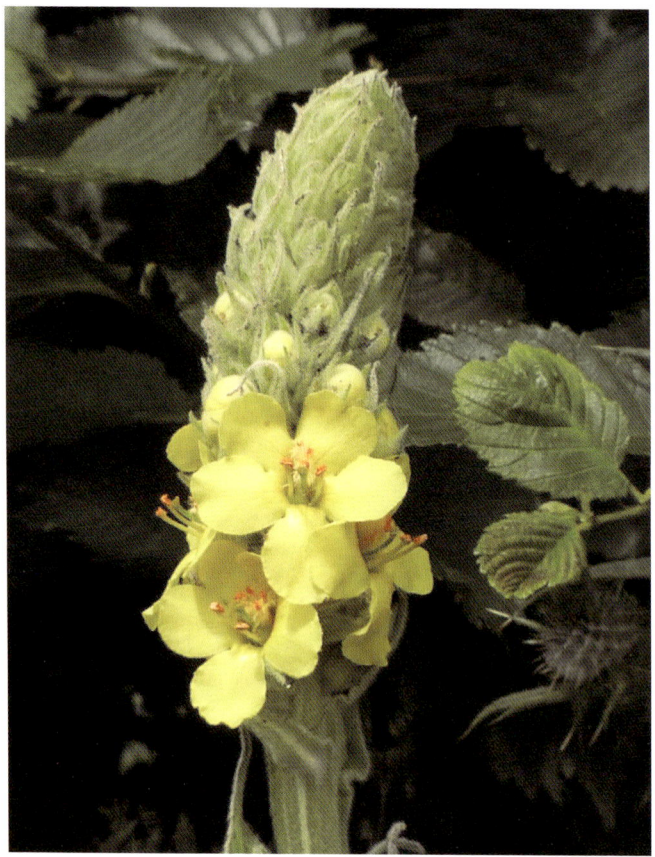

The last flowers to open are those at the tip. *Photo © NatureSpot / Graham Calow*

surprising as mullein favours well-drained, sandy soils rather than the heavy clay we have here in our garden. How astonished I was, therefore, when my husband said he had spotted one right on the other side of the garden, at the far end of the pond. How could it have arrived there? I have never seen any other mullein in the vicinity, despite my long country walks with our greyhound. The seeds can last for many years in the soil, however, ready to sprout when the land is disturbed. John had recently cleared some brambles to make a path by the pond. The newly arrived space and light could have prompted the recent growth. Perhaps this is the explanation. Although ours is not the best of specimens, nevertheless I will tend it carefully and collect the seeds to bring on the offspring in the greenhouse – well worth the effort as mullein is such a valuable herb.

There are many garden varieties of *Verbascum*. Beautiful though they are, they would find it hard to compete with our native mullein. Its five-lobed, lemon-yellow flowers are densely packed up the tall stalk, while its downy elliptical leaves are unusually distinctive. Rather than having a separate stalk, these have the habit of merging with the stem as far as the leaf below. As a biennial, the basal rosette appears first in year one, these leaves having winged stalks.

Folklore

'Mullein' is a corruption of *mollis*, which means 'soft' in Latin, referring to the downy leaves. As for *Verbascum*, this is derived from the Latin *barba* or beard, also indicative of the many hairs.

Some of the common names reveal both past superstitions associated with the plant, as well as practical uses. 'Aaron's rod' is perhaps the best known in the UK. According to the Old Testament, Aaron, the brother of Moses, had a staff which was endowed with magic powers, employed to good effect during the plagues in Egypt. 'Adam's flannel', however, is a bit more down to earth, reminding us that the soft leaves were used as toilet paper or nappies. 'Hag's taper' suggests something more sinister, linking the plant with witches' covens. This, however, is disputed in the literature, 'hag' meaning hedge rather than witch, mullein often being found in cleared land near a hedge. Nevertheless, the reference to taper is founded in reality: having highly inflammable leaves, especially when dried, entire plants were sometimes dipped in tallow and then set alight to be used as torches at a celebration or funeral.

Uses

Mullein is another wonder plant, rich in healing attributes. The mucilage gently soothes inflammation, especially when mucous membranes are infected. The glycosides support this, being also anti-inflammatory. The saponins are thought to provide the expectorant properties, helping to clear phlegm from the bronchial tubes. The flavonoids act as a gentle diuretic. Although further research needs to be carried out, laboratory trials indicate that infusions of the flowers have anti-viral properties.

A tea made from either the leaves or the flowers is a very long-standing traditional remedy for irritating coughs and colds and even the more serious illness of bronchitis. Herbalists over the centuries have seen how effective mullein is in clearing bronchial congestion. The plant has also been used to treat tuberculosis. A 19th-century physician, Dr Quinlan, prescribed an Irish remedy which involved boiling a handful of fresh leaves in two pints of milk and which was then strained and sweetened with honey. The patient was instructed to drink a cupful twice a day. A similar remedy was regularly used by cowmen for their cattle, earning the plant the name of 'bullock's lungwort'.

American pioneers considered that sitting on mullein leaves would cure piles. A more complex variation of this had been regularly used in Europe in the Middle Ages. A 15th-century Leechbook states:

> Take a pan with coals and heat a little stone glowing and put thereon the leaves of … mullein; and put in under a chair or under a stool with a siege, that the smoke thereof may ascend to thy fundament as hot as thou mayest suffer.

This sounds distinctly uncomfortable! Needless to say, it is no longer prescribed. However, there is some indication that the discomfort of piles could be eased with an oil infusion of mullein.

Modern herbalists have found that the flowers infused in oil make soothing drops to treat earache. As for the large leaves, these make an excellent poultice to ease a multiplicity of conditions, from an aching back, cracked ribs, swollen glands, to boils and splinters. See the remedy below.

Mullein is such a useful herb that it is well worth drying the leaves and flowers for later use.

Drying the leaves

If you have very sensitive skin, you may need to wear gloves because of the tickly hairs.

Pick the leaves in spring before the plant puts up its flower spike. Lay them out on paper in an airy place. Crumble them when dry and store in jars.

Drying the flowers

Pick on a sunny afternoon. Lay them out on paper or even better on a fine mesh to allow the air to circulate. Store in jars when dry.

Aaron's ear drops

You will need a smallish jar and some muslin for the preparation. Instead of dropper bottles, you could apply the remedy with a small teaspoon.

Mullein flowers
extra virgin olive oil

Fill the jar with freshly picked flowers, making sure they are perfectly dry. Cover them with the oil, then secure the muslin on top of the jar with a rubber band. This allows any moisture to evaporate. Leave on a sunny window ledge for about two weeks or until the colour has faded from the flowers. Every so often push the flowers down into the oil to make sure they are immersed. ♦ Strain carefully through muslin, excluding any watery residue. Using a funnel, pour the flower oil into sterilised dropper bottles. It will keep for up to three months in a cool, dark place. ♦ Two or three drops into the affected ear three times a day should help to relieve pain and soften any build-up of wax.

Mullein tea

1 rounded tsp dried or 2 tsp fresh mullein flowers
boiling water
a little honey

Put the flowers in a mug and pour on the boiling water. Sweeten to taste. Leave for 10 to 15 minutes. Strain before drinking. ♦ Mullein is not toxic, so the tea can be taken as necessary to relieve a hacking cough or a cold and to help ease breathing.

Adam's poultice

You will need a large, flat dish. Choose the leaves according to the size of area which needs to be treated. Have a hot water bottle to hand.

2 or 3 mullein leaves

boiling water

Lay the fresh leaves in the dish and pour on the boiling water just to cover. Leave a little while until they are cool enough to pick up. Lay on the affected area then keep warm with the hot water bottle. Relax and be patient until the healing ingredients have been absorbed into the skin.

Wildlife

How privileged we felt when three caterpillars of the mullein moth appeared in our garden – not on mullein, as it happens, but on their other food plant, figwort! They are quite beautiful with their yellow bands and black spots but also remarkably visible to hungry birds. It is unclear how many reach the adult stage as the moths are perfectly camouflaged when resting on a branch and therefore rarely seen. They are brown and black and look just like a piece of bark. In flight, during April and May, their wing span can extend to 50 mm/2 inches.

An even larger moth at up to 120 mm/4¾ inches, that can be a casual visitor to gardens in the late summer, is the death's head hawk moth. This is notable for the scull-like markings on the head of the adult. Beekeepers occasionally report seeing them entering hives, searching for sweet honey. The moth may often lay its eggs on mullein, but the yellow caterpillars are also partial to potatoes.

Common Nettle (*Urtica dioica*)

Nettle family (Urticaceae). Perennial. Pollinated by wind. Propagated by seed, rhizome and stolon. Edible if cooked. Medicinal.

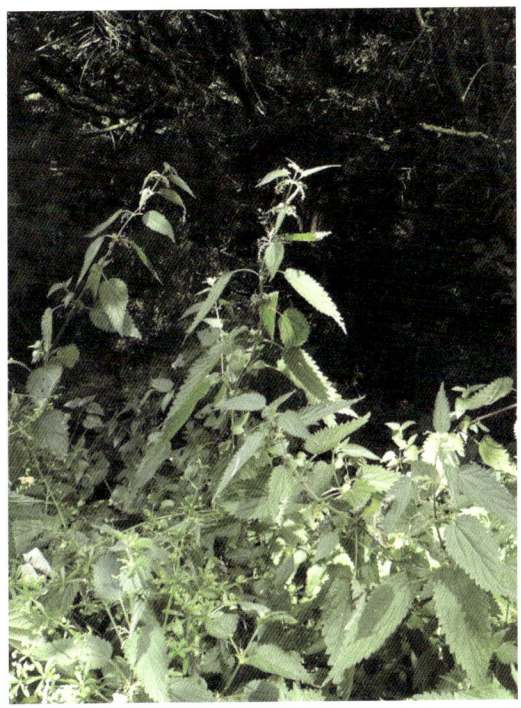

The common nettle is the bane of many gardeners, yet is so important for wildlife.

It always astonished me how my neighbour, born and bred in the countryside, could easily pull up nettles with her bare hands and think nothing of it. Asking how it was that she never seemed to be stung, she explained that you had to grip the nettles very hard so as to squash the stinging hairs. Some research into the matter showed that she was right. If the hairs are bent over they are unable to inject the histamine and other chemicals into the skin that cause the stinging sensation. The poet Aaron Hill (1685–1750) made up a verse about this which he scribbled on a windowpane:

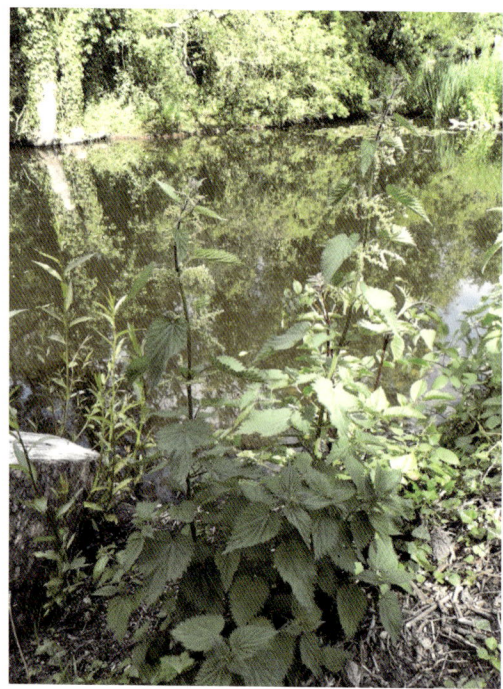
Even stinging nettles can look attractive in the right setting.

> Tender-handed stroke a nettle,
> And it stings you for your pains;
> Grasp it like a man of mettle,
> And it soft as silk remains.

Despite these assertions, I still have not had the nerve to test it out!

There is no difficulty in recognising the plant from its rather drab green, pointed, serrated, hairy leaves, set opposite each other on the angular, erect stem. Stinging nettle is dioecious, with distinct male and female plants. You can tell the difference from the flowers, which grow in upright panicles on the male plant but droop downwards on the female.

Some stinging nettles can grow very tall in summer, up to 2 m/7 ft, but then die back to the ground in winter. As anyone with a nettle bed will know, the plant sends out wide spreading rhizomes as well as stolons (runners) under the soil surface, ready to produce new shoots at the first warmth of spring or whenever the leaves are cut back. If you are planning to dig them out, you can identify the roots from their distinctive yellow colour. Nettles are often found in gardens as they like nitrogen-rich soil.

Folklore

As an all-pervasive weed, superstitions and tales involving the plant abound. Hans Christian Andersen told a fairy tale about a girl who had to make eleven shirts out of nettles for her brothers. This was to break the spell cast on them whereby they would turn into swans. As it happens, the strong fibre from nettle stalks makes a useful linen-like cloth, a process still current into the early 20th century. During World War I, cotton was in such short supply that German army uniforms were made from nettle fibres. Yet, as about 40 kg/88 lb of nettles are needed to make just one shirt, the poor girl in the fairy tale must have laboured many hours to pick enough!

The Ancient Greeks believed that nettle was an aphrodisiac and that the seeds, along with the roots of Narcissus, were effective against impotence. In the 15th century entirely the opposite point of view predominated, the seeds being recommended as a remedy against lechery: 'To avoid lechery, take nettle-seed and bray it in a mortar with pepper and temper it with honey or with wine, and it shall destroy it...' Gypsies in southern England regarded the leaves as a useful contraceptive, but the man had to put them in his socks! One wonders what the stinging did to his performance.

If you dream of nettles, this is a sign that you will be healthy and prosperous with a happy family life. If in the dream you are gathering them, then someone important thinks well of you. If, however, the nettles sting you, then disappointment and annoyance will come your way.

Uses

There was an old belief in southern England that it was unwise to use nettles as food, or for remedies, from May Day onwards. This seems to have been linked with the superstition that the devil would pick nettles to make his shirt on that day. Be that as it may, it is true that the tops are best picked young and fresh as the mature leaves contain tiny crystalline substances that are irritating and bitter. However, if you keep cutting the stalks back, tender new shoots will appear well into autumn.

Nettles are extremely rich in nutrients and are the basis of some of the very best natural remedies. In particular iron, which is easily absorbed into the system, is available in generous amounts, so people suffering from anaemia will profit from nettle soup or purée. Just two minutes of cooking will nullify the stinging hairs. For a tasty soup, follow any good spinach recipe and simply substitute nettles as the main vegetable.

Nettle ale

Before hops became the most popular ingredient for beer making, herbs were in regular use, with nettle being the clear favourite because of its characteristic flavour. It was also widely drunk as a remedy for rheumatism. Indeed, it contains anti-inflammatory polysaccharides and has painkilling properties.

Here in East Anglia, it was used as a treatment for consumption. As nettle contains the vitamins A and C, the ale would have given the patient's immune system a boost, helping to fight the disease.

Various good recipes can be found on the Internet.

Nettle Tea

2 tsp nettle tops (1 tsp if dried)
1 mugful boiling water

If you have no herbal tea in your cupboard, at least choose to stock nettle. Dry the nettle tops yourself (see below) or simply pick the young leaves and use fresh. ♦ Just pour the boiling water over the herb and infuse for 5 minutes.

This tea is a valuable all-round healer. Being rich in vitamins and minerals, it therefore makes an excellent spring tonic. If you rinse your hair with it you will be pleased with how it keeps dandruff under control and leaves a beautiful shine. Nettle tea stimulates the kidneys and is a natural diuretic, helping to flush out urinary tract infections as well as removing toxins from the system. At the same time, it dilates the smaller blood vessels and so improves the circulation – a boon to those who suffer from cold hands and feet. People with type 2 diabetes may find that it provides beneficial backup to their treatment by lowering blood sugar levels.

Drying the leaves

Wear gloves and pick the young plants well before flowering. Tie them into loose bunches to allow the air to circulate freely around them. By hanging upside down essential oils will drain into the tops. Leave in a dry, airy place, out of sunlight, for 3 weeks or until the leaves become brittle. Store in an airtight container in a dark place. Coloured glass is ideal.

Nettle root tonic

The roots of nettles are often prescribed by herbalists for older men, as a means of maintaining the health of the prostate. Anyone who has tackled a spreading nettle patch will know how tenacious the yellow roots can be. To dig them out, choose a day in the autumn, after rain preferably, when the ground is soft.

1. **Drying the roots**

Select the thickest roots and wash them well. Cut into pieces. Spread these out on a cake rack and leave in a warm place until fully dried.

2. **Making a decoction**

50 g/2 oz fresh nettle root (a little less if dried)
570 ml/1 pint water

You make a decoction first of all from fresh (or dried) root. Boil up the pieces in the water. Cover the pan and simmer for 20 minutes. Drain off the liquid and set aside until cool.

3. **Preserving the decoction**

Use Vodka, or any spirit will do. In a ratio of 3 parts spirit to 1 part decoction, pour into a large jar, adding a few root pieces. Leave for up to a month in a warm dark place, shaking from time to time, until the liquid has taken out the goodness of the nettle roots and changed colour. ♦ Strain through a sieve and pour into dark-coloured sterilised bottles. This should keep for a year or two. ♦ Take 1 tsp a day for maintenance of prostate health. **Warning: Not to be taken by women during pregnancy.**

Nettle tomato feed

The best feed for your tomatoes is easily made from nutrient-rich nettles. Being naturally high in nitrogen, it is an excellent fertiliser. You will need a large bucket with lid and water, plus some sort of weight that will fit in the bucket.

Wearing gloves, cut the nettles before flowering and crush the stems and leaves to speed up the process. Fill the bucket with these, put the weight on top and pour in the water to cover the nettles. Put the lid in place. You now have to wait three to four weeks for the feed to form. It will be far too strong to use neat, so dilute 1 part feed to at least 5 parts water, until it is the colour of tea. Your tomatoes will be delighted! ♦ You can keep on cutting the nettles and topping up the bucket to give summer-long fertiliser.

Wildlife

Several of our most distinguished butterflies and moths rely on nettle as a food plant for their larvae, in particular the colourful peacock with its striking 'eyes' and the prettily patterned small tortoiseshell, as well as the comma with scalloped edges to its wings.

Among the moths, angle shades, which looks just like a dead leaf, will appreciate your nettle patch, as will the dot moth (grey, but easily identifiable by the white patch on each wing), and also the pale buff ermine.

If you have dark outbuildings, then they may well be harbouring the mouse moth during the daytime. Not only are these mouse-coloured but, if aroused, will scamper away in a mouse-like fashion.

Common Ragwort (*Jacobaea vulgaris*)

Daisy family (Asteraceae). Biennial. Pollinated by insects. Propagated by seed. Poisonous.

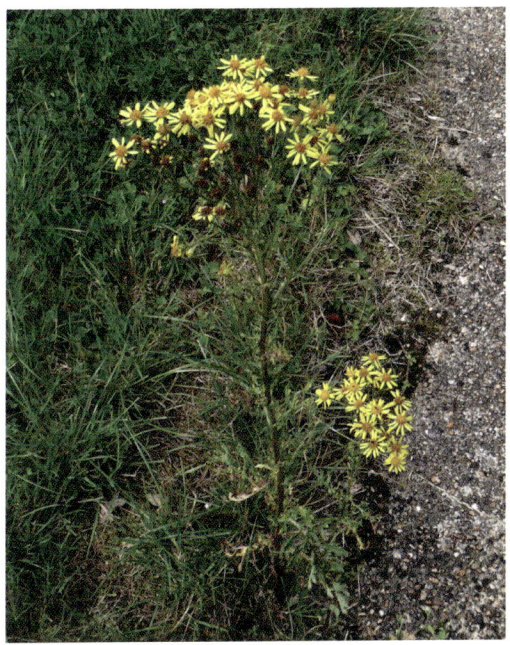

Common Ragwort is toxic to horses, but as we are not riders, it can grow safely in our garden.

This is the most unwanted of all weeds amongst farmers. Horse owners in particular detest it and exterminate it with ferocity. There is some justification for this as it is poisonous to animals. However, horses will instinctively avoid it, no doubt deterred by its acrid smell. Nevertheless, it is wise to be cautious as it can be a problem if inadvertently mixed with hay.

My husband recalls his youth when fields were brightened by its sunny yellow flowers. In amongst the petals and raggedy leaves you could see the most striking orange- and black-striped caterpillars, known as 'cinnabars', the sort that small boys used to delight in putting in empty jam jars and keeping as 'pets' until turning into chrysalises. In the wild, these will normally spend the winter just below the surface of the soil or safely hidden in leaf litter. In the late spring, red-and-black cinnabar moths emerge, also poisonous, the vermilion (or cinnabar) dots and stripes warning off birds and lizards. It is extraordinary that the alkaloid poisons in the plant do not kill either the caterpillars or the moths but are stored in their bodies to act as a chemical defence against any predators.

Folklore

One of the old English names for ragwort is "stammerwort", referring to the common belief that it could be used to treat stuttering.

However, according to the Irish, the plant is really a fairy horse in disguise. Be very careful not to tread on ragwort after sunset therefore. It is said that, if you do, a horse will spring up from the roots of the crushed plant and gallop off with you. You must certainly never burn ragwort, because the fairies will have nothing to ride on and will be very angry with you and bring you all sorts of bad luck.

In the Hebrides it is believed that the fairies use the plant for shelter and protection at night during rough weather. When they want to travel from one island to another, they will invoke the ragwort horse to carry them there. Witches, too, favour this form of transport at midnight.

There have thus been strong associations with horses through the ages. The name 'Jacobaea' is derived from St James, the patron saint of horses. Folk names for the plant include Jacoby, St James wort or James' weed. This could be because ragwort is usually in full flower on St James' day, 25th July.

Uses

Common ragwort is not recommended as an internal herbal medicine as the pyrrolizidine alkaloids are toxic to the liver. These active compounds are, however, still considered by some herbalists to be useful in poultices or as salves to reduce inflammation or bring boils to a head. Gerard, writing in the late 16th century, says: 'It is much commended, and not without cause, to helpe olde aches and paines in the armes, hips, and legs, boiled in hogs grease to the forme of an ointment.' Since such remedies applied to the skin could be absorbed into the system, I think I would rather not try them, even if I were able to find a tub of hog's grease in my local supermarket!

In the past, the plant has been used to produce dyes, in particular green and orange. Because the stems are very tough, rope has been made from them and even baskets. The Scots sometimes dried ragwort for thatching.

Wildlife

I prefer to give the beautiful cinnabar moth a chance. Unlike the local farmers, John was positively thrilled when two common ragwort plants appeared in our garden, one emerging from a crack next to the house and the other by our front path. We decided to save some seeds to sow on our meadow, hoping for some of these stunning caterpillars and moths next year. If ragwort is destroyed, then so too are these fascinating little creatures as they depend on this plant for nourishment. Their only other food source is groundsel which contains similar alkaloids.

This is not the only moth using ragwort as a food plant. More than thirty other species favour it, along with twenty species of fly, several beetles and various aphids and bugs. The nectar is known to be particularly sweet and rich, attracting a wide variety of pollinators. Among the moths, the tawny speckled pug is notable as it is common and widespread and may well visit your garden. Its red, brown and grey patterned wings extend to 23 mm/1 inch and it flies during the height of summer.

If you are fortunate, the pretty small copper butterfly may lay its eggs on your ragwort. These are greyish-white and are usually laid singly on the underside of the leaves. The male adults can be quite aggressive, seeing off any other insect competitors and then returning to their flower-head perches, once again on the look-out.

Selfheal (*Prunella vulgaris*)

Dead-nettle family (Lamiaceae). Perennial. Pollinated by insects. Propagated by stolon or seed. Medicinal.

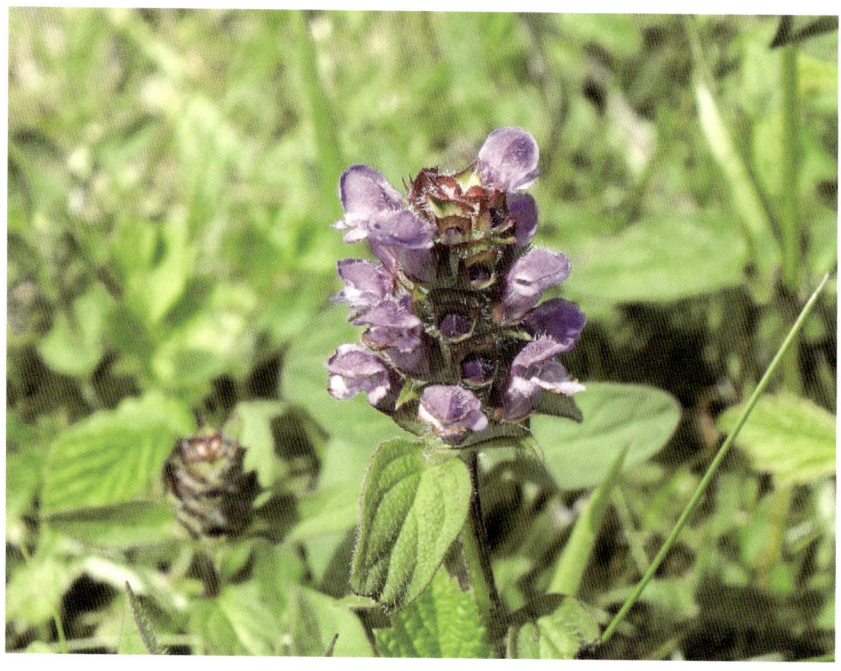

As the name suggests, selfheal is a beneficial medicinal herb. It will even tolerate a certain amount of mowing.

This sturdy plant lasts surprisingly well in grass, even when mown or grazed, its deep violet petals betraying its presence. Surrounding these are the bracts which are attractively copper tinged. It thrives in our damp meadow and even turns up in our lawn, its creeping habit seemingly resisting the mower. As a perennial, it roots itself from the stem, creating patches within the grass.

The flowers appear together in rings of six at the head of the plant, each with five petals. The bases of these are joined to make tubes. The upper two lobes form a 'hood', while the lowest is hook-like in profile. It is this which has earned the plant the popular names of 'hook-heal', 'sicklewort' or 'carpenter's herb'. When seen from the front it can give the impression of an open mouth, with the two small side petals suggesting swollen glands. According to the Doctrine of Signatures, the plant should therefore be suitable for the healing of throat problems, as well as for cuts and wounds. You will see that the leaves are occasionally somewhat toothed along the edge but are generally oval and pointed.

Folklore

Some people used to believe that selfheal was such a powerful herb that it must have been sent by God to cure every disease and banish the devil. During the witch hunt, women used to plant it in their gardens to keep away the inquisitors.

The Druids certainly had great faith in it and would carry out an elaborate ritual before drying the herb. When the dog star was rising and the moon was in a dark phase, they would go out to search for it. They would then cut the plants with a sickle and hold them up in their left hands while chanting an incantation.

Uses

In the case of selfheal, the healing qualities suggested by the Doctrine of Signatures turn out to be true! Modern research shows that selfheal has anti-viral properties by having the capacity to prevent viruses from replicating. It is known to be effective in the treatment of feverish colds and 'flu, sore throats, mouth ulcers and also herpes. Early herbalists had learned of its efficacy from experience. Culpeper recorded that the juice of selfheal 'when mixed with honey of roses, cleanses and heals all ulcers in the mouth and throat, and those also in the secret parts'.

Selfheal is also a natural antibiotic and has even been shown to be useful in the treatment of tuberculosis. Not only does it speed up the healing of cuts and wounds, it prevents them from turning septic.

Selfheal bath oil

A few drops of this oil in your bath will soothe and soften your skin.

Selfheal leaves and flowers

cold-pressed olive oil

few drops rose oil

Pick sufficient selfheal leaves and flowers to fill a sterilised glass jar. Chop up before placing in the jar, then pour the olive oil over to cover them and add the rose oil. Secure a piece of muslin on the top with a rubber band. ♦ Put the jar on a sunny window ledge and every so often stir gently, pressing down the leaves and flowers. Leave for up to 4 weeks until the colour of the plant material has been completely absorbed into the oil. ♦ Strain and bottle.

Selfheal lip balm

Not only excellent for easing the discomfort of dry lips, this salve will help to speed up the healing of cold sores. It can also be used for small wounds, burns and bites.

First make the infused oil as described above.

190 ml/1/3 pint infused selfheal oil

1 tbsp clear honey

1 tbsp grated beeswax

Put the oil in a pan and place on a low heat. Stir in the honey and beeswax until it melts. ♦ To test the consistency of the balm, spoon a couple of drops into cold water. If it forms into a ball, the salve will be thick, whereas if it spreads over the surface it will be thin. Add oil or beeswax accordingly. ♦ Pour into small, wide-mouthed sterilised jars and secure the lids. The balm should last up to a year.

Selfheal tisane

As a natural antioxidant and immune stimulant, this tea is a good choice for feverish colds and 'flu. It is also efficacious as a gargle. Chinese herbalists generally harvest the plant when it has finished flowering and is just becoming brown. The flowering tops can also be dried for later use.

2 flower heads selfheal, fresh or dried
275 ml/½ pint boiling water
1 tsp honey

Place the selfheal in a mug. Pour on the boiling water, stir in the honey and leave to stand for 10 minutes. Strain before use.

Wildlife

Selfheal is often recommended for wildflower meadows as it is very appealing to pollinators. A variety of insects will visit the flowers for nectar, including bumble bees and butterflies. In our garden the white butterflies, large white, small white and green-veined white, seem to be particularly drawn to them.

The larvae of various species of moth use selfheal as a food plant, consuming the seeds and flowers, one of which is the shaded pug. Although this pale grey, mottled moth flies from dusk onwards, it can easily be disturbed during daytime, so you may notice the adults during June or July. Among other insects the shiny, rather rounded leaf beetles can also be found feeding on selfheal.

Garden birds will of course take advantage of this feast of insects, especially during the breeding season when there are so many hungry mouths to feed. Later, tree sparrows can be seen pecking among the grass in search of the seeds.

Prickly Sowthistle (*Sonchus asper*)

Daisy family (Asteraceae). Annual. Pollinated by insects, especially hoverflies. Propagated by seed. Formerly medicinal. Edible.

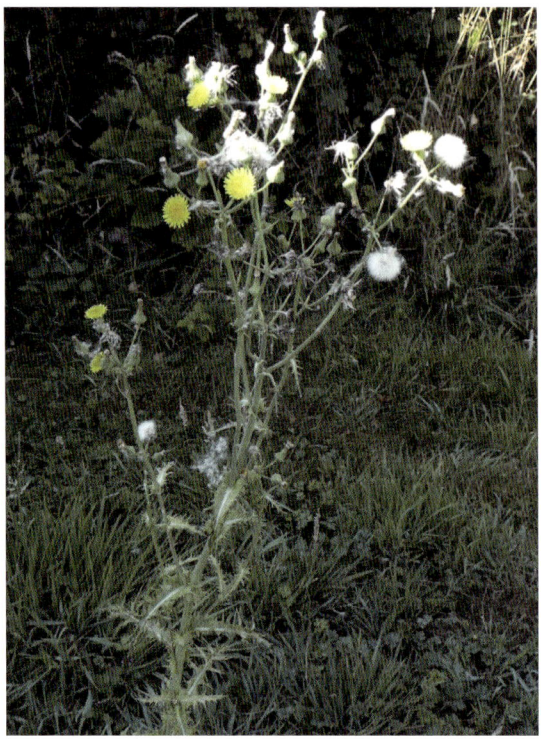

Prickly sowthistle has traditionally been used as a potherb. Pigs really do find this plant most appetising, despite its spiny leaves.

When a tall, somewhat prickly looking plant with pale yellow flowers established itself at the back of one of our borders, I was unsure of its identity. I therefore asked my neighbour, always brimming with information about anything local to East Anglia, what it could be. He scratched his head for a moment, looked far off across the field for inspiration, and then declared, ''T is 'n't aint!' Puzzled, I waited for an explanation, but he simply nodded and repeated the phrase. Then I cottoned on – he was telling me the popular name of the plant, meaning that it looks like a thistle but is not one.

The yellow heads of ray florets of the prickly sowthistle indicate that it is akin to the dandelion. After flowering has finished, the seeds float away on small hairy parachutes. If you do not want this 'weed' in your garden, be aware that after you have pulled it up and left it on the ground the plant will continue to mature and release seeds. A single plant can produce any number from 5,000 to 40,000! These are a gift for birds, however, which love them.

Folklore

One of sowthistle's most magical powers seems to have been to offer strength to those in need. For example, if a Welshman were in a hurry, he could place it under his hat and would then be able to run without tiring. Horses could likewise be assisted if several plants were tied to their tails before ploughing. An Anglo Saxon legend relates that hares can cure themselves from excessive heat by nibbling the herb.

Most astonishing, however, was the ability of sowthistles to reveal hidden treasure, or even to open locked doors. Such stories are to be found in particular in Italian folklore.

Uses

The stem is angled and will ooze a whitish, milk-like latex when cut. It is perhaps for this reason that herbalists used to recommend the plant for lactating women, suggesting that the flow of milk would thereby be increased. Culpeper thought that it had 'great medicinal virtues', that it was 'cooling and good against obstructions', with an effect that was 'mild and aperient'. Despite these apparent assets, it is not currently prescribed by herbalists. However, as the common name of sowthistle suggests, pigs do still benefit from eating the leaves and seem to relish them.

The whole plant is quite soft, including the prickles and the leaves, which spiral up the stem. These are in fact edible and make an interesting addition to a salad. The young ones taste the best. They can also be cooked like spinach.

Wildlife

It is worth considering that sowthistles attract hoverflies, predators of garden pests. At the same time aphids find the plant appealing. The presence of sowthistle may be helpful in luring them away from cherished garden flowers.

If you find moths fascinating, as I do, then leave a few sowthistles at the rear of borders which will offer nourishment to the larvae of several varieties. In particular those of the shark macro-moth depend almost exclusively on *Sonchus* for their food supply and the adults will often search in gardens as well as other open spaces for this plant. The moth is quite large and can spread its wings up to 52 mm/2 inches, flying in June to July. If at rest on stones it virtually disappears, being a stone-coloured grey-brown itself.

Several species of fly carry the name *sonchi*. For example, if you see purple swellings on sowthistle leaves they will contain the larvae of a gall midge named *Cystiphora sonchi*. Then there is a gall wasp called *Phanacis sonchi*. Its larvae live and feed in galls on the stem. There is no doubt that sowthistle has considerable wildlife value.

Spear Thistle (*Cirsium vulgare*)

Daisy family (Asteraceae). Biennial. Pollinated by bees and butterflies. Propagated by seed. Sharp spines.

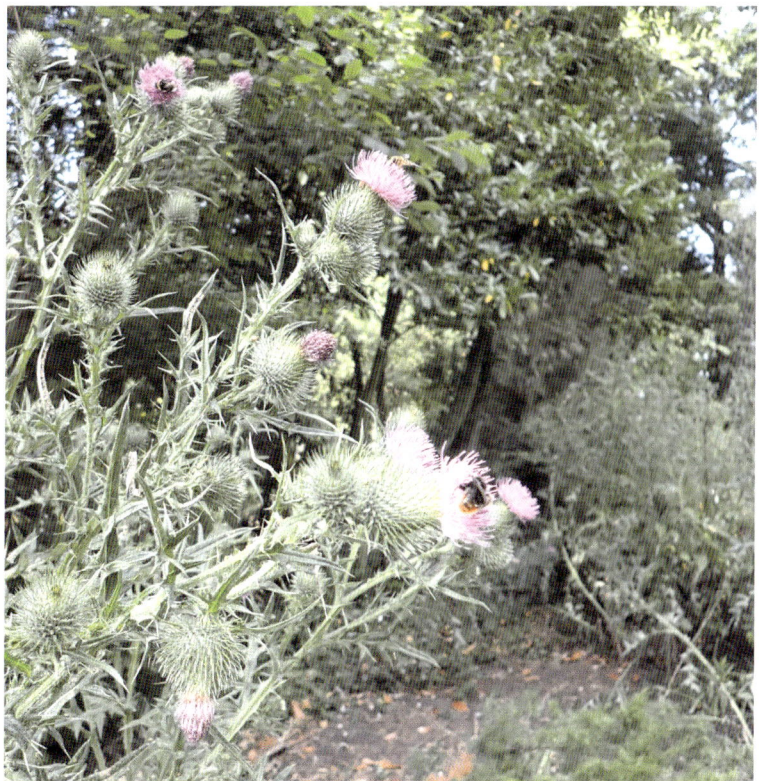

Farmers loathe spear thistle due to its amazing ability to survive all extermination attempts. However, in the right place in our garden this 'weed' can look truly majestic.

This imposing plant is regarded by farmers as a pernicious weed. As cattle wisely avoid its prickly leaves, it proliferates on grazed land. Despite rigorous use of herbicides, its ability to survive is astonishing, made possible by the fluffy down which carries the seeds a considerable distance. Birds too help with this distribution. Spear thistle certainly favours our flower beds and

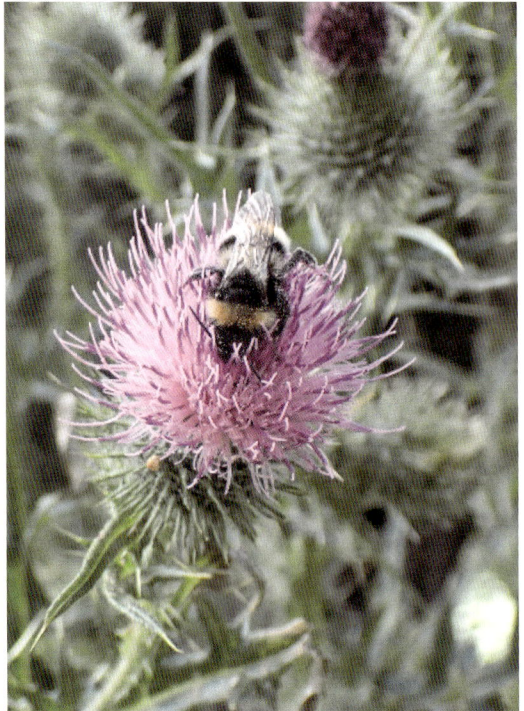

Many insects benefit from the rich nectar.

the wilder corners of our garden, but we find it essential to decide which plant to keep and which to cut so as not to be overrun by it. Since it grows on average to 1.5 m/5 ft, often more, it looks splendid towards the back of a border where its spiky leaves provide an architectural statement.

An ancient rhyme gives advice on how to control thistles:

> Cut thistles in May, they'll grow again one day,
> Cut thistles in June, that will be too soon.
> Cut thistles in July, they'll lay down and die.

Anonymous

Last year we were too busy to keep on top of our large garden and a considerable number of thistles escaped the loppers until the seeds had set.

This meant laboriously gathering the downy fluff before the wind had wafted it in every direction. Now that it is July it would make good sense to do some thinning as the rhyme suggests. Very strong, thick gloves are necessary as the pointed 'spears' on the end of the leaves can easily draw blood.

Indeed, the plant is prickly throughout, with pointed leaf lobes and barbs along the winged stem. Even the bracts are bristly. Once established, it is not easy to dig out as it has a deep taproot. It strikes me as astonishing that such a majestic plant should grow from such a minute seed. However, being a biennial, it does take two years.

Folklore

The purple flower heads, composed of a compact cluster of tiny, tubular florets, each positioned at the end of side stems, are very familiar to us as the emblem of Scotland. Legend tells us that, during the 13th century, an attack by Norsemen on the west coast of Scotland was averted one night when a barefoot invader accidentally trod on a prickly thistle and yelled out in pain, thus warning the encamped Scots of their approach. Whether or not this is true, the spear thistle, with its dignified bearing, fierce resilience and astonishing ability to survive, seems to be a thoroughly appropriate symbol for the Scottish people. Some individuals declare that it is not the spear thistle but the silvery 'Scotch' or cotton thistle which is the emblem. However, this is unlikely as *Onopordium acanthium* is not a native of Scotland.

Another interesting story, probably apocryphal, tells us how the spear thistle found its way to America. As the fluffy down is so soft, it used to be gathered to stuff pillows, cushions and mattresses instead of the more expensive feathers. A certain emigrant Scottish minister took with him his down-filled bed only to discover that in America there was no shortage of feathers. So it was the seeds from his abandoned mattress that established the plant on the other side of the Atlantic!

Uses

No doubt the prickly aspect of spear thistle discouraged any therapeutic use. Gerard, however, asserts that if the roots are boiled in wine and then either consumed or made into a poultice, they 'take away the ranke smell of the body and arme-hole'. Before the days of mass-produced deodorants, digging up the long root while at the same time avoiding the 'spears' was perhaps worth the effort, but needless to say this is not prescribed by present-day herbalists!

Wildlife

If you love to see both birds and butterflies in your garden, then allow one or two spear thistles to grow. Finches adore the seeds and you may be lucky enough to attract colourful goldfinches. Blue tits also favour them. Many butterflies feed on the flowers, including skippers and fritillaries, also the ringlet and more common meadow brown. The nectar is a rich adult food source.

Caper Spurge (*Euphorbia lathyrus*)

Spurge family (Euphorbiaceae). Biennial. Pollinated by insects. Propagated by seed. Irritant. Poisonous.

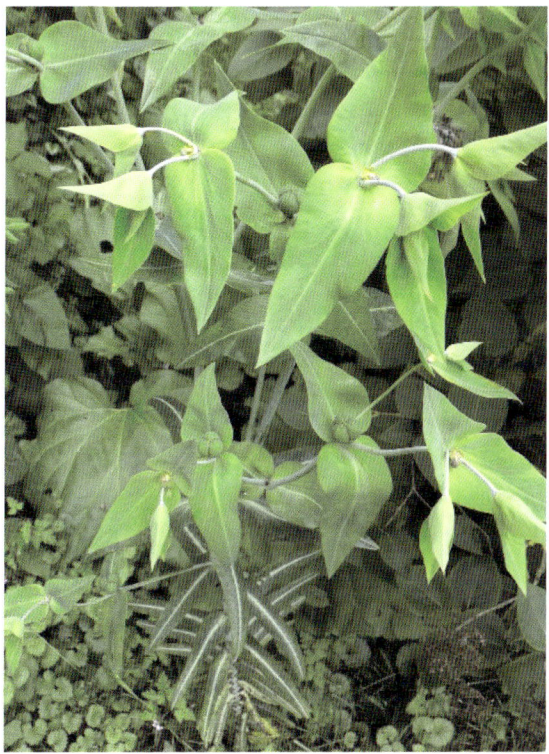

One of the most imposing of 'weeds', caper spurge is appreciated by gardeners with a mole problem as it is reputed to deter these animals.

It is always especially thrilling when a plant I have never seen before suddenly appears in our garden, most particularly one as strikingly unusual as caper spurge. A statuesque 120 cm/4 ft tall, its stout stem is generally beige coloured with dark blue-green, pointed leaves either side, each with a pale green stripe down the centre. They give a spiky appearance. The upper leaves are ovate and lighter in colour, while the flower heads are a greenish-yellow. These are extraordinary, having neither petals nor sepals; rather each flower is either male or female resulting in an extremely economical method of reproduction, the male having just the stamen and the female the pistil.

The seeds are encased in prominent globular capsules of three divided sections, each delineated by a brown band. It lies to one side, opposite clusters of pollen-coated anthers and three styles emerge from the top. These pods are similar in appearance to capers – hence the name – but beware! These are extremely poisonous, as indeed are all parts of this plant, including the milky latex in the stem. Always wear gloves when handling it and never let it anywhere near your eyes as it has been known, in extreme cases, to cause blindness.

It was clear from the wild spurges contentedly making their homes in our garden that this was a family of plants that would do very well here. So I decided to try out a garden variety in our one and only dry, rather stony border where little else seemed to thrive. I chose *Euphorbia cyparissias* which produces a mass of lime-green flowers in the early summer. What a show! If you are feeling more adventurous you might try 'Fireglow' (*Euphorbia griffithii*), with its dramatic orange-red flower clusters and reddish stripe down the middle of each leaf. Both are hardy.

Despite the handsome appearance of *Euphorbia*, you may decide not to have it in the garden if there are children or pets nearby.

Folklore

A long-standing common name for caper spurge is 'mole plant', having the reputation, like petty spurge, of being anathema to these little animals, especially if the seeds are put down their holes. It is also thought that moles may be deterred by the toxic chemicals in the roots of the plant. However, this certainly fails to work in our garden as moles happily continue to dig their runs, leaving their heaps on our lawn, much to my husband's annoyance.

Less usually, the plant has been referred to as 'petroleum plant', due to the high levels of hydrocarbons it contains. Perhaps in the future it may be grown as a biofuel.

Uses

Like all spurges, it is a purgative, this one being particularly vehement, no doubt the result of the body's urgent need to rid itself of such a vicious poison. Gerard warns against it: 'these herbes by mine advise would not be received into the body'. Beggars, rather pathetically, used to employ its irritant action to create sores in their skin in the hope of eliciting extra sympathy from passers-by. The main folk remedy was to use the milky latex to burn off warts, but on no account should this be attempted.

Wildlife

There is something rather curious about the seeds of this plant. Each has a small fleshy outgrowth that appears to be attractive to ants. It seems that these insects will take the seeds away, thus increasing their chances of successful germination elsewhere. Although the pods open explosively, this sends their contents only a few metres distance. The ants significantly increase their range of dispersal.

Great Willowherb (*Epilobium hirsutum*)

Rosebay Willowherb (*Chamaenerion angustifolium*)

Willowherb family (Onagraceae). Perennials. Pollinated by insects, especially bees. Propagated by seed. Medicinal.

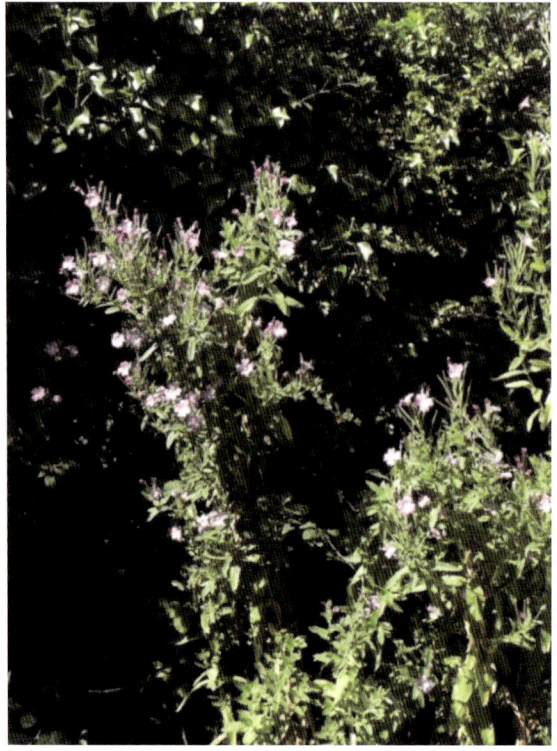

Here great willowherb grows in a characteristic clump. Willowherb nectar is a nutritious food source for bees.

Close inspection of the four notched petals reveal that the two upper ones are slightly larger than the lower two. The shallow roots of willowherb spread sideways under the soil, putting up new stems here and there, forming the characteristic clumps. The slender, spear-shaped leaves, green

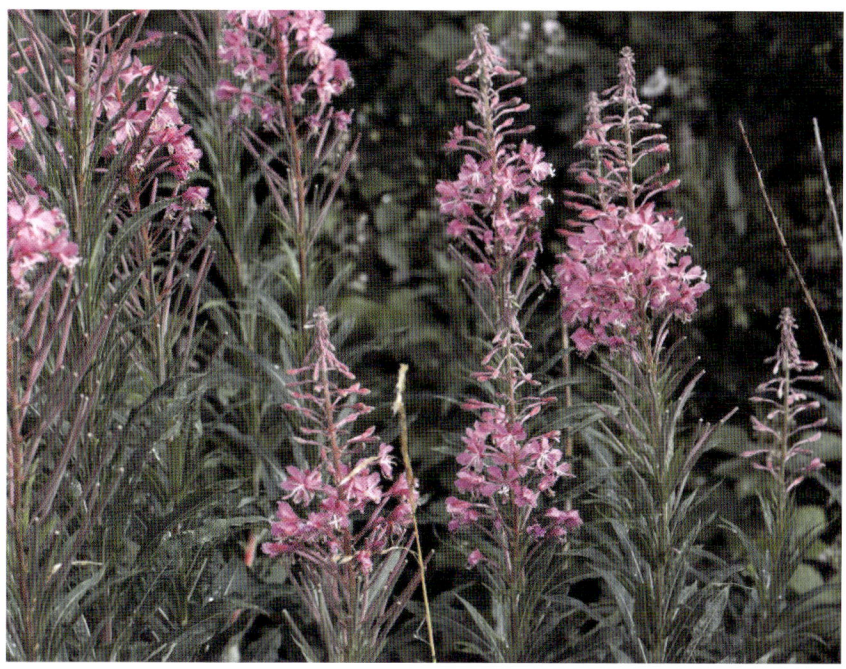

The tall flower spikes are a characteristic feature of rosebay willowherb. *Photo © NatureSpot / David Nicholls*

on the upper side and slightly silvery beneath, grow alternately up the straight, hairy stem, which can be as much as 2 m /6½ ft tall.

The seeds are astonishingly prolific, with up to 100,000 per plant. You will notice the fluffy down in the autumn that will carry the seeds a considerable distance, wafted along by the breeze. Once on the ground, they will survive for a great many years, lying dormant in the soil, ready to sprout up when the conditions are right.

Folklore

Once a scarce woodland plant, two recent nicknames reveal the secret of the current successful spread of rosebay willowherb: 'bombweed' and 'fireweed'. After the fires and bombs of two World Wars, this plant established itself in the cleared sites, having no competition from other plants and evidently favouring the ash as a growing medium. With a tendency to group together, the tall magenta flower spikes might also have provided a visual reminder of the flames. It is not surprising that London adopted it as its county flower.

Uses

Research in 2016 at Montana State University concluded that the therapeutic potential of extracts of willowherb was remarkable. This is due to the presence of compounds known as polyphenols, which are very beneficial to human health. Not only are these anti-inflammatory, anti-allergic, anti-microbial and anti-viral, they also act to moderate certain immune responses making them more effective in combating disease.

The most potent constituent of the polyphenols capable of doing this is oenothein B. It activates the lymphocytes, those white immune cells that patrol the lymph system, including the natural killer (NK) cells which attack 'foreign' invaders and unwanted cancer cells. Supplements containing oenothein B have been shown to be helpful in treating prostate disorders. That said, due to the complex effects that oenothein B has on immunity, further research is needed to understand fully how this works precisely.

Exciting too are studies that indicate that polyphenols have an anti-aging effect and are helpful in preventing the cognitive deterioration associated with Alzheimer's disease and dementia. Bearing in mind that many of us are living longer, a supplement that promotes mental health in old age would be truly wonderful.

The astringent and tonic actions of willowherb are well recognised. If patted on to the skin, it can relieve irritations and help to cure acne. So far, all the indications are that willowherb extracts are quite safe to take.

Fireweed tea

Current herbal medicine suggests that this tea, made from the dried leaves, is a suitable remedy for urinary problems, diarrhoea and heavy periods. When used as a mouthwash or gargle it soothes ulcers or sore throats. One folk tradition assures us that it can cure hiccoughs, but I have not tried it!

1. **Drying the leaves**

Pick the leaves before flowering on a warm morning after any dew has evaporated. Simply spread them out on paper and leave in an airy, shady place. Turn them over from time to time until they are crisp. Store in an airtight glass jar.

2. **Preparing the tea**

Dried leaves of rosebay willowherb
boiling water

Put 4 or 5 leaves into a mug, pour on the boiling water and allow to stand for 5 minutes. Strain before drinking if you prefer. ♦ Use as a mouthwash or gargle until the condition improves. Drink up to 3 mugs per day for internal complaints.

Willowherb syrup

The syrup is excellent for sore throats.
15 rosebay willowherb flower spikes
425 ml/¾ pint water
3 tbsp honey (naturally anti-bacterial)
juice ½ large lemon

Remove any insects and pick the flowers off the spikes. Put in a pan and add the water. Boil up, then reduce the heat, cover and simmer gently for about 10 minutes. Take out the flowers and add the honey and lemon juice. The colour should be pink. Boil up again and simmer for 5 minutes. Turn off the heat and allow to cool. ♦ Pour into a sterilised bottle and seal, preferably with a cork. Store in the fridge. It should last some months. Discard if it ferments. ♦ Take 1 tbsp 3 or 4 times a day (less for children).

Wildlife

Rosebay willowherb supplies rich nectar for honey production. So, do allow a few to grow in your garden as they will attract bees and other insects, which in turn pollinate our crops. Great willowherb, although less showy, is equally beneficial. The plants are easy to pull up if you find that you have too many.

Hedge Woundwort (*Stachys sylvatica*)

Dead-nettle family (Lamiaceae). Perennial. Pollinated by bees and flies. Propagated by seed and rhizome. Medicinal.

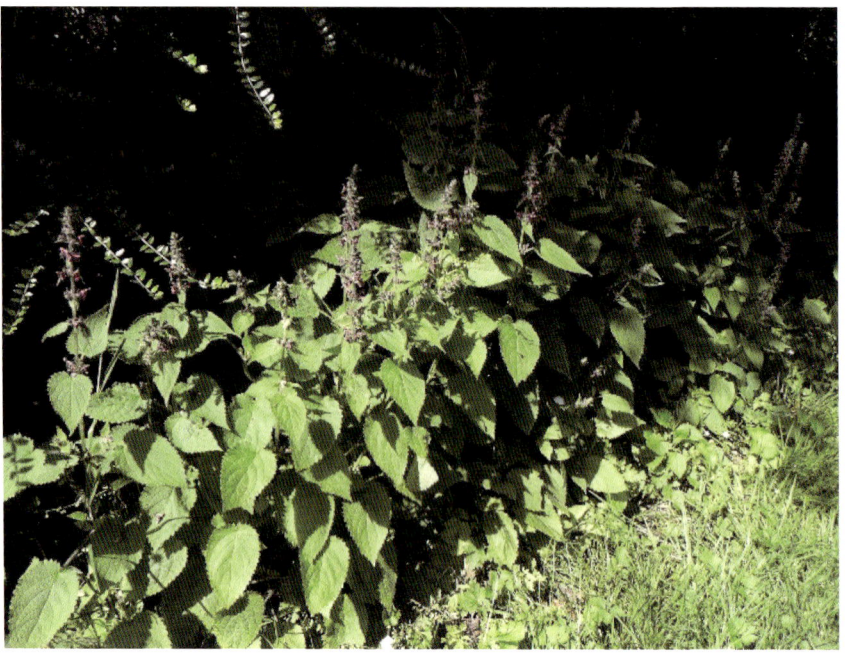

The acrid smell of woundwort belies its value as a precious medicinal herb.

Most herbals when describing woundwort emphasise its abominable smell as being 'strong and astringent', 'bitter and disagreeable' or even 'pungent and foetid'. Personally, I certainly find it distinctive, although not so very unpleasant as I can detect tangy, lemony hints. At any rate, it is a flourishing 'weed' in our garden and very happy in moist, shady places. Not only do the seeds pop out very effectively when each calyx tube dries and contracts but the plant also sends out rhizomes under the soil to produce offspring.

The purple flowers, in whorls around the stem, are in fact very pretty with hooded upper petal and attractive white markings on the lower lip.

The hairy, serrated leaves, however, although an elongated heart-shape, are less likeable and predominate visually. For this reason, I tend to restrict hedge woundwort to the more out-of-the-way corners of our garden. It is important to allow it some space though, not only for its considerable medicinal value but also because bees and long-tongued flies are very attracted to it.

Folklore

Because woundwort is such a powerful healer, most folklore connected to the plant consists of traditional remedies, some of which are described here. However, according to Thomas Green, author of *The Universal Herbal of 1820*, toads are reputed to be charmed by the plant and can be found sitting under it. There could be some truth in this, as woundwort has a liking for damp, shady places, as do toads.

Uses

Hedge woundwort, true to its name, has been valued for centuries as a wound healer. John Gerard, the Elizabethan herbalist, describes how he cured a shoe-maker's servant who had attempted suicide:

> First, he gave himselfe a most mortall wound in the throat, in such sort, that when I gave him drinke it came forth at the wound, which likewise did blow out the candle: another deepe and grievous wound in the brest with the said dagger, and also two others in Abdomine.

It is most surprising that this poor man survived long enough to present himself to the herbalist! The remedy was comprised of four handfuls of woundwort boiled up with hog's grease and olive oil from which 'plaisters' were made and applied to the injuries:

> The which mortall wounds, by God's permission, and the vertues of this herbe, I perfectly cured within twenty daies.

Scientific analysis has shown that woundwort contains the compound betonicine, which is a haemostatic, in other words stops the flow of blood. The plant is also a styptic, a property which assists with the binding of body tissues. In addition, it is naturally antiseptic and anti-bacterial.

Woundwort ointment

For any deep wounds you must of course seek medical advice, but for minor cuts and abrasions this ointment can help to speed up healing. To ease aches and pains, you can make a plaister from it by first melting the ointment in a bain-marie, then spreading it thickly on to a bandage. This is then wrapped around the hurting limb and left for up to two days to allow the herb to penetrate.

150 ml/¼ pint almond or walnut oil

15 g/½ oz grated beeswax

75 g/3 oz woundwort leaves, minced

small, sterilised jars

The woundwort leaves are best picked when tender, just before flowering. Have a couple of small, sterilised jars ready. ♦ Using a bain-marie, put the ingredients into the inner pan and cover with a lid. Fill the outer pan with water up to the level of the oil and bring to the boil. Reduce heat and allow to simmer for one hour. Top up as necessary. Take off the heat, remove the lid and stir from time to time while the mixture cools. ♦ Before it sets, spoon the ointment into the jars, cover with lids, then label with description and date. It should keep in a cool place for up to three months.

Woundwort eyewash

Because of its naturally antiseptic and healing qualities, this infusion is recommended by herbalists for conjunctivitis and sties. You will need an eye bath.

1 rounded tsp fresh woundwort leaves and flowers, crushed (or 1 level tsp dried)

275 ml/½ pint boiling water

Pour the water over the herb and allow to infuse for 10 minutes. Strain very carefully through muslin. ♦ Use as an eye wash when just tepid.

Woundwort is also antispasmodic, so if drunk as a tea, it will help to ease stomach cramps. The plant is not toxic.

Wildlife

Bees in search of nectar alight on the lower lip, then crawl up the petal tube, becoming dusted with pollen as they pass the stamens that lie in the hooded upper lip. A few plants had sprung up right next to our lavender bush, so I was intrigued to observe that the bees favoured the woundwort at least as much as the lavender, if not more so.

It is one of the host plants for caterpillars of the Adonis blue butterfly and various moth species, including speckled yellow moth, small rivulet and beautiful golden Y. However, you may spot the predatory bronze shield bug making a meal of the caterpillars. This gleaming insect is often found on woundwort.

Yarrow (*Achillea millefolium*)

Daisy family (Asteraceae). Perennial. Pollinated by insects, including hoverflies, wasps and butterflies. Propagated by seed and rhizome. Medicinal.

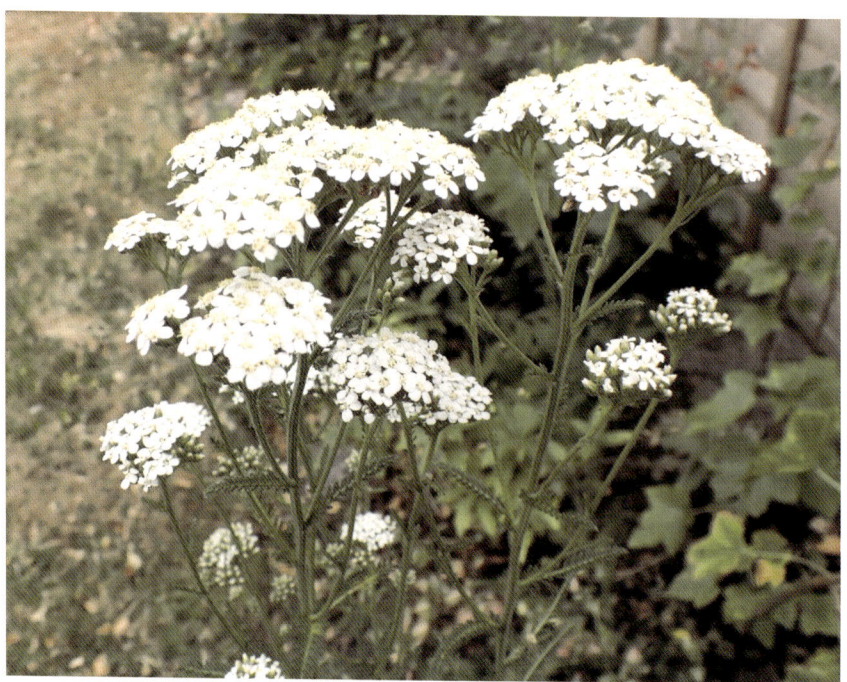

This beneficial medicinal herb is also reputed to have protective powers.

Yarrow has always been warmly welcomed into my borders as this 'weed' seems to be a fine companion plant. As long as I have prevented it from taking over, it appears to enliven sickly neighbours. This, apparently, is due to secretions from its creeping rhizomes. After the flowers have finished, it is a beneficial addition to the compost heap as it is rich in nitrates, phosphates, chlorides of potash and lime and also copper.

Personally, I find the plant most attractive. Yarrow is immediately identifiable by its ferny leaves that spiral around the sturdy and downy, furrowed stem. The many small flowers cluster together densely to form flattish heads. In the centre of each flower are white, disc-shaped florets. These are surrounded by several outer petals, generally five, which sometimes have a pinkish hue. Pinching the leaves or flowers produces a distinctive aroma with a hint of sweetness that is also a little sharp. Depending on the situation, the plant can grow as tall as 100 cm/40 inches, but it can also survive a certain amount of cutting and can make a short feathery sward. Those in our garden tend to reach around 65 cm/25 inches.

If yarrow is obviously happy in your garden, this is an indication that the many showy cultivars will do very well, though they will generally prefer a sunny, well-drained position. *Achillea* 'coronation gold' has striking yellow flower heads that retain their colour when dried, making a cheerful winter decoration.

Folklore

The modern name seems to derive from the Anglo Saxon for the plant, *gearwe*. As for the scientific name of *Achillea*, this refers to the Greek hero of Homer's Iliad, Achilles. According to legend, he used yarrow to heal his soldiers' wounds during the Trojan War. Hence the common names of 'soldier's woundwort', 'knight's milfoil' or *herba militaris*.

The plant was always believed to be strongly protective. It would be hung in a tool shed, perhaps in a superstitious attempt to avert accidents or to heal any cuts should they occur. At the same time, it was thought to deter thieves, which seems somewhat unlikely! Nevertheless, it earned another popular name – 'carpenter's grass'.

A bunch of the flowers would be tied to a baby's cradle, meaning that the child would grow up to have an even temperament. This idea of docility perhaps comes from the observation that cattle become more amenable if yarrow is planted in their meadow grass. Indeed, there is evidence that the herb is particularly good for them, being rich in minerals. The following incantation, translated from the Gaelic, also promotes the idea that even just picking the plant will have a beneficial, calming effect:

> I will pluck the yarrow fair
> That more benign will be my face,

> That more warm shall be my lips,
> That more chaste shall be my speech …

Yarrow was also associated with love and romance. The flowers would be put into a bride's posy, which was thought to bring seven years of blissful happiness. Thus, in the West Country it achieved yet another name – 'seven years' love'. For a vision or dream of one's future spouse, an ounce of yarrow should be sewn in a flannel and placed under the pillow. At the same time, the following verse should be spoken:

> Thou pretty herb of Venus' tree,
> Thy true name it is Yaroow;
> Now who my bosom friend be,
> Pray tell thou me to-morrow.

From Halliwell's Popular Rhymes

Uses

Yarrow has been regarded as an outstanding medical herb since time immemorial. Moreover, modern herbalists still list it amongst the most useful, especially as a wound healer and for female problems. If you have the space near the house, it is well worth transplanting some of these 'weeds' here, having them to hand for instant first aid. Pharmacological studies have shown the plant to have many other properties, being anti-inflammatory, anti-spasmodic and sedative.

Its ability to stem the bleeding from cuts as well as to thin out clots appears to be contradictory, yet this dual capacity has been very well authenticated over the years. In effect it can regulate the blood flow. Its ancient name of 'nosebleed' testifies to its ability to stop this annoying problem, while claims were made that it could also do the opposite. Here in East Anglia a girl concerned about her boyfriend's fidelity would tickle the inside of her nose with a leaf and say:

> Yarroway, yarroway, bear a white blow;

If my love love me, my nose will bleed now.

There is, of course, the possibility that East Anglian young men were not often faithful! However, the leaves bruised, then rolled up into a ball and stuffed up a nostril are most effective in curing a nosebleed. My husband suffers from these from time to time, especially if stressed, and we have discovered this to be a quick and easy remedy. Equally, applying the leaves can speed up the healing of wounds by curtailing the blood flow. It is perfectly safe to crush the leaves and place in or on a cut as they are naturally antiseptic.

Yarrow is certainly one of the best herbs for female problems. As an anti-spasmodic, it helps to ease menstrual cramps and thereby reduce heavy flow. At the same time the salicylic acid (constituent of aspirin) contained in the plant will relieve the pain. By simply chewing one of the ferny leaves, quick relief can be achieved. Sipping a tisane made from the aerial parts is also helpful. I wish I had known about this easy remedy as a young woman, having suffered the agonies of dysmenorrhea. If taken really hot, yarrow tea can also induce perspiration and thereby help to lower the fever of 'fluey colds.

Toothache can be mollified by biting on a bunch of the leaves. As long ago as Elizabethan times, the physician John Gerard had noted its efficacy: 'Most men say that the leaves, chewed, and especially greene, are a remedy for the Tooth-ache'.

Milfoil tea

This has several benefits. Not only does it help to relieve feverish colds and alleviate menstrual problems, but it can also act as a digestive aid and be used to clean wounds. Ideally, pick the aerial parts when the flowering tops are just coming into bud. These can be used fresh or hung in an airy place and dried for making the tea during the winter months.

3 tsp dried yarrow
275 ml/½ pint boiling water
½ tsp honey

Pour the water over the herb and leave to infuse for at least 10 minutes. Sweeten with the honey. Strain and sip in small amounts three or four times a day. **Warning: Do not use if pregnant or breast feeding. In rare cases an allergic reaction can occur in very sensitive individuals.**

Staunchweed ointment

This is an old East Anglian remedy, reputed to be excellent for the rapid healing of cuts and grazes and also of any bleeding beneath the skin as in bruises or piles. Dig up the yarrow plant and use very fresh.

1 whole yarrow plant
a little water
purified lard

Wash the roots very well then chop every part of the yarrow into fine pieces. Put into the water and boil up until it becomes a pulp. When cool, push this through a sieve or refine in a blender, then mix into the lard at a ratio of about 2:3 to form a smooth ointment. ♦ Keep in the fridge. Apply and cover with a bandage as necessary.

Wildlife

I have often observed how attractive yarrow flower heads are to insects. All sorts of beetles will alight there, as will hoverflies, ladybirds and various butterflies. The plant is therefore a real asset to any wildflower garden. It is interesting that, as a companion plant, it does attract beneficial insects, such as predatory wasps that prey on insect pests, using them as food for their larvae.

It has been noted that several species of bird, such as the starling, will pick yarrow with their beaks and carry it to their nests as a soft lining. It has been discovered that this discourages the growth of parasites. How ever did the birds find this out? Laboratory tests have shown that the oil from the plant will kill the larvae of mosquitoes.

AUGUST

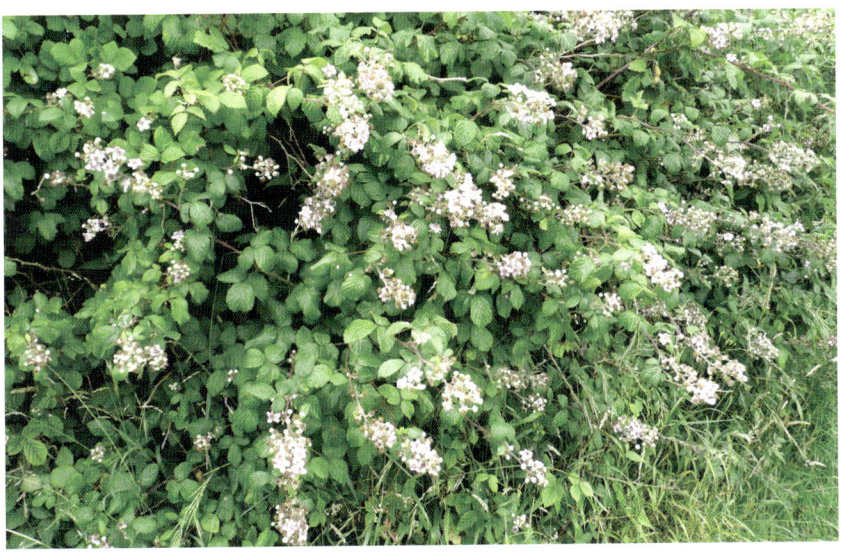

Brambles are now fully in flower and alive with buzzing bees and other insects making the most of the nectar.

When we first moved into our house we were deeply involved in updating the interior and the garden was left to grow as it pleased. Marking our western boundary, there was a hedge which had been neatly trimmed. At the time we took little notice of it. Since all of our energies were subsumed by DIY activities, we were scarcely aware of the hedge putting up healthy new shoots until one spring it produced an impressive display of white flowers. These were such a joy that we decided to leave the stems long with just an occasional trim. Moreover, this high hedge not only provided extra privacy, it now gave us good protection from prevailing south-westerly winds.

That August I happened to be walking along the path on the far side of the hedge about to visit my neighbour, when I noticed something shiny and red dangling among the profusion of green leaves. Lifting up some of the lower branches, I was amazed to see a great many more hanging in clusters. They were wild cherry plums! Choosing a really ripe one, I took a bite and my mouth was filled with the most intense and truly delicious plum flavour. Avoiding the wasps, which were already taking a considerable interest in these tempting fruits, my neighbour and I had soon filled two large bowls. Over the next couple of weeks, we had made scrumptious crumbles and pies and put the leftovers in the freezer. Despite our harvesting, there were still a great many plums left for the wildlife, especially those that we were unable to reach.

Since then, I have taken a great interest in hedges and became involved in a hedgerow survey for our county, identifying and recording the various species. In this area of intensive farming, the hedges provide vital food stores and nesting places for birds and small mammals. They also act as safe 'corridors' along which such creatures can scamper, joining up different habitats. I learned that the flowers and fruit of our native species will only form on second- or third-year growth. Therefore, if new twigs are persistently cut back, the hedge will be unproductive. It was pure chance that we had allowed our plum hedge to grow. How delighted we were with the outcome! Every few years we give it a careful prune to keep the growth vigorous. We much enjoy sharing its rich crop with the birds and insects.

As for the other unbidden arrivals, buddleja is by far the most spectacular, now fully in flower. On one sunny afternoon I counted seven small tortoiseshell butterflies relishing its sweet nectar. This lifted my spirits hugely as this butterfly has suffered marked declines recently.

Red Bartsia (*Odontites vernus*)

Broomrape family (Orobanchaceae). Annual. Pollinated by insects, especially bees. Propagated by seed. Formerly medicinal.

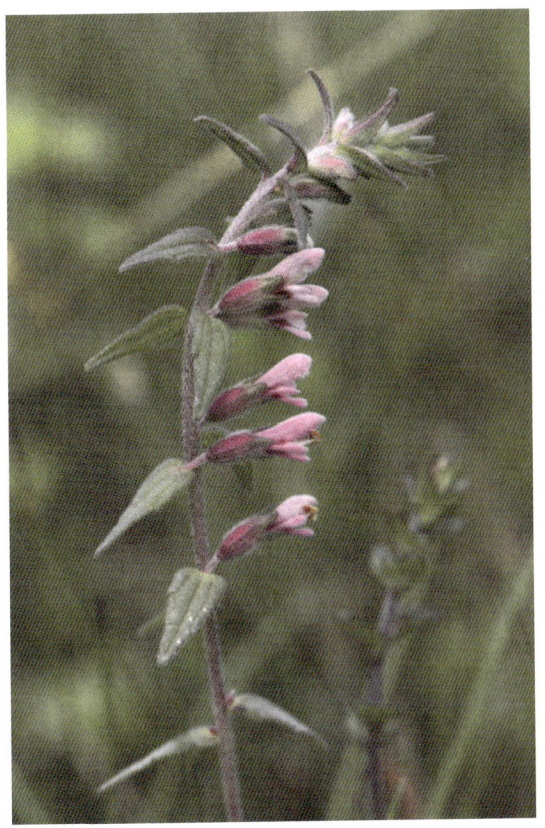

You are unlikely to see red bartsia in your garden unless you have a rather dry stony or waste patch. *Photo © NatureSpot / David Nicholls*

One day, I almost thought we had acquired some heather on the overgrown end of our gravelly drive. How could that be? Our garden is hardly a moorland habitat. It was only after checking in my wildflower book that I recognised it as bartsia, which has deep red, two-lipped flowers in leafy, one-sided spikes, the lower lip having three lobes. The leaf-like bracts are purple tinged, as are the stalks. In the south of Britain, these tend to bend over a little to form an arch, while the northern variety has more upright stems. The whole plant is no more than 30 cm/12 inches high. Being semi-parasitic, this plant can grow on waste ground with low fertility, feeding off the nearby roots of host grasses for extra nutrients. No wonder that it had been attracted to that stony site in our garden.

Folklore

In ancient times it was once used as a cure for toothache, apparent from the scientific name of *Odontites, odons* being Greek for tooth.

Uses

It is nowhere to be found in recent herbals.

Wildlife

This plant is crucially important for the survival of the macro-moth barred rivulet (*Perizoma bifaciata*) as its larvae feed on red bartsia seeds. You may see the adult flying near a lighted window in July or August. Its wing span is 26 mm/1 inch, featuring dark grey and white horizontal wavy markings with some brown colouring towards the head. The larvae are pale beige with grey stripes along the back and black spots each side. Barred rivulet will spend at least one winter as a pupa before emerging.

Besides some carder bees and wasps, the solitary bee *Melitta tricincta* feeds on nectar and collects pollen exclusively from red bartsia. It occurs generally in southern England.

Butterfly-bush (*Buddleja davidii*)

Figwort family (Scrophulariaceae). Deciduous shrub. Pollinated by butterflies. Propagated by seed. Potentially medicinal.

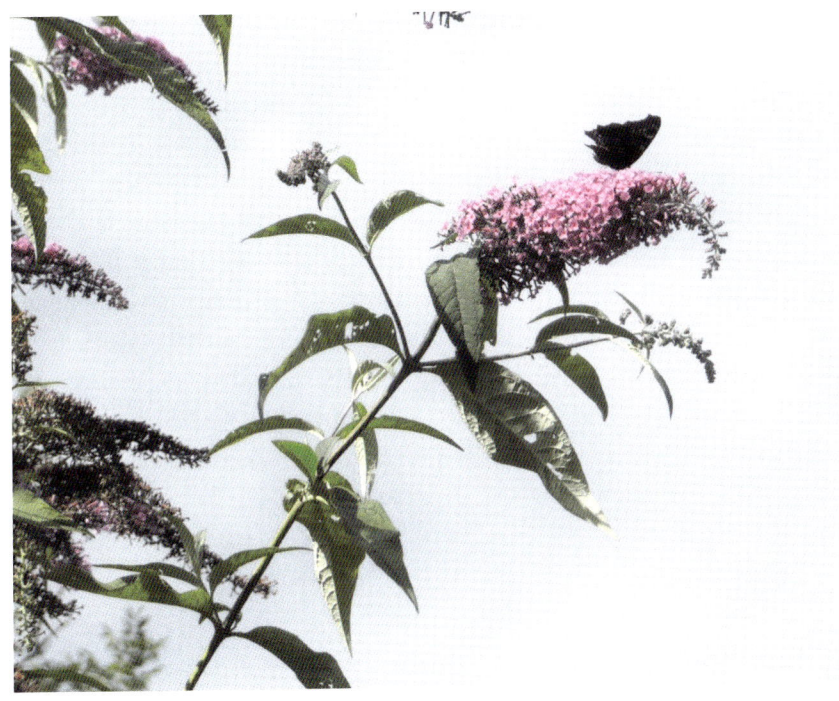

Many small mauve or lilac flowers form the sweet-smelling inflorescences of buddleja, which are so attractive to butterflies.

As most gardeners know, this shrub is famous for the way in which the beautiful fragrant spikes of lilac flowers attract butterflies, thereby earning it the name of 'butterfly-bush'. However, it might just as well be called 'railway bush' due to its success in colonising the railway network! I have often been astonished at how it manages to cling on to the dry shingle and old walls and masonry along the tracks, wondering how the roots obtain sufficient water to survive. In fact, it is very good at conserving moisture due to the downy hairs covering the long, lance-shaped, grey-green leaves. These protect the stomata, or pores, thus reducing evaporation.

None of the many species of buddleja is native to Europe, rather they are endemic to Asia, Africa and the Americas, favouring the stony, open ground of mountain tops. The weed *B. davidii* is in fact a garden escapee that was introduced to Britain from central China in the late 19th century. It is named after a French missionary and botanist Père Armand David, who first came across it when visiting Hubei province in 1887. He saw its potential as a garden plant.

The shrub is now listed as 'invasive', but I have to say that I was happy indeed when one sprang up spontaneously in a sunny position next to our pond, anticipating the many butterflies that would be attracted by its honey-scented perfume. This is hardly a dry situation, but it flourishes nevertheless and benefits from substantial annual pruning in winter. I am so captivated by this beautiful shrub that I am planning on having an avenue of butterfly bushes, so I will be taking cuttings in September. Indeed, this may not be necessary as the thousands of seeds are very easily dispersed by wind due to their winged shape, so it is likely that baby buddlejas will soon be appearing spontaneously.

Folklore

Because butterfly bush was introduced to Europe at such a late date, there are no long-standing traditions associated with it. However, it is interesting that buddleja is one of the few plants that can tolerate the calcium in mortar. After World War II it helped to brighten the rubble of devastated buildings and so also became known as the 'bombsite bush'. Another nickname is 'summer lilac', due to the similarity of the flower spikes.

Uses

Although now well naturalised to Europe, the species has been here too short a time for any medicinal tradition to have developed. In its indigenous settings, the leaves have been made into poultices and applied to wounds to assist with healing.

More recently, research at King's College, London, has shown that the roots, which have a peppery smell, in fact possess anti-fungal properties. It is thought that these act to protect the plant. It may be that they can be extracted and used in human medicine.

Wildlife

The inflorescences, which grace the ends of the long, arching branches, are formed from a great many tiny mauve to lilac flowers, each tubular with an orange centre. The sweet perfume attracts the most spectacular butterflies onto our buddleja, including red admirals, peacocks, painted ladies, small tortoiseshells and commas. It is such a pleasure to observe these colourful fragile creatures. Bees and moths also delight in feeding on the nectar.

Cherry Plum (*Prunus cerasifera*)

Rose family (Rosaceae). Deciduous tree. Self-fertile; also pollinated by insects. Propagated by seed or suckering. Edible fruit.

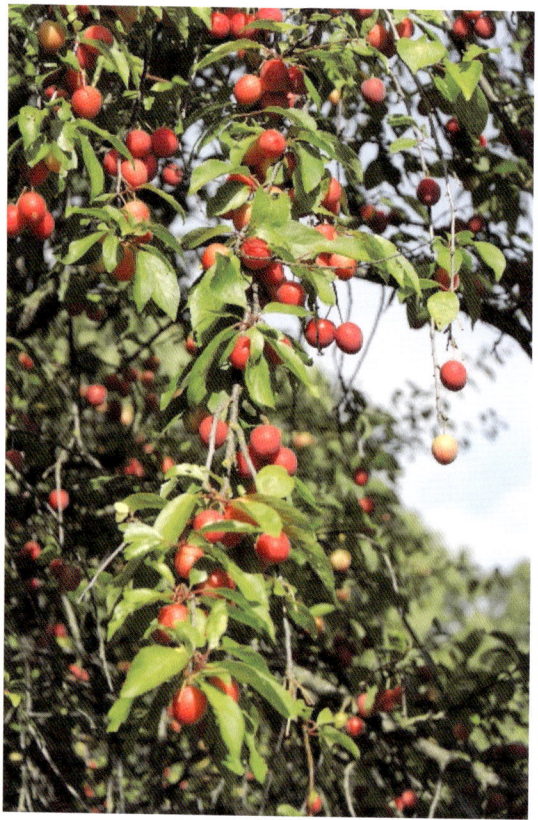

The round fruit of cherry plum, a deep red when ripe, have an intensely delicious flavour. *Photo © An-d, CC BY-SA 3.0, Wikimedia Commons*

THE FRUIT

The botanical name *cerasifera* means 'bearing cherry-like fruits', but in fact the plums are a little larger than a cherry and, when ripe, deep purple in colour. They are described as a drupe, having a single seed or stone.

Folklore

It is said that if you dream of picking ripe plums, then that is a sign of good health. If, however, the plums are green then you could be facing illness among family members. Dreaming of rotten plums on the ground warns you to watch out for disloyal friends and lovers. Even worse, if you see yourself gathering them, then this could foretell of a future marked by destitution.

Uses

Harvesting our wild plums is one of our greatest pleasures in August as you will have gathered from the introduction to this month. They are mouth-wateringly delicious simply stewed with honey and added to breakfast muesli or with custard as a dessert. If you want to keep their goodness for longer, however, then this jam is a winner.

Wild plum jam

1.4 kg/3 lb cherry plums
1 kg/2¼ lb sugar
425 ml/¾ pint water

Have ready 5 jam jars, washed and heated for at least 5 minutes in a moderate oven. Pick the stalks off the plums and give the fruit a rinse. Cut each open then put in a pan with the water and simmer until soft. Remove the stones. ♦ Meanwhile, pre-heat the oven to 180°C/350°F/gas mark 4. Put the sugar into a bowl and place in the oven to heat through. ♦ Add the hot sugar to the fruit and stir gently, leaving on a low heat until the sugar is totally dissolved (about 15 minutes). Then boil up rapidly for 10 minutes. Test for setting by spooning a little onto a cool plate. ♦ Turn off the heat, skim off any scum with a perforated spoon, then pour the jam into the hot jars. Seal immediately with waxed paper and cover the jars. Enjoy!

Wild plum Compote

Add to your muesli for a nourishing breakfast. By including a rounded tablespoon of live yoghurt, digestion will be improved and nutritional value increased, particularly in the form of calcium.

500g/1 lb 2 oz cherry plums

knob of butter

1 tsp ground cinnamon

1 tbsp honey

275 ml/½ pint boiling water

Wash the plums, cut in half and take out the stones. Melt the butter in a pan, then add the cherry plums. Sprinkle in the cinnamon and stir in the honey, adjusting for sweetness as necessary. Pour in the boiling water, put the lid on the pan and simmer gently over a low heat for about 15 minutes.

Wildlife

As soon as the plums are ripe, a swarm of wasps will descend on them, so it's a race as to who will get there first to enjoy the luscious fruit. While I am always happy to share our produce with wild creatures, pickers need to keep their fingers safe from stings. Fruit-eating birds, such as blackbirds, will also eagerly join in with the competition for the plums.

Broad-leaved Dock (*Rumex obtusifolius*)

Knotweed family (Polygonaceae). Perennial. Pollinated by wind. Propagated by seed and root cutting. Edible. Medicinal.

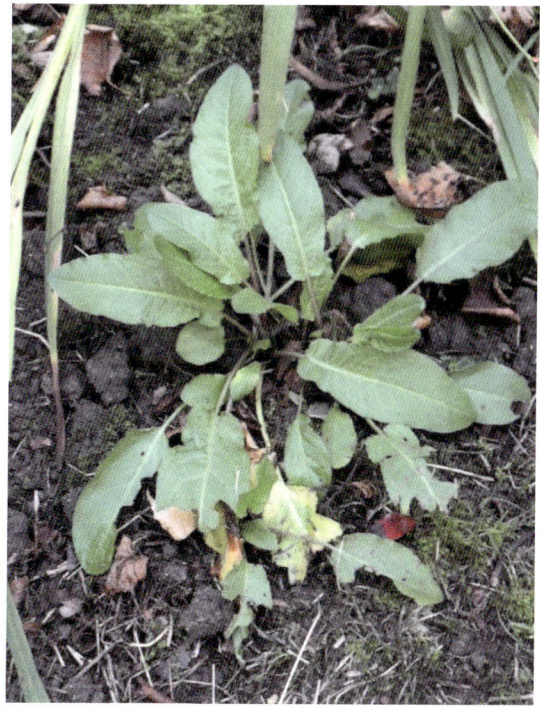

Dock is an important food plant for the larvae of many moths, as you can see from the nibbled leaves.

This perennial weed truly is the bane of gardeners. If allowed to mature, then it is extremely difficult to dig out due to the length of its taproot, which can reach down to almost 1 m/3 ft 3 in. Moreover, if it should break as you attempt to pull it out, any pieces left in the soil will produce yet another specimen. If you do not want this rather common plant in your garden, then keep a look out for seedlings and hoe them up quickly. You will be able to recognise the young rosette of oblong, mid-green leaves, often with two distinctive lobes at the base. If this tenacious plant defeats

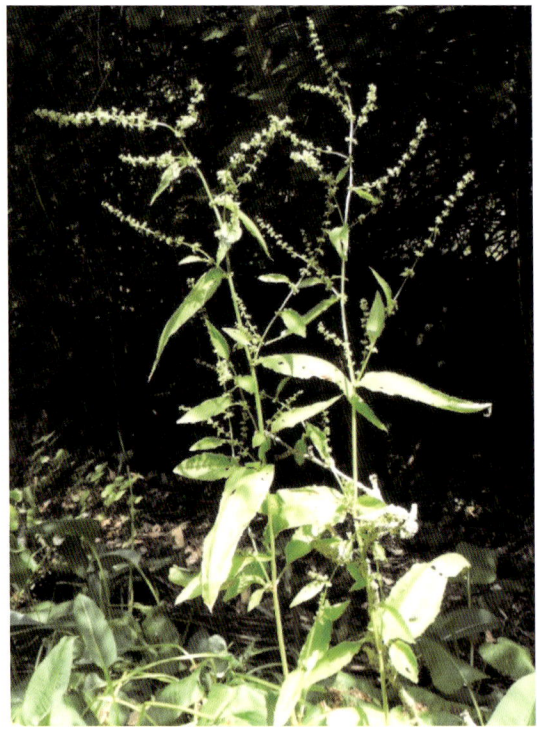

A mature dock can produce many thousands of seeds.

you, then persist in repeatedly cutting off the crown of leaves. Unable to photosynthesise, it will eventually die.

Not only will dock reproduce itself from a piece of root but will also scatter a great many seeds. The similar curled dock (*Rumex crispus*), which has spikes of densely packed flowers, has been known to distribute up to 30,000 from one large plant! The seeds of *R. obtusifolius* have evolved into a three-sided shape with toothed 'wings', allowing them to disperse widely, by either water or wind, or by attaching themselves to animal fur. Moreover, they do not have to be fresh to germinate. Seeds found on excavated sites have been shown to be as old as fifty years, yet half were still able to sprout. So beware! If you have ever had dock in your garden, the likelihood of seeds lying dormant in your soil is rather high.

Broad-leaved dock can grow quite tall, its main branching stem frequently achieving a height of 1.3 m/4 ft. The broadest leaves are at the base, those on the stem being narrower and placed alternately. Some of the lower ones may have reddish stalks, the large leaves slightly wavy. It can therefore easily be confused with curled dock whose distinctive feature is the waviness of its oblong leaves.

The small, somewhat nondescript flowers are mostly hermaphrodite, rising in spikes above the leaves and arranged in many whorls around the stems. They are greenish in colour but turning red as the plant ages.

Folklore

There are some strange superstitions surrounding dock and young women. If an unmarried girl is searching for a husband, she should take some seeds of the plant and walk to a lonely place half an hour before sunrise on a Friday. She must then sow the seeds and chant the following rhyme:

> I sow, I sow,
> Then, my own dear,
> Come here, come here,
> And mow and mow.

A man will then appear to her carrying a scythe. He will be her future husband. To prevent her becoming barren, she must tie some dock seeds to her left arm. It seems from such tales that these seeds were associated with fertility.

Uses

Dock is well known as a good remedy for nettle stings, as the traditional rhyme reminds us:

> Nettle out, dock in,
> Dock remove the nettle sting.

As country children, we were often stung by nettles, but I can't say that I found the rubbing on of dock leaves particularly soothing. Maybe I should have spit on it first. Scientific tests have shown that the enzymes in saliva encourage the release of various anti-inflammatory properties carried within the leaf.

Here in East Anglia a soothing remedy was made from the roots. After digging them up and washing them, they would be boiled in water and the liquid bottled. This was then applied to any irritating skin condition, including rashes from infectious diseases such as measles, to insect bites or dermatitis. Herbalists may still prescribe this treatment. It was also taken internally as a cure for boils. Similarly, an infusion of the seeds would be a soothing remedy. Culpeper in the 17th century thought it was better to boil the roots in vinegar, which 'helpth the itch, scabs, and breaking out of the skin, if it be bathed therewith'.

Before the advent of refrigerators, the large leaves were used to help preserve butter, either by wrapping it up or else by putting the butter in a dish of water and laying the leaf over it. This led to the popular name of 'butter dock'.

While the leaves are edible, they are nevertheless high in oxalic acid, like rhubarb, in particular those of curled dock. You may like to pep up a salad with the sharp taste of dock by adding a few leaves, but this is not recommended for people with conditions such as kidney stones, gout or arthritis.

Wildlife

As a child, one of my favourite 'pets' was the caterpillar of the garden tiger moth called 'woolly bear'. This has long, dark brown hairs and a characteristic orange-red stripe. I would put it carefully in a jam jar with some dock leaves and await with impatience its amazing transformation into a chrysalis.

This is by no means the only caterpillar that relies on dock. It is the food plant of the larvae of many other moths, including buff ermine, common marbled carpet, mottled beauty, ghost moth, angle shades, emperor, mouse moth and lesser yellow underwing. The pretty small copper butterfly also depends on this plant. Despite being considered a 'weed', dock has its place. If your garden is a reasonable size, then allow one or two to grow in an out-of-the-way corner. Birds simply love the seeds, especially finches.

Hedge Mustard (*Sisymbrium officinale*)

Cabbage family (Brassicaceae). Annual/biennial. Pollinated by insects, including butterflies. Propagated by seed. Edible. Formerly medicinal.

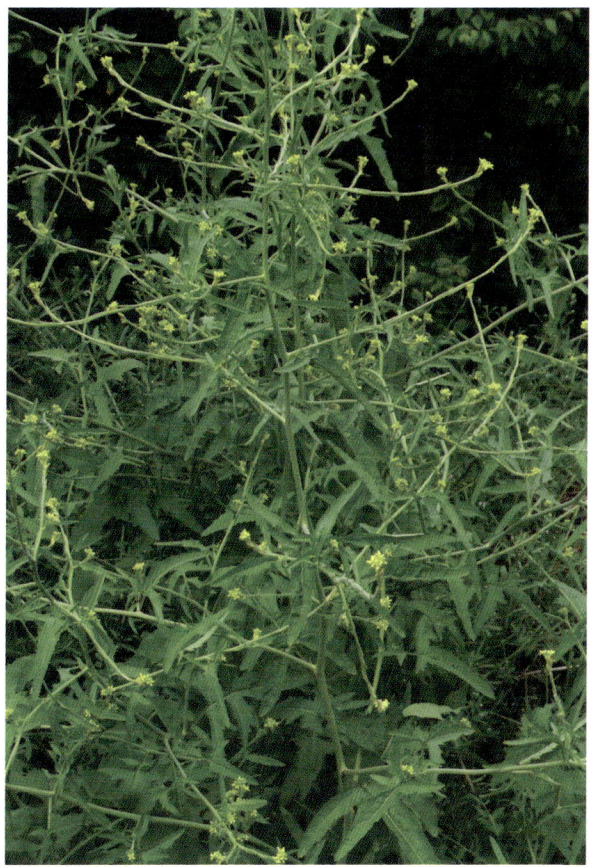

Hedge mustard may look rather insignificant, but the tangy leaves provide vital nourishment for the caterpillar of the pretty orange-tip butterfly.

I have to admit that, in my view, this is not the loveliest of weeds, but it is a curious plant. With its thin wiry stems and minute yellow, four-petalled flowers, it has a somewhat neglected air. Its alternative common name of 'wire weed' suits it well. It is almost as if it was abandoned by its maker half-way through the design process. Certainly it favours rough, unloved corners of the garden, especially where the ground has been disturbed. As regards height, its stem and branchlets can grow to almost 1 m/3ft 3in, but generally somewhat less.

It is described in wildflower books as an annual but can also act like a biennial, its basal rosette of deeply lobed leaves over-wintering in the soil. The upper leaves are rather different, being long and arrow-like, but often the purplish stems can look quite bare, the tiny, bristly, downward-pointing hairs hardly visible.

The long pods, each containing around 15 seeds, stand erect, close to the stem, splitting from the base for dispersal. One plant can easily produce up to 3,000 seeds. These are remarkably tenacious. Seeds up to 30 years old, found in excavations, have been known to germinate successfully. Young plants may appear in either autumn or early spring.

Folklore

In the early 17th century, at the time when Nicholas Culpeper was a practising astrologer-physician, it was still believed that the sun, moon and planets governed different parts of the body. It was also thought that there was a strong association with the various herbs, so that they were most effective if gathered when their particular planet was visible in the sky.

Culpeper believed that hedge mustard was ruled by Mars, which in turn governed the arteries. It is difficult to work out from this why he thought that it was 'good in diseases of the chest and lungs'. Perhaps it was really the piquant taste of the leaves that gave him this idea.

Uses

Farm animals usually turn their noses up at hedge mustard, yet some European communities value the tangy flavour of the leaves in a salad or to perk up a stew. The seeds are sometimes ground to produce a mustard-like paste and used as a condiment.

The Ancient Greeks believed that the plant was a useful antidote to all sorts of poisons, and many later herbalists have agreed with them, including Culpeper. In France it was commonly referred to as the 'singer's plant', being made into a syrup to cure a sore throat. It seems that it was also recommended to actors. The 17th-century French dramatist Jean Baptiste Racine said that it was 'good for all diseases of the chest and lungs, hoarseness of voice … for all other coughs, wheezing and shortness of breath'.

I have yet to hear of a modern performer who relies on this remedy. Indeed, today's herbalists rarely prescribe it. Occasionally a concoction of the juice and flowers is suggested as a revitaliser or to alleviate bronchitis and stomach ailments.

Wildlife

Despite its skinny, straggly appearance, hedge mustard is an important food plant for several Lepidoptera, most particularly the charming orange-tip, one of my favourite butterflies. These do well in our garden. To help them, I allow some hedge mustard to grow near a compost heap. The butterflies readily lay their eggs at the base of a flowerhead. Apparently, the caterpillars are attracted to the rather bitter, cabbage-like flavour of the leaves.

Black Nightshade (*Solanum nigrum*)

Nightshade family (Solanaceae). Annual. Pollinated by insects. Propagated by seed. Poisonous.

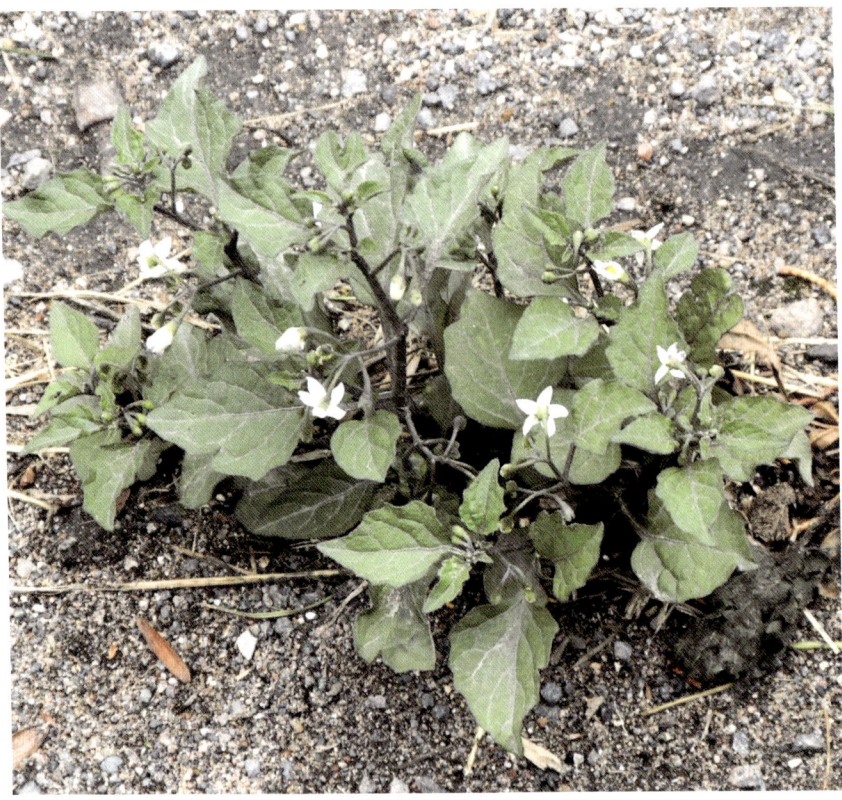

Black nightshade often appears in gardens, thriving well in rich soils. The unripe berries, however, are very poisonous. *Photo © NatureSpot / Graham Calow*

If you have a vegetable garden and enjoy growing peas and beans, the chances are that you will find the straggly stems of black nightshade sharing the richly nitrogenous soil. Like bittersweet, the white petals of the star-like flowers are turned backwards, although not quite to the same degree. In the centre of each is a protruding clump of stamens bearing bright yellow anthers. You will see that the flowers grow in clusters on short stalks and that the green leaves are pointed, some with wavy edges. This annual plant can gain a height of about 70 cm/2½ ft. After flowering, round fruits are formed, first green then turning black – hence the name.

Folklore

The name *Solanum* is thought to derive from the Latin *solamen*, meaning solace or relief. It seems that it was believed to have soothing qualities. In Europe, leaves of black nightshade would be scattered into cradles to calm babies, while over the other side of the Atlantic American Indians took it for insomnia. They were well aware of its strongly sedative and narcotic properties, at the same time apparently disregarding its dangers.

Uses

It seems astonishing that, considering all parts of black nightshade are poisonous to humans, it has traditionally been prescribed as a medicine. To be fair, Culpeper is a little cautious, saying 'it must be used moderately', although claiming that it is 'in no way dangerous, as most of the Nightshades are'. He recommended it for cooling 'hot inflammations' of all kinds. While it is no longer used as a herbal remedy, extracts of black nightshade form the basis of certain drugs, in particular for the relief of gastro-intestinal irritation. Experiments with mice have also demonstrated that *Solanum nigrum* has certain anti-cancer properties.

The unripe green berries are particularly poisonous, containing the most glycoalkaloids, including solamargine, solasonine and solanine. Eaten in considerable amounts, especially by children, they could be fatal, with symptoms of fever, vomiting, diarrhoea, hallucinations and ultimately respiratory failure.

After reading of its potentially disastrous effects, particularly to children, you may decide **to discard this weed**, despite its pretty flowers!

Wildlife

If you examine the leaves, you may see some small beetles, rather rounded in shape with a beautiful metallic sheen, often with a red or green hue. These are leaf beetles. As the name implies, both the larvae and adults of these beetles will feed on the leaves of black nightshade.

When the berries are fully mature birds will eat them, as will small rodents. They seem to know instinctively that they are much less poisonous when they are a deep purple-black. The seeds seem to be unharmed after passing through the digestive systems. Indeed, it is thought that this process may speed up germination. At any rate, it is a very effective way of dispersing the seeds.

Nipplewort (*Lapsana communis*)

Daisy family (Asteraceae). Annual. Pollinated by insects; also self-fertile. Propagated by seed. Edible.

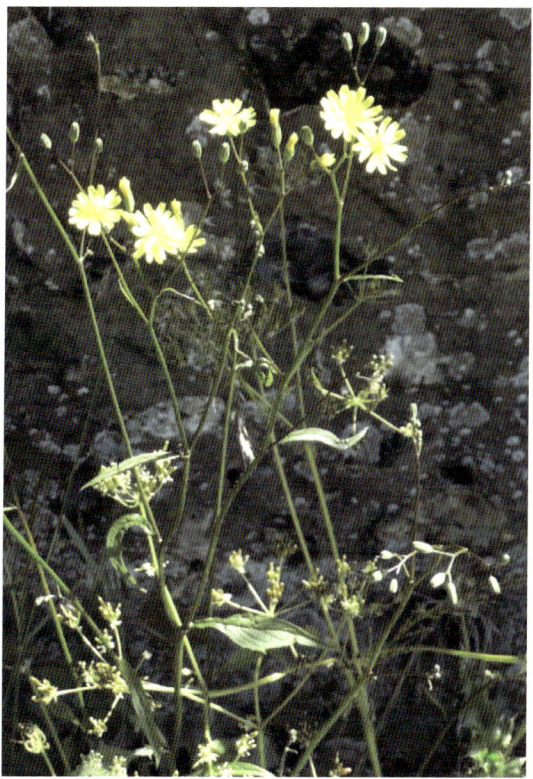

Nipplewort is a common annual 'weed' which may well arrive wherever you have been digging the garden over.

As nipplewort tends to pop up in disturbed ground, it is likely that this annual wild flower will intrude into your garden, especially if the soil is heavy. You will recognise it by its rather spindly but upright branching stems, up to 1.2 m/4 ft tall, and its small, lemon-yellow florets that only open in bright sunshine. Despite its name, there is no milky latex but rather a clear sap.

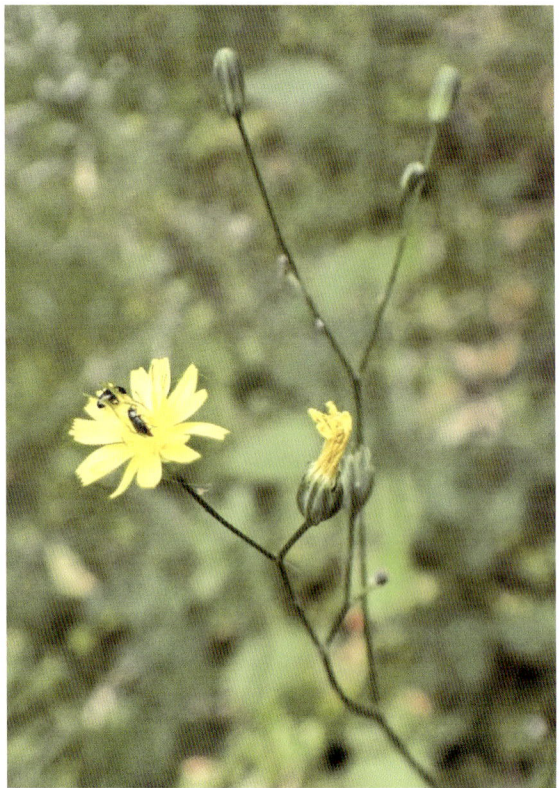

Hoverflies are particularly attracted to this plant.

Although a relative of the dandelion, the seeds have no parachutes. Seeds are formed in pods and their dispersal depends on gusts of wind or an obliging animal passing by. They can, however, be numerous, with the average of around 1,000 per plant. For this reason you may prefer to pull it out, which is very easy as the roots are shallow. Alternatively, you can simply cut it before seeding and use the upper, edible leaves in salads.

Folklore

The 17th-century physician and botanist, John Parkinson, boasts of having given the plant its English name. In his *Theatrum Botanicum; or an Herball of Large Extent* of 1640 he writes: 'Camarius saith that in Prussia they call it Papillaris, because it is good to heale the ulcers of the nipples of womens breasts, and thereupon I have intituled it Nipplewort in English.' However, the name may have been in use before that, simply because the buds look rather like nipples. The scientific name is derived from *lapsane*, the edible herb used in ancient Rome.

Uses

Although it is thought to be calming and antiseptic, the plant is no longer in general use as a herbal remedy.

Wildlife

On a warm sunny day, when the flowers are wide open, hoverflies will gather around them and feed on both the pollen and the nectar. Drone flies, those honey bee mimics, will also be attracted to nipplewort. These, along with other smaller insects, will pollinate the plant.

If any rabbits are passing by, they will much enjoy nibbling on the lower leaves.

Pellitory-of-the-wall (*Parietaria judaica*)

Nettle family (Urticaceae). Perennial. Pollinated by wind. Propagated by seed. Pollen an irritant. Medicinal.

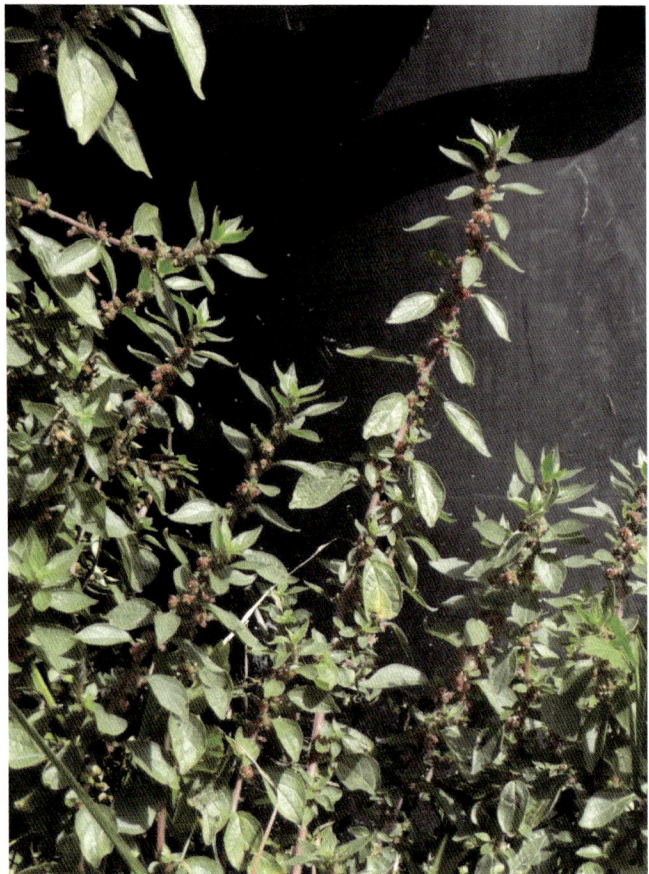

People suffering from breathing conditions may not want pellitory-of-the-wall nearby as it can provoke asthma attacks. Here it helps to disguise a dustbin.

This unassuming little 'weed' may be found growing in the cracks of old walls or stone buildings. Although native to the British Isles, pellitory-of-the-wall must have been rare here in East Anglia before it was colonised by humans as there are few suitable natural rocky outcrops. Today it is mainly found in the places where we live rather than in the countryside. It is not surprising that it was given the name *Parietaria* as it is based on the Latin *paries* for 'wall'. How it discovered the remains of an 18th-century brick wall here in our garden is a mystery – but there it is.

At first one notices the small darkish green, downy, oval leaves and red stems. These are slightly sticky to the touch. Closer inspection reveals the tiny, white flowers which cluster in the leaf axils. Brushing against the stamens will cause them to spring up and scatter the pollen. Unaware of the risk to asthma sufferers, I was rather astonished when a friend grabbed a handful of the plant and ripped it up, exclaiming, 'Ugh, you don't want that in your garden, surely!' So be careful if you or your family suffer from allergies as pellitory can bring on hay fever and asthma attacks. If this is the case, you may not wish to have this plant in your garden.

Folklore

Housewives of the past have found pellitory to be an effective cleaner of both glass and copper. In fact, it contains sulphur and potassium nitrate. If burnt it produces a powerful smell, which was often likened to hell fire. As a result, the belief arose that it would drive away the devil!

Uses

A good way to avoid the pollen problem is to pick the plant for herbal use. In the 17th century, Culpeper wrote with admiration about pellitory, praising its effectiveness for many ailments from 'an old and dry cough' to expelling 'the stone or gravel in the kidneys or bladder', to easing 'the pains of the mother', 'the pains of the teeth' and the noise in the ears, to cleansing 'foul rotten ulcers … and running scabs or sores in children's heads', while helping to 'stay the hair from falling off'!

Today its medical uses are limited mainly to a tonic for the kidneys and bladder. It does appear to help dissolve stones and relieve cystitis by increasing the flow of urine and reducing inflammation. It also lessens any fluid retention. William Salmon, writing in 1693, described how, when a youth and 'the hope of life but small' on account of the 'dropsy' (oedema), a syrup of pellitory taken morning and evening evidently cured him entirely.

Syrup of pellitory

Pick the herb when in bud. Rather than pull it from the base, just snap the stem in half, allowing the remainder to grow back.

50 g/2 oz chopped pellitory

850 ml/1½ pints water

450 g/1 lb honey or sugar

Put the pellitory and water into a pan and bring to the boil. Reduce the heat, cover and simmer gently for about 20 minutes. Strain into a jug. Put the liquid back into the pan and continue to simmer, but uncovered, so that it reduces by about half. Add the honey or sugar while stirring to make the syrup. Simmer for a little longer. ♦ Pour into sterilised bottles. The syrup should keep for at least 6 months unopened. Store in the fridge once opened. ♦ Take 3 tsp up to 6 times a day (adults); 1 tsp 3 times a day (children).

Wildlife

One of our most beautiful butterflies is the red admiral. The favourite host plant for its caterpillars is the nettle. As a non-stinging species of Urticaceae, pellitory is a relative of the nettle, so red admirals will also seek out this plant for the sustenance of its larvae. If you love butterflies but hate nettles, then pellitory might offer a solution.

Procumbent Yellow Sorrel *(Oxalis corniculata var. atropurpurea)*

Wood-sorrel family (Oxalidaceae). Perennial. Pollinated by insects. Propagated by seed, bulbil and stolon. Edible. Medicinal.

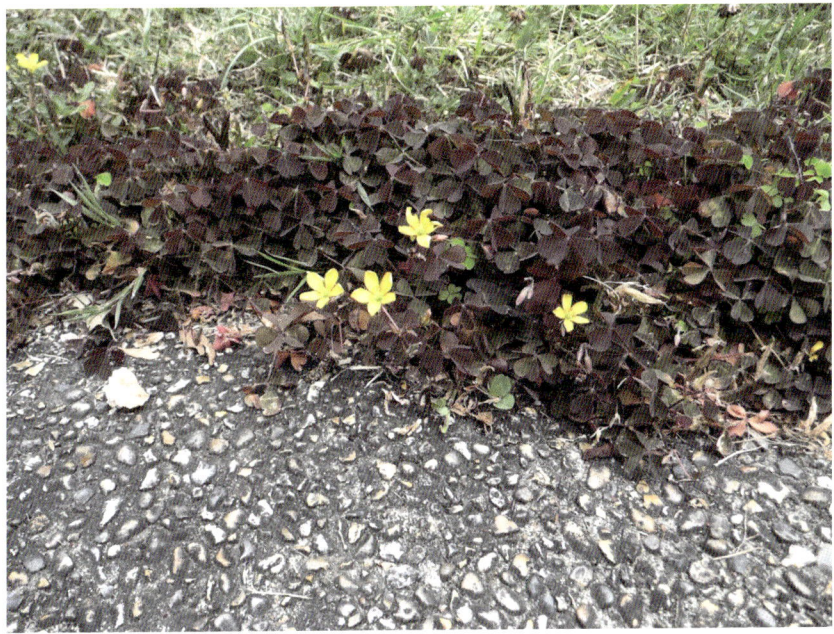

Yellow sorrel is not only attractive but is worth having to hand for treating insect bites.

This pretty creeping 'weed' freely decorates the ground around our front door, establishing itself in paving cracks as well as a nearby sunny border. It certainly enjoys a dry and warm site and spreads easily via its underground bulbils and from seeds that are ejected with some force from bursting pods. It will also root where stems touch the ground at the nodes. I struggled to give it a correct identification as it was excluded from some of my wildflower reference books. This could be because it was evidently introduced to the British Isles and is therefore not strictly speaking native.

Yet, further investigation led me to discover that it has been recorded wild here as long ago as 1770 and was actively cultivated in Britain at least 50 years before that. With an interesting bitter taste that earned it the name of 'sour-grass', yellow oxalis was valued as a condiment and for its therapeutic properties.

'Sleeping beauty' is certainly an apt common name as there is a delicacy to the clover-like leaves and five-petalled flowers, borne on slender, fragile-looking stalks. Moreover, the recumbent habit belies the fact that new leaves and flowers can 'awaken' at many points. Those that plant themselves in between our paving stones have trifoliate leaves of a deep purple colour, making a striking contrast with the yellow flowers; those in the border, however, have larger green leaflets. The purple variety is certainly my favourite and welcomes me as I step out into the garden.

Folklore

It is rather odd that so little folklore surrounds yellow sorrel, bearing in mind how common it is. Perhaps this is because its origins are not European but thought to be Asian. Certainly, the Chinese knew long ago that copper was one of the trace elements to be found in the plant. As revealed by the 15th-century text 'Precious Secrets of the Realm of King Xin', the plant was used to locate underground copper deposits. How successful this was is unknown.

Uses

Modern analysis has shown that the plant is a good source of vitamin C. The 19th-century herbalist William Kemsey had some justification, therefore, to 'use it in all hot diseases'.

The flowers have a pleasant, acidic flavour. However, as the leaves contain oxalic acid which can bind up the body's calcium, they should be used in salads only in moderation.

It is a beneficial plant to have nearby in summer as the leaf juice is naturally anti-bacterial and makes a helpful treatment for insect bites.

One other reason for its cultivation was the yellow dye produced from the whole plant.

Wildlife

The wide-open, yellow petals invite attention from passing insects seeking nectar. Small wild bees are likely to stop by as are flies and hoverflies. I have often seen little black beetles investigating the plant, readily crawling right inside the flower looking for nectar at the base of the petals where there are orange markings.

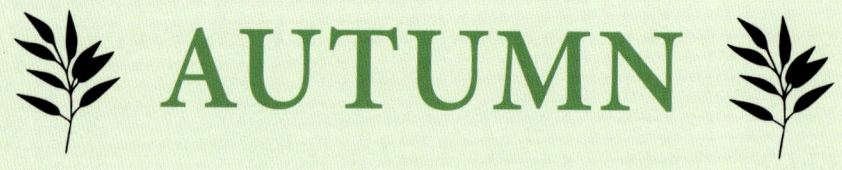

AUTUMN

When frosty kiss of Autumn in the dark
Makes its mark
On the flowers, and the misty morning grieves
Over fallen leaves;
Then my olden garden, where the golden soil
Through the toil
Of a hundred years is mellow, rich, and deep,
Whispers in its sleep.

'Mid the crumpled beds of marigold and phlox,
Where the box
Borders with its glossy green the ancient walks
There's a voice that talks
Of the human hopes that bloomed and withered here
Year by year, –

Dreams of joy, that brightened all the labouring hours,

Fading as the flowers.

Faint and far away their ancient griefs appear:

Yet how near

Is the tender voice, the careworn, kindly face

Of the human race!

Let us walk together in the garden, dearest heart,

Not apart!

They who know the sorrows other lives have known

Never walk alone.

From 'Autumn in the Garden' by
Henry van Dyke (1852–1933).

SEPTEMBER

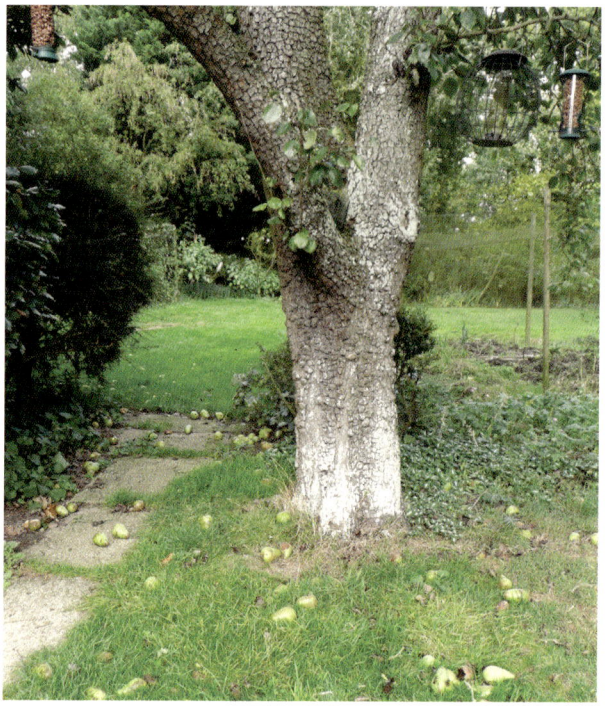

Our ancient pear tree produces fruit prolifically. Its windfalls are readily pecked by blackbirds and later provide fructose for the beautiful peacock butterflies.

It is already the middle of the month and we have just returned from a holiday in the south of France where we enjoyed three weeks of unremitting sunshine. From time to time we worried about our garden: would there be enough rain to plump out the vegetables? We need not have worried. A quick tour of the plot confirmed that my courgettes had turned into enormous marrows, that there was a splendid row of cabbages ready to pick and eat and that the broccoli had sprouted tender flowery heads. By contrast, in Mediterranean regions there has been no rain for a whole month, and my eyes had grown used to burnt-out grass and parched trees already withdrawing sap from leaves which have turned brown and dropped off prematurely.

As I take my first tour of our little patch I am struck by the lushness and the intense green of this English garden! It may be a typical wet September day that could well be described as dreary, but everywhere nature boasts its productivity. Blackberries gleam dark and enticing in the hedgerows, competing with the red hawthorn berries and scarlet rose hips for attention. Windfall apples and pears lie on the ground ready to be collected and turned into pies and crumbles. As for weeds – they have taken the opportunity provided by our short absence to establish themselves in totally new places. An area cleared for some low-growing shrubs to provide shelter for small amphibians and other animals beside our pond has suddenly become packed with a wide variety of wild flowers. A cursory survey of the emerging leaves and young plants tells me that hedge mustard, bristly oxtongue, hawkbit, groundsel, goosegrass, chickweed, dandelion, buttercup, plantain, primrose, forget-me-not, thistle, nettle, herb-Robert and rosebay willowherb are among the many species that have already set down roots. I now have the dilemma of deciding whether to turn this into a wildflower patch rather than a shrubbery!

Blackberry (*Rubus fruticosus* agg.)

Rose family (Rosaceae). Semi-evergreen shrub. Pollinated by bees and butterflies. Propagated by seed and biennial rooting stems. Edible berries. Medicinal.

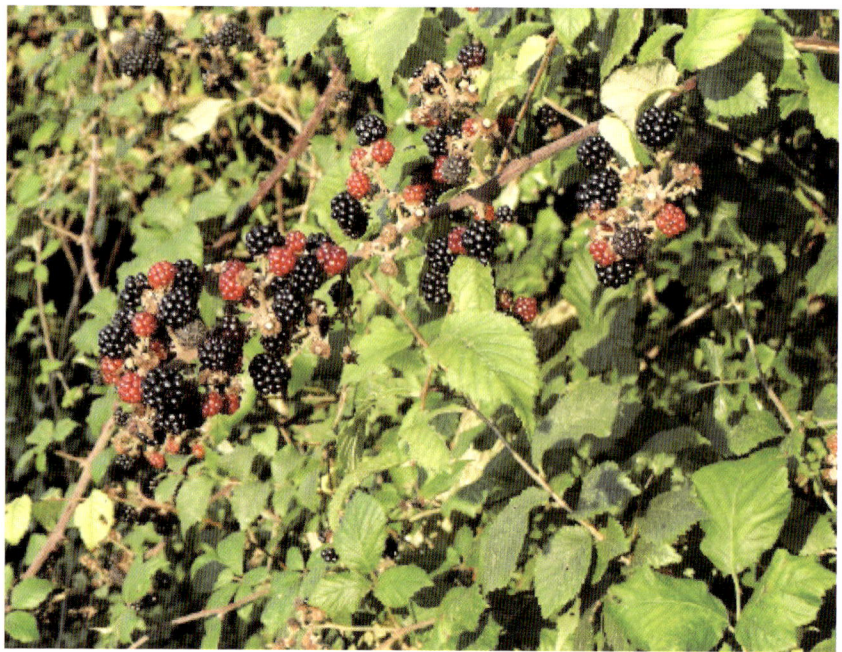

If you can find space in your garden for brambles, not only will you benefit from the delicious fruit but will also be providing a haven for wildlife.

Much of my weeding time in our rambling country garden is spent trying to get the brambles under control. They have the nasty habit of getting their roots down right next to my favourite shrubs, so it's impossible to dig them up without causing damage to garden plants. The best option here is to cut them at the base which at least slows them down. At this time of year, I must catch the newly sprouted long, curving canes before they touch the ground and re-plant themselves. Even if young roots have already formed it is not too difficult to pull them out. This gives me a great feeling of satisfaction! Yet, our wild blackberries have the most delicious flavour, so it is just as well that they often become well established before I reach them.

Needless to say, strong gloves are essential for lessening the damage to oneself caused by the thorns. Even so, because these are recurved, or backward-leaning, it is all too easy for one's clothes to become caught by them. I have often had patiently to detach myself from their clutches, carefully lifting away the prickly stem. It is the thorns that enable them to climb up other bushes and trees, and I have frequently had to pull down many metres of rambling branches.

Folklore

The prickly characteristic has left a significant imprint on the folk psyche, the stems often being referred to as 'lawyers' because of the difficulty in escaping from them! At a more recent date, they had romantic associations, offering an excuse to gentlemen to disentangle the long dresses of lady friends. There is a delightful poem by the Pre-Raphaelite Thomas Woolner called 'My Beautiful Lady', which describes just such an event. Here is a stanza:

> Or maybe that some thorn or prickly stem
> Will take prisoner her long garment's hem:
> To disentangle it I kneel,
> Oft wounding more than I can heal,
> It makes her laugh, my zeal.

Despite the inevitable scratches and prickles, I have always found the picking of blackberries a real pleasure. Perhaps this relates to our hunter-gatherer past when the women folk would have ventured out in groups to find nuts and berries for the community. We know that they have been collected and eaten for thousands of years, seeds having been found in the stomach of a Neolithic man dug up at Walton-on-the-Naze in Essex. These days it is a more solitary pastime, an occasional gatherer to be seen by a country lane with an inverted walking stick pulling down the entangled branches.

Whenever I go blackberrying I search the bushes for the full, shiny, deeply coloured fruit, often at the end of clusters, as these are the sweetest. Each of the 'drupelets', which compose the fruit, lose this shine when a little old and past their best. In fact, folk tradition tells us that we should never pick them after Old Michaelmas Day (10th October) as the devil spoils them by pissing on them! He was apparently furious at falling into a prickly bramble bush, having been kicked out of Heaven by St Michael. Modern science would explain this in more pragmatic terms: the cooler, damper weather of October may cause moulds to develop on the fruit which might not be good for the health. Having picked blackberries after this date myself, I have noticed that they have generally lost their firmness and can be quite mushy. This has left me with hands stained purple. Perhaps it was thought that the Devil's piss would be this colour!

Uses

When ripe, raw blackberries are rich in antioxidants that offer protection to the body's cells, thereby helping to prevent disease. They contain as much as 35% of daily value per 100 grams of vitamin C, 35% of the essential mineral manganese, 25% of vitamin K and 21% of total dietary fibre. They are also a useful source of vitamin A and folic acid (a B vitamin). At the same time, the leaves are high in tannins with astringent properties. Without question, this plant has many health-giving aspects and has been used for centuries in various treatments and remedies. I have selected those that can be backed up by science. Those that cannot are rather obvious, such as crawling under the arching stems to cure boils or whooping cough or encouraging the growth of one's hair by cutting off the tips and putting them on the bramble shoots. I am left wondering whether one suffers total hair loss if the bush is dug up!

John Gerard, the Elizabethan physician, records that the berries 'heale the eies that hang out', which conjures up rather a startling image to the modern reader. However, the fruit is certainly good for the general health of the eyes because of the vitamin A content. It has also been discovered more recently that the deep purple pigment contains anthocyanins, which, like vitamins A and C, are potent antioxidants that protect cells from damage.

Anecdotal evidence suggests that blackberries, like blueberries, guard against degeneration of the macular at the back of the eye, a condition that can eventually lead to blindness. Moreover, the pips are high in ellagic acid that has anti-cancer properties, so it makes sense to refrain from spitting them out. Many hundreds of observational studies have shown that diets rich in these nutrients reduce the risk not only of cancer but also of heart disease, cataracts, Alzheimer's and arthritis. So, next time a bramble plants itself in your garden treasure it for its healing powers and cultivate it.

Blackberry and apple jelly

Vegetarians prefer agar agar to gelatine as it is made from seaweed rather than from animal products.

570 ml/1 pint apple juice
2 tsp agar agar flakes
grated rind and juice of 1 orange
225 g/½ lb fresh blackberries
1 dessert apple, cored and sliced
small carton of soya cream

Pour the apple juice into a pan and heat. Stir in the agar agar until the flakes are dissolved. Add the rind and juice of the orange. Arrange the blackberries and apple slices in a bowl and pour the jelly mixture over them. Leave to set. ♦ Serve with soya cream.

Blackberry leaf tea

This can be made very simply with the fresh leaves, preferably when they are young. Because it has styptic qualities, the tea is very good for alleviating diarrhoea. Culpeper knew this from experience, saying in his *Herball* that the leaves 'do much bind the belly'. When lukewarm, it can be used as a mouth wash to help heal ulcers or gingivitis, or as a gargle to soothe a sore throat. Folk medicine recommends it also as a rinse for minor skin problems.

handful of young blackberry leaves and shoots
2 cups boiling water

Wash the leaves and tear them into pieces. Place in a pot and pour on the boiling water. Allow to infuse for 5 minutes.

Blackberry syrup

I have on a bookshelf an ancient copy of Mrs Beeton's *Household Management*, which belonged to my grandmother. Along with telling the reader what the upper housemaids' duties are, or how many items you should have in your silver tea set, it does contain some excellent recipes which are worth a try, even if the amount of ingredients is sometimes excessive. I have adapted this recipe but retained the principle of using a bain-marie, because this concentrates the juice and thereby the nutrients and gives an intense flavour.

450 g/1 lb blackberries
450 g/1 lb honey
1 tbsp cold water
small glass of brandy

Put the berries, honey and water into a fire-proof pot or jar with a lid. Stand it in a large saucepan and surround with boiling water. Allow to simmer for 2 hours. Strain off the juice. Put into a pan (either enamel or stainless steel) and simmer gently for 20 minutes. Stir in the brandy. ♦ Pour into sterilised bottles and store in a cool, dark place. ♦ Take a teaspoon of the syrup when necessary to ward off colds or ease a sore throat.

Wildlife

We are happy to share the produce of our brambles with the birds. Other wildlife also benefits from the blackberry bush, not only for the food it supplies but also for the cover offered by the entangled, low-growing stems to small mammals and amphibians. The leaves are an important nutritional source for various caterpillars, while many butterflies can be seen visiting the pretty white or pink flowers for nectar, including the small tortoiseshell, comma, gatekeeper, speckled wood and peacock. The pollen is also attractive to bees. If you wish to provide a wildlife haven in your garden and have time to do rigorous pruning and training, then consider including the native bramble.

Black Horehound (*Ballota nigra*)

Dead-nettle family (Lamiaceae). Perennial. Pollinated by insects. Propagated by seed and division. Medicinal potential.

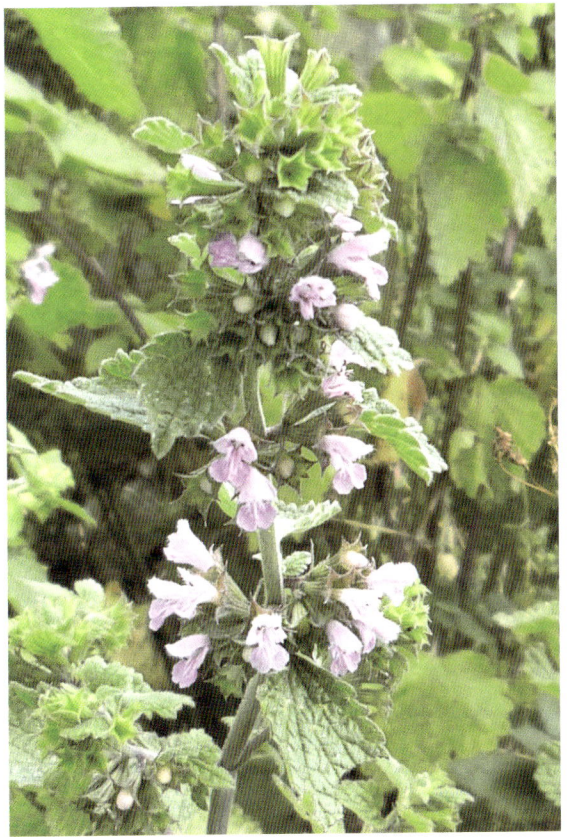

Despite its foetid smell, black horehound was once grown as a medicinal herb.
Photo © NatureSpot / Graham Calow

Try picking this plant and then taking a sniff. Ugh! It is well known for its foetid, mouldy smell, sometimes compared to stale perspiration. At any rate, it has earned the common name of 'stinking Roger'. Even cattle are put off by the odour and avoid eating it, despite its prevalence around hedgerows and field borders and its liking for disturbed ground, especially close to human habitation.

It is certainly partial to our borders, sometimes providing a little welcome ground cover, and will flower well into autumn, long after others have ceased, tolerating quite low temperatures. I personally find the plant quite attractive, if a little straggly. The mid-green leaves are rounded or heart-shaped and toothed, rather downy and with distinctive patterns of veins. The pinkish-purple flowers peep out from leafy whorls, the upper petal notably prominent and hooded. The lower petal is divided into three, with two smaller lobes either side.

Folklore

Why describe it as 'black'? This is unclear, but it could be because the seeds are black or, more likely, because the leaves turn black when dried and then used medicinally. As for 'horehound', this most probably comes from the Old English *har* meaning 'downy', while 'hound' could be a corruption of *hune* for 'plant'. 'Ballota' is derived from the Greek word *ballo* meaning 'to reject' – and one sniff tells us why!

Uses

Black horehound has been used as a remedy for various complaints since ancient times. Indeed, it goes way back to Dioscorides, *c.* 40–90 AD, the Greek physician and botanist who wrote an encyclopaedia of herbal medicine. He recommended it as a cure for the bite of a mad dog, as did Culpeper, who is more generous about the plant's odour, describing it as having 'a keen and earthy smell'. Despite this disagreeable factor, it was often grown in herb gardens, harvested when in flower and then dried for use in syrups. Culpeper thought highly of it using it not only for cleansing 'foul ulcers' but also for treating 'hysteric and hypochondriac affections'. At the same time he advised caution, suggesting that 'it ought only to be administered to gross phlegmatic people, and not to thin plethoric persons'.

It is no longer a favourite of modern herbalists, although it is sometimes prescribed for coughs, nausea or motion sickness, or mild sleep disorders. Indeed, there are verbascoside compounds in the flowers which have a sedative effect. Moreover, black horehound is known to contain antioxidants, so it clearly does have therapeutic properties. There has been some excitement recently with the discovery that the flavone tangeritin, normally present in the peel of tangerines and other citrus fruits, is found in this plant. It seems to have anti-cancer properties as it will selectively kill off leukaemia cells while leaving normal ones alone. There is an indication that it could also be helpful in the treatment of Parkinson's disease. Clearly, this is a plant with medicinal potential.

Wildlife

Sometimes when digging in the garden I have come across a small, white caterpillar with a brown head and have often wondered what it was. I now see that it could well have been the larva of either a ghost moth or perhaps the common swift moth. These live underground and feed on the roots of small herbaceous plants, such as horehound and those of grasses. The adult male ghost moth is a pure white – hence the name. The female, however, looks quite different, having creamy-yellow forewings with orange markings. She is also larger with a wingspan of up to 70mm/2¾ inches. They fly in the summer. The larvae are unusual in that they overwinter twice, so that the full life cycle takes two years to complete.

The common swift moth is somewhat smaller and more muted in colouring, but its brown wings provide good camouflage, so it is less likely to be picked off by a bird. This one flies in the late spring.

You might notice that newly emerging leaves on the tips of black horehound stems are rolled over tightly. The reason for this is that the fly *Contarinia ballotae* has formed a gall here. If you open it up, the small, white larvae are likely to jump out.

Dogwood (*Cornus sanguinea*)

Dogwood family (Cornaceae). Deciduous shrub. Pollinated by insects, including bees and butterflies. Propagated by seed and cutting. Formerly medicinal.

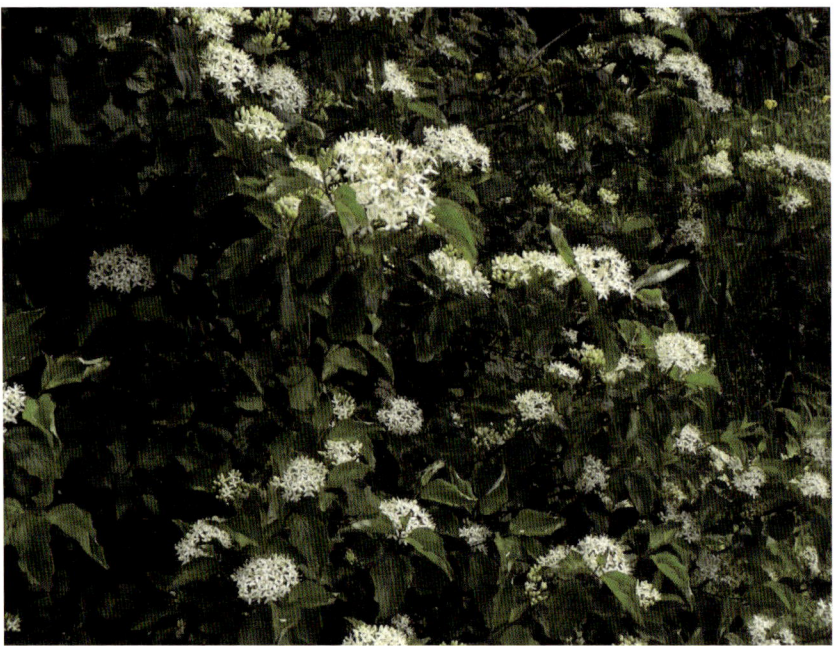

The creamy-coloured flowers of dogwood are most attractive and a magnet to many insects which benefit from the sweet nectar.

I am not entirely sure whether our dogwood can be classified as a 'weed' as this shrub was already growing very energetically by our pond when we first arrived here and may or may not have been deliberately planted. However, it is certainly the native variety, with attractive red stems and clusters of creamy-white flowers in summer after which black berries are produced in September. Not long afterwards the leaves put on a spectacular show, matching the stems in colour. There are many similar specimens in hedges surrounding local fields, so it could well have been planted with the help of a visiting bird. At any rate, we do have to keep it under control

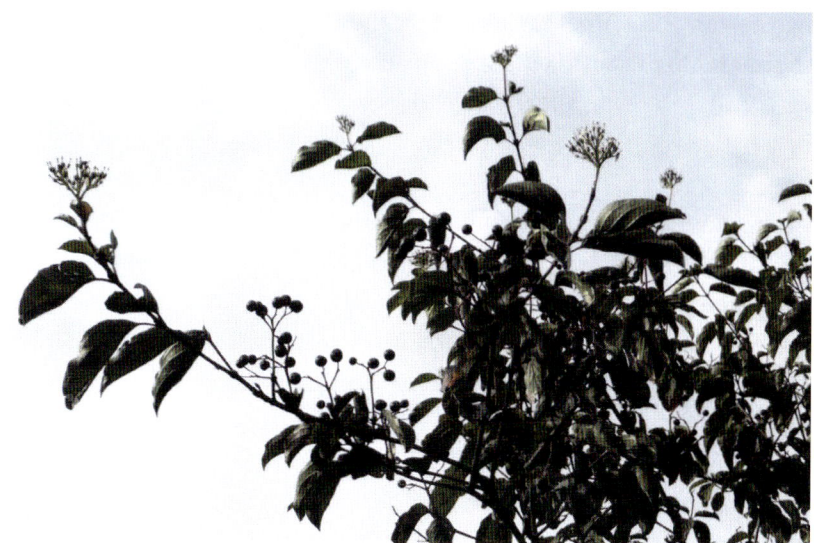

Our garden birds hungrily devour the black berries. Clearly, they find them very tasty!

as it has a spreading habit and tends to send up shoots under the adjacent grassy path that leads into our meadow, and these we have to dig up.

Gardeners choose to plant varieties of this genus particularly for their deep red stems (the botanical name comes from the word *sanguis,* Latin for 'blood'), which add warm colour to a winter border.

Folklore

There was a famous dogwood tree that grew on the Palatine Hill in Rome. According to Plutarch, it was believed to have been the javelin thrown by Romulus from the Aventine Hill which penetrated the soil and subsequently took root. It seems to have become some sort of talisman, offering safety to the city. Unfortunately, the bush was accidentally felled while Julius Caesar was in power. Perhaps this was an omen that Roman luck was running out!

Children have traditionally had great fun with the oval leaves. Each child carefully picks a large leaf. Then he or she holds the ends and pulls the leaf very gently apart. Fine elastic tissues of latex are left between the two halves. The winner of this game is the one who can produce the longest strands without causing them to break.

Uses

American pioneers used to bite off a twig and then clean their teeth with it. The leaves and bark when smoked have a narcotic effect and native American Indians were well aware of this.

The origin of the common name, however, is lost in the mists of time. It seems to have nothing to do with dogs but may be a corruption of the old word 'dag', referring to some sort of a skewer or spike. John Evelyn, writing in the 17th century, confirmed that it made the best skewers for butchers because 'it does not taint the flesh'. Indeed, the wood is dense, strong and flexible and has been prized for the making of rims in basketry and for the very first tennis rackets, as well as for the forming of loom shuttles and handles for tools. It was also sometimes the choice for making long bows. Chaucer, referring to it as a 'whipple-tree' in *The Knight's Tale*, indicates that it was a practical means of linking a horse-drawn cart to the harness. It may still be used to make old-fashioned canes or for fine inlays.

Wildlife

I like to think of our dogwood as a protective tree. It offers shelter to many of our little songbirds. They fly here for safety after pecking at some seeds, fat or crumbs which we put out for them on the nearby bird table. At this time of year, they gorge on the berries, stripping the bush clean. In the spring, the leaves are an important food source for the larvae of the splendid emperor moth, grey with prominent eye spots, the female having a 7.5-cm/3-inch wingspan. You may be lucky enough to see one if your garden is close to heathland.

Elder (*Sambucus nigra*)

Moschatel family (Adoxaceae). Deciduous shrub. Pollinated by insects. Propagated by seed. Berries edible when cooked. Medicinal.

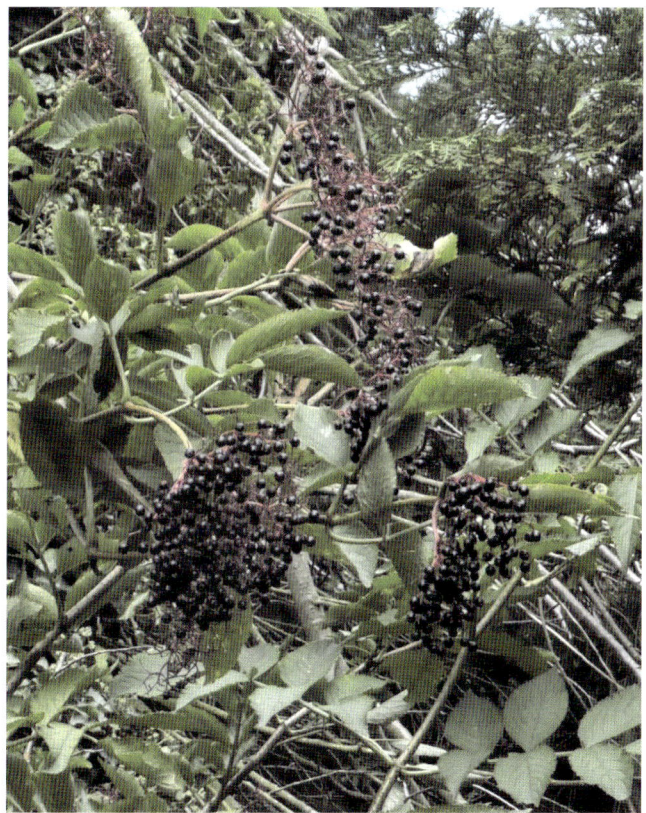

Elderberries, when ripe, are extremely nutritious for both humans and birds, and can help to sustain the immune system.

THE BERRIES

Readers who have dipped into this book each month will already have read about the folklore and wildlife of the elder tree during its flowering period in June (see pp. 142-5). September is the time when it produces clusters of deep purple berries, which, like the flowers, are rich in health-giving nutrients. Birds seem to know this instinctively as they feed on the berries voraciously. It is noticeable that they wait until the fruit is very ripe. Humans should take this as good advice as the seeds and raw, especially unripe, berries, along with the bark and leaves, contain the cyanogenic glycoside sambunigrin, which is potentially toxic if taken in significant doses. In other words, they can cause diarrhoea. It is better, therefore, to consume the berries in a syrup (see below) when they can be extremely beneficial, especially in alleviating the symptoms of colds and 'flu. You will find that excessive secretion of mucus is reduced, and the remedy is therefore very effective in treating sinus infections. The purple colour tells us that anthocyanins are present, which shorten the duration of infections. Research in Israel has suggested that they may alter the surface of the virus, so that it is unable to take hold. Like the purple pigment found in blackberries, this helps to protect the eyes from damage due to age and too much exposure to sunlight.

As flavonoids, especially quercin, are found in the plant, be aware that if you are taking other antioxidants, such as vitamin C, the effects may be increased. This is also true of some antibiotics and decongestants. Elder can give a real boost to the immune system. It is well worth keeping a bottle of syrup in the cupboard, therefore.

Elderberry syrup

Pick the berries when ripe and a deep purple colour. You can easily strip them from the stalks with a fork. The addition of cinnamon to the syrup will not only add a spicy flavour but the essential oil is naturally antimicrobial and antioxidant, so the therapeutic effects of the elderberries will be enhanced.

450 g/1 lb elderberries

275 ml/½ pint water

175 g/6 oz unrefined caster sugar

stick of cinnamon

½ lemon, sliced

Use glass medicine bottles. First sterilise these by washing in very hot water, then drying in the oven on a low temperature for at least half an hour. ♦ Put the ingredients into a stainless steel or enamel saucepan. Bring to the boil and simmer gently for 20 minutes. Strain through a fine sieve or muslin and pour into the bottles. Allow to cool and screw down caps. ♦ For colds and 'flu or a sore throat, take 1 tsp neat several times a day. Alternatively make a soothing drink by adding hot water.

Healthy elderberry dessert

This is not only a delicious, fruity dessert with a strong flavour but it will also help to keep those autumn colds at bay.

1 pear, peeled and chopped
400 g/14 oz elderberries
50 g/2 oz sultanas
3 tbsp clear honey
2 tbsp sherry
150 ml/¼ pint yoghurt

First stew the pear in a little water until soft and mushy. Strip the elderberries off the stalks with a fork. Put them into a saucepan with a small amount of water and bring to the boil. Simmer until tender. Press through a sieve. Return the berry purée to the pan and, over a gentle heat, stir in the sultanas, honey and stewed pear. ♦ When the purée is cool, add the sherry and yoghurt and mix together.

Autumn Hawkbit (*Scorzoneroides autumnalis*)

Daisy family (Asteraceae). Perennial. Pollinated by hoverflies, bees and butterflies. Propagated by seed. Formerly medicinal.

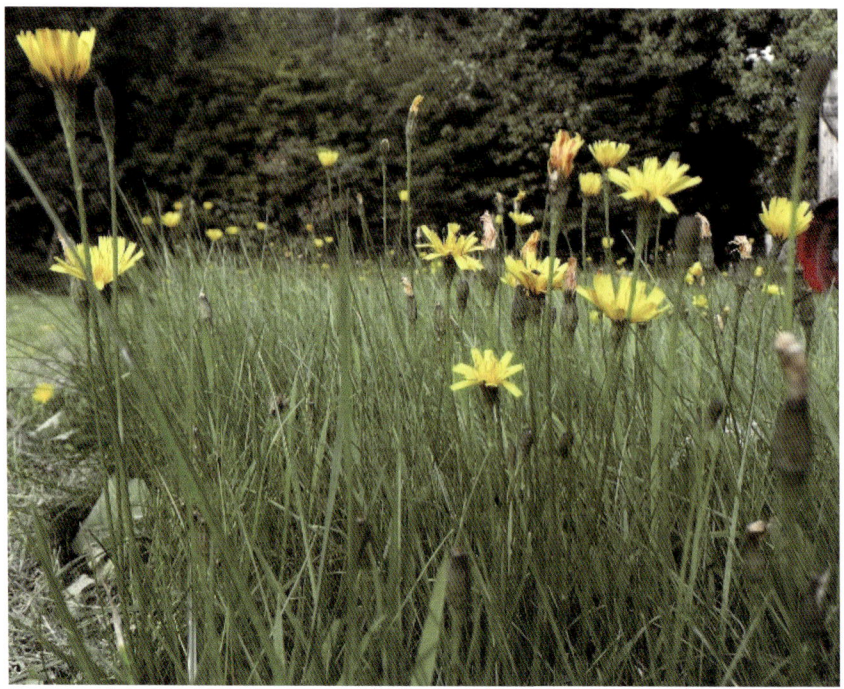

Autumn hawkbit can be a useful 'weed' in the garden as it attracts hoverflies whose larvae feed on aphids.

Our driveway is a pebbly one, the far end of which has become overgrown. This area is right next to our large pond, so any sort of herbicide to reduce the weeds is out of the question as we know that even the least toxic, based on pyrethrum, will be harmful to aquatic life. Moreover, we share our garden with protected great crested newts and are committed to providing them with just the right kind of habitat. With their spotted orange bellies, these creatures are unmistakable. The only option, therefore, is to mow the space from time to time and use it as parking for visitors.

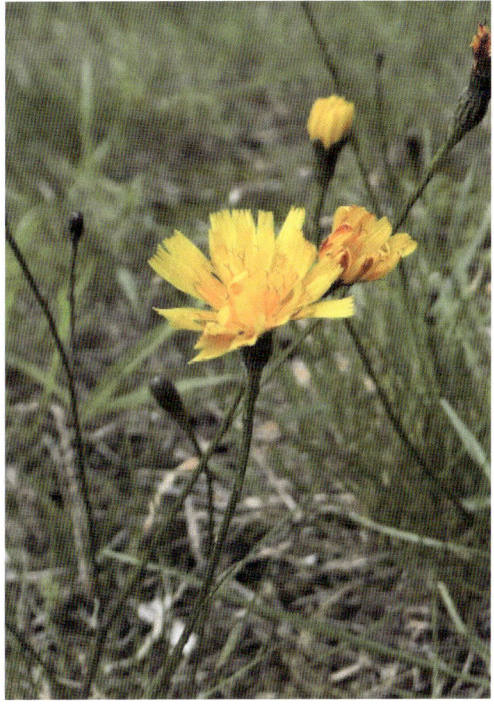

If you look underneath the flower heads, you will see that the outer rays are striped deep orange to red.

As these plants are perennials, you will see the flattish rosette of green leaves all year. These are lance-shaped with deeply toothed margins. New leaves start to push up from the centre in the spring. Each autumn some bright, little, yellow flowers appear, apparently tolerating the mowing. They look somewhat like dandelions but with a more open display of petals, which, from their squared-off edges, seem as if they have been neatly trimmed with scissors. I can therefore identify the plant as autumn hawkbit.

Folklore

I was mystified by the name and wondered about its origin. In this countryside area of eastern England we sometimes see sparrowhawks, a bird which is generally loathed by local people because it is known to kill songbirds. However, the numbers are extremely small compared to the devastation caused by pet cats and motor vehicles, both of which cause the death of literally millions of birds every month. A sparrowhawk landed in our garden recently and demolished a pigeon. I had the privilege of watching this magnificent bird of prey at close range through the window and was struck by its startlingly beautiful yellow eyes.

Perhaps, therefore, the association of the colour had something to do with the name of the flower, but this failed to explain the second part. Why would a hawk bite a flower? After some investigation I discovered that in former times country folk believed that hawks ate this flower in order to improve their eyesight!

Uses

Despite the fact that this is a common wild flower that grows easily in a variety of places, ours enjoying the open ground and short grass, herbalists appear to have been silent about its possible therapeutic benefits. Perhaps this is because it has been overshadowed by the profusely growing dandelion.

Wildlife

The late flowering of this hawkbit is important as a food supply for autumn butterflies, bees and other insects. As with all members of the Asteraceae, it is the small wild bees that particularly benefit from the nectar. I also notice how hoverflies are attracted to this plant, insects that are very useful to us gardeners as the larvae feed on aphids. It is clearly a 'weed' to be encouraged. If this flower appears spontaneously, then allow it to flourish in short grass to provide late-season nectar.

OCTOBER & NOVEMBER

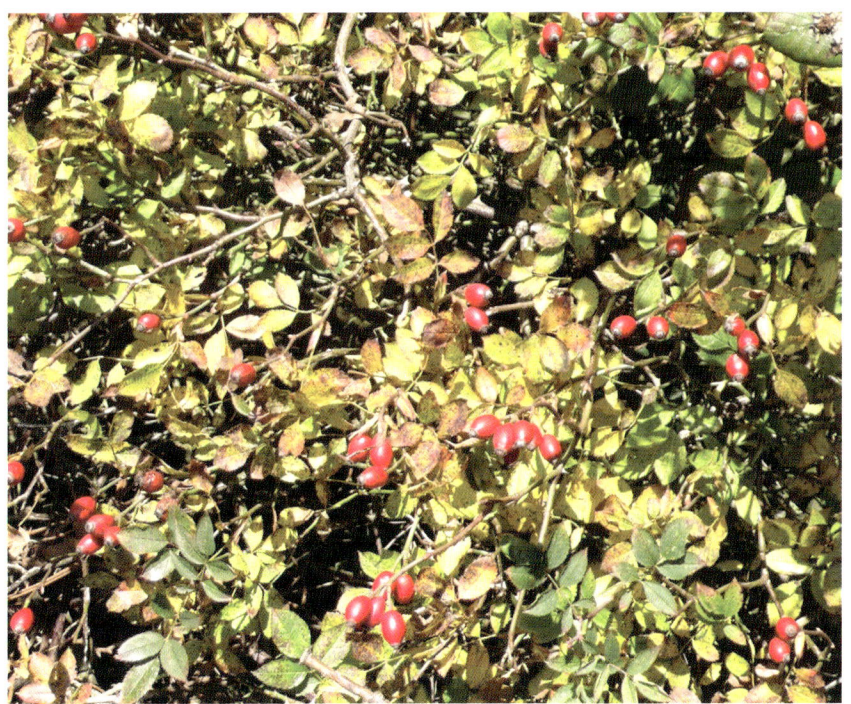

Rose hips fill the hedgerows, providing autumn nourishment for birds.

Much as I groan inwardly at the thought of the dark, cold days ahead, nevertheless, I find the golden sun and long shadows of autumn utterly bewitching. The mornings are glorious, misty, with fine cobwebs spread over the grass, all decorated with dew drops sparkling like tiny diamonds.

By the middle of October, we have already had a ground frost and plenty of persistent showers which have soaked well down into the earth. The soil is now pleasingly friable and easy to work. It is therefore a good time for weeding.

Part of our home is constructed from former stables and a coach house, and adjacent to this is an attractive semi-circle of cobbles, or rather I should say 'was' as these have become almost totally overgrown. Clearing this area has now become a necessity. We avoid any sort of spraying as even the mildest weed killer can cause havoc with the life in our pond, so it must all be done by hand. I start by pulling up handfuls of long grass, only to discover that their roots are deeply buried in a mat of moss, entwined about with the long strands of hop trefoil, a sort of yellow clover. Some of these are a good 60 cm/2 ft or more long, embedding themselves between the cobbles every so often with a succession of roots. There is plenty of clover elsewhere on our lawns to provide nectar for bees, so I decide that much of the trefoil will have to go for the sake of clearing the cobbles. I know that the blackbirds will benefit as I have watched them on many occasions pecking at the juicy worms that reside among the stones in the damp cracks.

It is surprising how much soil has collected around and beneath the roots of the weeds in a relatively short time, brought up by the action of busy worms. I ask my archaeologist husband whether the soil is simply building up or whether the cobbles are actually sinking. He assures me that it is a mixture of the two and goes on to describe an experiment which is being carried out to determine how quickly artefacts become buried through natural actions. Such knowledge helps with the dating of some sites. Be that as it may, the weeds and soil together that I am removing will make a fine contribution to my compost heap.

In a warm, sunny spot right next to the wall I notice a slight movement. It's a minute newt, perhaps just 5 cm/2 inches long, hardly visible, its brown colouring merging so completely with the soil. Each little leg has four perfectly formed 'toes'. At this time of year, the newts are leaving the pond and looking for somewhere to hibernate. As I watch, this tiny specimen slides under a cobble and disappears.

By the end of October there is little new to report, apart from the delightful arrival of primroses, pre-empting spring. This has been a recent phenomenon, no doubt due to global warming. Amazingly, several other flowers manage to hang on well into November, even after sharp frosts. A stately hogweed still displays corymbs of white flowers, though now a little faded, at the same time as the successful production of many hundreds of large seeds. Sow thistles continue to show off their bright yellow flowers. A tour of the warmest corners reveals pinpoints of pink as clusters of black horehound make an effort to open their snap-dragon lips. Nearby, nipplewort has kept its flowers, although a little straggly, and there is even the odd daisy. Together they offer last-minute vital nectar to any insects that have managed to survive the cold and damp. So I chose not to pull them up.

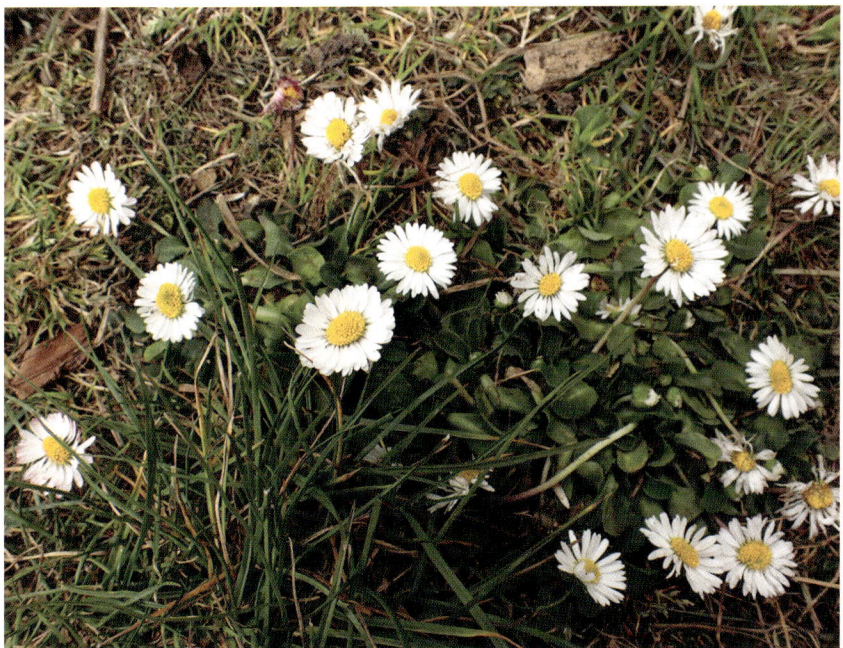

Daisies can appear at any time throughout the year if conditions are favourable.

Blackthorn (*Prunus spinosa*)

Rose family (Rosaceae). Deciduous shrub. Pollinated by insects. Propagated by sucker and seed. Edible. Medicinal.

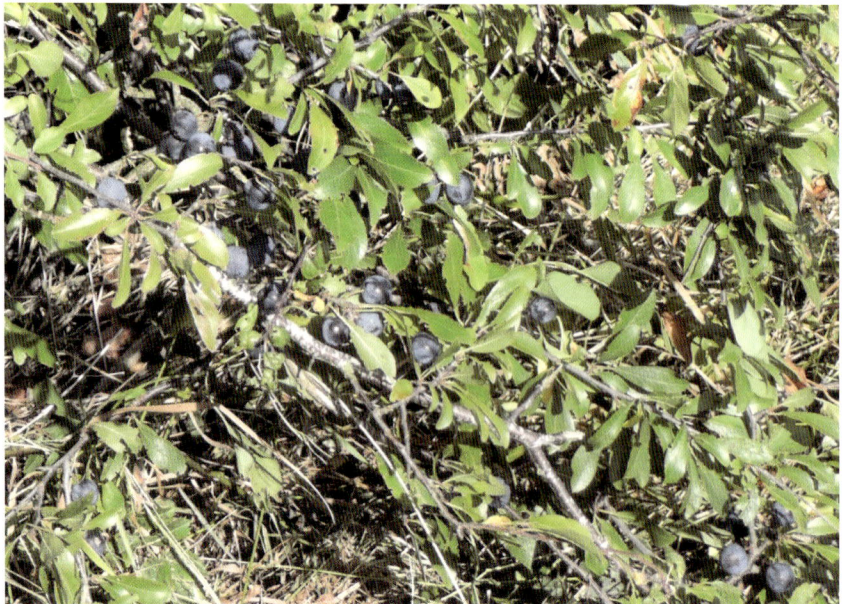

Although horribly bitter when raw, the fruit of blackthorn makes flavoursome jams and jellies. Adding the sloes to gin is a well-known country custom.

THE BERRIES

In a productive year, the sloes, fruit of the blackthorn, hug the stems of the shrub in tight clusters. Their dark blue skins are generally covered in a distinctive grey bloom, signifying the presence of natural yeast. This, together with the tannins in the juice, tells us that it is an ideal fruit for wine-making. In the autumn my husband gathers pounds of sloes from the wild blackthorn bushes around our pond, and each year he refines his recipe for the rich red wine that they produce. Holding a glass of the clearing wine up to the light, sniffing it and swirling it around before checking the taste for subtle improvements becomes a regular winter ritual in our kitchen.

Folklore

The blackthorn has already been discussed at some length during its flowering season in April (pp. 34-7). There I mention something of the superstitions that surround the shrub, in particular those involving the sharp thorns and early flowers. Yet there seems to be no prohibition against bringing the succulent fruit into the house.

In the West Country it was thought that sloes were an excellent cure for warts. First, you cut open a sloe then rub it over the wart to allow the juice to penetrate. To be sure of the remedy working you must finally throw the fruit over your left shoulder.

A common country belief is that if the blackthorn bushes are heavy with fruit in the autumn, then a bad winter is forecast.

Uses

Apart from several good recipes and remedies, one of the main uses for the unripe juice has been as a dye. The colour is a deep slate-blue and is indelible, needing no mordent. It was therefore ideal for marking linen, surviving multiple washes without fading.

The making of sloe gin in the autumn has remained a favourite country custom to this day. The only recommendation is to wait until after the first frost before picking them. Culpeper advises us in his *Complete Herbal* of the early 17th century that sloes are 'not fit to be eaten until mellowed by the frost', as they are 'of a sour austere taste'. Indeed, they are! I was foolish enough to pick a tempting-looking sloe and try to eat it raw. The first bite filled my mouth with a taste so bitter that it dried my tongue and set my teeth on edge. However, the addition of plenty of sugar or honey makes the fruit perfectly palatable and brings out the luscious flavour. Treated thus, it makes excellent jams, jellies and syrups.

Herbal medicine most often recommends the sloe as a cure for sore throats and to alleviate mouth ulcers or bleeding gums, as the fruit is rich in vitamin C. Culpeper even suggests that it 'can fasten loose teeth'. This seems somewhat unlikely, although boiling up the sloes and using the liquid as a gargle has been a common remedy in our local area until very recently.

Sloes are reputed to stimulate the appetite if a syrup is made from the juice and taken before meals.

Sloe gargle and cough remedy

The addition of honey to the juice, rather than sugar, increases the therapeutic effect, as honey has both a soothing and anti-bacterial action.

450 g/1 lb sloes
½ lemon, chopped
175 g/6 oz clear honey

Put the ingredients into a stainless-steel pan and add double the volume of water. Bring to the boil and simmer for about half an hour or until soft. Strain off the juice, allow to cool and store in the refrigerator for up to a week. ♦ To make a syrup to soothe coughs, follow the above method but reduce the amount of water so that it just covers the fruit. Take 1 tbsp as necessary. ♦ For use as an appetiser, take 1 tbsp before meals.

Sloe gin

Remember to pick the sloes after the first frost when they will be 'bletted' or softened.

450 g/1 lb sloes
225 g/½ lb sugar
gin

Rinse the sloes, then prick them with a sharp skewer. Mix with the sugar. Half fill a clean, empty bottle with the sweetened fruit. Fill up the bottle with the gin, seal and store. Every so often give the bottle a shake. With luck the liqueur will be ready just in time for Christmas.

Wildlife

Despite the bitterness of the sloes, the birds will readily eat them, especially thrushes, blackbirds and starlings. To help their survival, therefore, we make sure that plenty of the fruit is left for them after gathering what we need for ourselves.

The dense thickets formed by the blackthorn bushes provide perfect nesting places, while the thorns offer protection from predators.

Dog-rose (*Rosa canina*)

Rose family (Rosaceae). Deciduous shrub. Pollinated by insects. Propagated by seed or cutting. Edible. Medicinal.

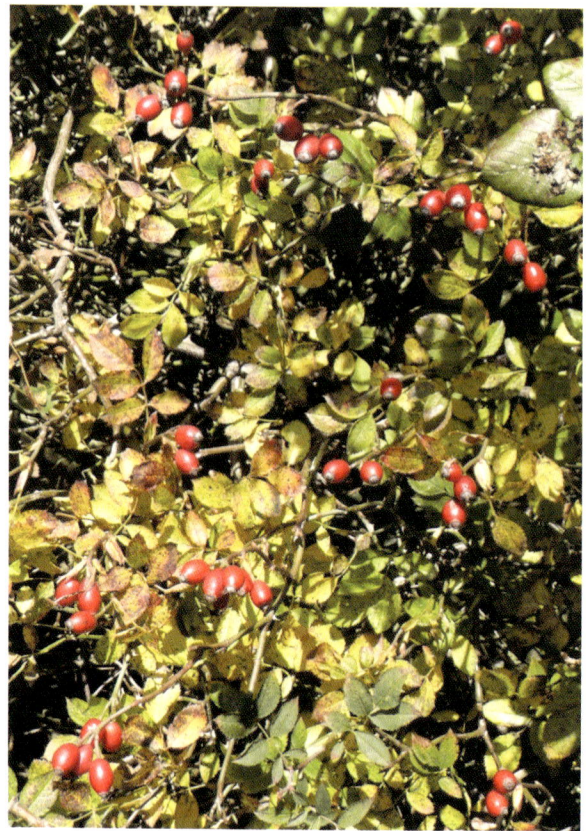

Rose hips contain copious amounts of vitamin C and other antioxidants. Do not despise the common dog-rose therefore. It is well worth picking the hips and making an immune-boosting syrup.

The dog-rose plant has already been discussed in detail under June (pp. 136-9) when the roses are blooming. The autumn, however, sees the production of its valuable fruit.

THE HIPS

I am old enough to remember collecting the orange-red rose hips as a child in the 1950s for National Rose Hip Syrup, which was initiated during World War II to provide the population, in particular children, with essential vitamin C, at a time when importing fruit such as oranges was extremely hazardous. As my legs were still very short and the rose hips seemed to flourish mostly at the top of hedges, I suspect that my mother did more collecting than I did. However, the 3d, i. e. threepence in old money, per pound in weight we were paid made a valuable contribution to my pocket money and I felt immensely proud to be earning something.

Folklore

Mischievous country children have for centuries used them as a very effective itching powder. By tip-toeing up behind someone, the hairy seeds could be dropped down the back of the neck and cause both aggravation and amusement. Children referred to them as 'itchie-backs' or 'cow-itches'.

Uses

Rose hips are particularly rich in vitamin C, containing more than either citrus fruits, sweet peppers or raw broccoli. There is as much of this vitamin in 30 berries as there is in 40 oranges. Yet this is by no means the only nutrient available from rose hips. Vitamins A, B, D, E and K, iron, calcium, antioxidants and fatty acids are all to be found in the berries. It is not at all surprising, therefore, that they have long been associated with considerable health benefits.

There has recently been some good news for the sufferers of the debilitating condition of rheumatoid arthritis. Research conducted in Germany and Denmark showed that a remedy made from rose hips reduced discomfort from painful, swollen joints by forty per cent, a result which surprised Professor Willich who supervised the study in Berlin: 'It's a tough disease, which makes it all the more remarkable to find such beneficial effects from this remedy.' It has been known for some time that the antioxidant flavonoids in rose hips have anti-inflammatory properties. Indeed, the treatment has been used to good effect by sufferers of osteoarthritis. As long ago as the mid-17th century, the physician Nicholas Culpeper knew from experience that this plant had the capacity to 'mitigate the pains that arise from heat, cool inflammations, procure rest and sleep'. He also knew that it 'comforts the heart'. Modern explanations make it clear that the antioxidant vitamins A, C and E in the fruit, together with the flavonoids and the pectin, which is a soluble fibre, all protect against heart disease as well as cancer and work to support the immune system. Including pectin in the diet has been shown to reduce blood cholesterol levels. Yet this is not the only cholesterol-reducing ingredient in rose hips: the plant sterols which are present have the same effect. These work because they are similar on a molecular level to real human cholesterol and so block absorption into the bloodstream. There is no question that the rose hip is a wonder-berry!

Rose hip syrup

It is best to collect the hips after the first frost when they are a little softer, so October is a good month for this. During the preparation of the hips, make absolutely sure that you have got rid of all the irritating hairs that surround the seeds.

As the syrup is a good source of vitamin C, just two teaspoons a day will help to keep colds and 'flu at bay during the winter months. By adding some water, it can also be used as a cordial. The cinnamon will not only add flavour but also enhance the health-giving effects as the oil is naturally anti-bacterial. I recommend making this with honey rather than sugar as it, too, has antiseptic properties and will help to soothe away coughs.

450 g/1 lb rose hips

1.25 litres/2 pints water

2 sticks cinnamon

225 g/½ lb clear honey

After picking, wash the hips thoroughly, then roughly crush them. Put them in an enamel or stainless-steel pan and add the water and the cinnamon. Without covering, bring to the boil then turn down the heat and allow to simmer gently for 20 minutes. ♦ Arrange some muslin in a sieve and strain carefully, if necessary repeating until the juice is clear. ♦ Return the juice to the pan and stir in the honey. Simmer for a further 10 minutes. Pour into hot sterilised bottles and seal immediately. ♦ The syrup will keep in the refrigerator for up to 10 days once a bottle is opened but can be stored in a cool dark place for a year if left sealed. ♦ Dosage for children is 10 ml/2 tsp per day. Double for adults.

Wildlife

During hard winters rose hips can be life-savers for many birds. Although fieldfares prefer worms, if the ground is frozen they will use the available fruit. Having crossed the North Sea to visit us, they are likely to be very hungry and may well turn up in your garden if you are in a rural area.

If your garden is mature, with tall trees, then you may also see blackcaps. In spring they will sing high up and may choose to nest in dog-rose, especially if there are few bramble bushes available. In the autumn and winter, they will gorge on berries; rose hips are a clear favourite.

We always used to have greenfinches in our garden, but a nasty disease significantly reduced their population. A good supply of nourishing rose hips can aid their recovery, especially in late winter. Unfortunately, the flailing of hedges in the countryside strips them of berries, making life much harder for fruit-eating birds.

Garden berries can help to compensate. The tough seeds of rose hips pose no problems for greenfinches as they have remarkably strong beaks.

Hawthorn (*Crataegus monogyna*)

Rose family (Rosaceae). Deciduous shrub/small tree. Pollinated by beetles and flies. Propagated by seed. Edible.

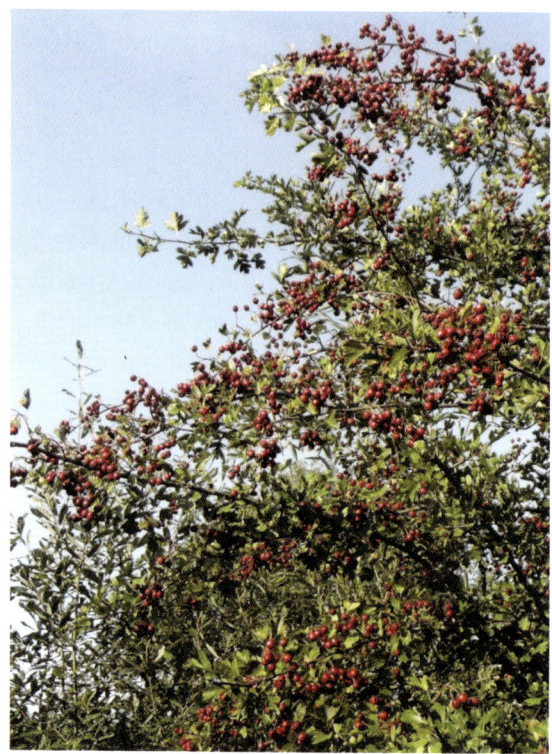

Haws are known to contain flavonoids that have a protective effect on the cardiovascular system. The berries are a vital source of nourishment for birds and small mammals.

THE BERRIES

Before reading this section, turn back to May (pp. 91-6), where you will find detailed descriptions of the attributes of this plant when in flower together with its folklore and uses. By the time October has arrived, our hedgerows are dotted with the small, round, intensely red berries of hawthorn and the birds are having a feast. As with sloes, they are thought to be more palatable after the first frost that acts to soften them. Those haws that have not been eaten on the tree eventually fall to the ground. Here they are appreciated by ground-feeding birds, especially those that thrive on fallen fruit, such as blackbirds. Small mammals, including mice and hedgehogs, will also make the most of this treat.

Uses

This wild variety of hawthorn, the one most commonly found in Britain, contains a single seed and the flesh is not particularly juicy. Despite this, the berries have been used as a food since pre-historic times and the seeds have been discovered at various archaeological sites in both Europe and North America.

As far as a healthy heart is concerned, the haws contain the same chemical constituents as the flowers and are therefore also beneficial. You may recall that it is the flavonoids which give protection to the blood vessels.

To extend the usability of the haws they can be successfully dried by spreading them out in a warm airy place. To re-constitute, cover with cold water and leave for 24 hours. They make excellent jams, jellies and syrups.

Haw chewy

If a small piece is chewed each day, it will help to reduce 'bad' cholesterol. The ginger enhances this effect.

450 g/1 lb hawthorn berries

3.5 cm/1½ inch piece root ginger, chopped

175 g/6 oz brown sugar

water

juice ½ lemon

Put the berries, ginger and sugar into a stainless-steel pan and add half the volume of water. Bring to the boil, then simmer on a low heat for 15 minutes. Cool, add the lemon juice and mash to a pulp. Press through a coarse sieve. ♦ Pour into greased baking trays no deeper than 1 cm/½ inch and dry in a low oven for about 2 hours.

When cool, cut into small squares. ♦ The chewy can be stored in an airtight container in the refrigerator for 3 to 4 weeks.

Haw syrup

Helpful for circulatory problems, especially in the elderly, and reputed to relieve tightness in the chest.

450 g/1 lb hawthorn berries

425 ml/¾ pint water

clear honey

Put the berries and water into a stainless-steel pan and bring to boiling point. Allow to cool, mash, then leave for 24 hours. Boil up again and simmer to reduce. Turn off the heat when the berries have finally lost their red colour. Strain. Return the juice to the pan and add an equal amount of honey. Boil rapidly and pour into sterilised jars. ♦ Take 1 tsp a day or use as a flavouring.

NB. Hawthorn recipes are not suitable for children nor for pregnant or breast-feeding women.

Common Ivy (*Hedera helix*)

Ivy family (Araliaceae). Evergreen climber. Pollinated by bees, wasps and butterflies. Propagated by seed and stolon. Mildly toxic.

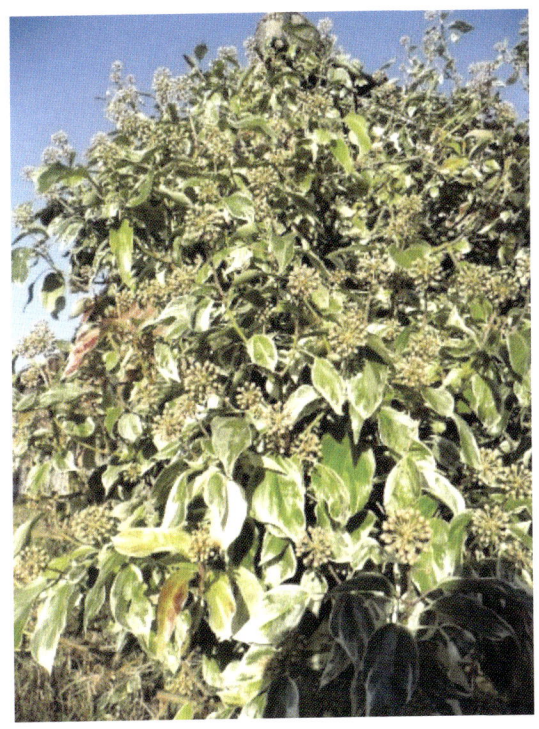

Common ivy is disliked by many householders as it 'attracts flies' and is thought, erroneously, to damage trees.

There is a delightful description of ivy in Gerard's *Herball* of 1596:

> The greater Ivie climbeth on trees, old buildings and walls: the stalkes thereof are wooddy, and now and then so great as it seemes to become a tree; from which it sendeth a multitude of little boughes or branches every way, whereby as it were with armes it creepeth and wandereth far about: it also bringeth forth continually fine little

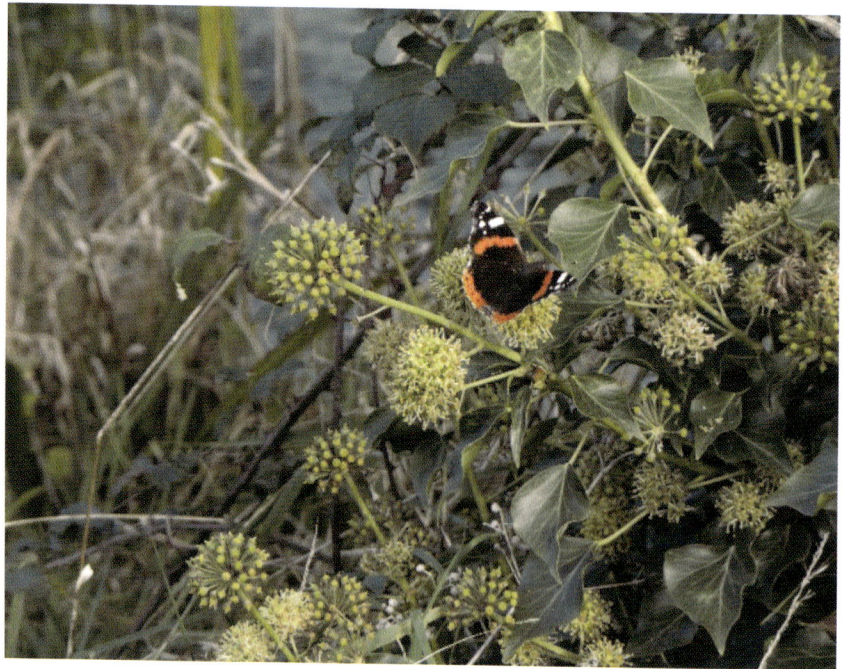

A red admiral takes advantage of the late nectar.

roots, by which it fastneth it selfe and cleaveth wonderfull hard upon trees, and upon the smoothest stone walls.

Here in our garden ivy flourishes magnificently, obviously at home in our somewhat cold, damp clay, spreading vigorously both under our trees and shrubs and up their trunks and stems, not to mention its desire to decorate the walls of our house. Much of my weeding time, therefore, is spent pulling this plant out of our perennial borders and off our house walls.

People often complain about ivy, believing that it strangles trees, but does it really? Some years ago I decided to run my own test. At the northwest corner of our garden two silver birches had planted themselves at the same time and were quite young when we first moved here. Ivy had already begun to fasten itself to their stems, so I pulled it off one but allowed the other to continue to climb. Now, twenty-five years later, both birches are fine trees, and both equally healthy despite one being thick with ivy. My husband's view is that *Hedera helix* clings particularly persistently to wood that is already dead, giving the impression that it has suffocated its host.

A chat with a tree surgeon threw more light on this problem. Ivy in fact is not a parasite and does not draw sap from a tree, merely using it as a support. Its main roots might, however, if very large, compete for nourishment with the tree's roots. It can only be a danger to its host if it grows so large that it overtakes the tree's crown and obscures the sunlight. At this stage it can also cause the tree to be top-heavy, making it vulnerable in a gale.

As this plant grows so profusely in our garden, I am constantly on the look-out for a pair of shiny, dark-green rounded leaves on a reddish-brown, upright stem. When so young, they are very easy to pull out. Later the leaves become deeply lobed on non-flowering stems but are ovate and unlobed where flowers are produced.

Folklore

The ivy plant, with its climbing and entwining habit and glossy, dark evergreen leaves, seems to reside deep within the human psyche. In ancient times it was associated with Bacchus, or Dionysus, who was depicted crowned with an ivy leaf wreath. It was considered to be a 'cool' plant that lessened the heat of the grape vine. Images of it were subsequently placed outside taverns to advertise the liquor sold within.

In the early Christian tradition ivy symbolised immortality and was laid in coffins to represent the new life to come. It then became associated with Christmas and was incorporated into decorations. It also has romantic associations. The Victorians in particular loved it when trailing over summer houses and bowers, offering private retreats and secret corners in the garden.

Uses

What sort of therapeutic value does the plant have? It is odd that the leaves are mildly toxic to humans, yet, according to farmers, sheep and cattle will sometimes seek these out if feeling unwell and will apparently benefit from them. The leaves are known to contain active elements which have both expectorant and antispasmodic properties and could, in theory, be helpful in clearing the lungs or relieving rheumatism. Such remedies are, however, no longer recommended as consuming the leaves can cause a seriously upset stomach. Nevertheless, it might be worth considering the external application of ivy leaves in the form of a poultice to discourage both corns and verrucas, as described below. Anecdotal evidence of its effectiveness in these respects is given by Richard Mabey in his *Flora Britannica*, among others. It is said that if you put the leaves under the sole of the foot and inside the sock, verrucas will drop out after about two weeks, but that seems rather optimistic.

Ivy vinegar

This is a folk remedy for corns. If you drip the mixture carefully on to the corn, keeping clear of the surrounding skin, at least twice a day, the corn should disappear in two to three weeks.

Handful ivy leaves

275 ml/½ pint vinegar

Crush the leaves and place in the vinegar. Pour into a bottle or jar and cover tightly with a cork or lid. Allow the leaves to steep in the vinegar for at least two days.

Wildlife

Ivy is very beneficial to wildlife, its shiny evergreen leaves providing safe cover for small birds, such as the blue tit, for roosting and nesting, and a hibernation site for the striking brimstone butterfly. The little pipistrelle bat will also find a roosting place in a well-established ivy plant.

Additionally, it is one of the favourite food plants of the caterpillar of the beautiful, large swallow-tailed moth. You will have great difficulty spotting the larvae, though, as each looks exactly like a twig and is perfectly camouflaged. On a warm July evening, however, you may be rewarded by seeing the fluttering yellow wings with distinctive pointed 'tails' of the adult moth as it is attracted to a lighted window.

In winter the black berries, too bitter for humans to enjoy, are devoured eagerly by birds, especially wood pigeons and doves. In late September and early October, the sweet-smelling nectar from the greenish yellow, somewhat knobbly-looking, flower heads attracts bees, wasps, butterflies and many other insects which stock up on sugars before the cold weather. This autumn I have been captivated by the number of red admiral butterflies on our flowering ivy. On a warm evening I have also been able to admire the herald moth enjoying the nectar. The pretty holly blue butterfly depends on ivy for its food too, laying its eggs in the flower buds which, along with the developing fruits, the caterpillars then feed on.

So, how much should one keep ivy under control? My decision is not to allow it to creep up our house walls as they can otherwise suffer from damp, but to leave some under trees in our small woodland area where it provides useful ground cover, apparently not minding the lack of light. Otherwise I allow it to ramble over hedges where it flowers profusely and, to a certain extent, around sturdy tree trunks. By making such choices, both gardeners and wildlife can live alongside each other.

WINTER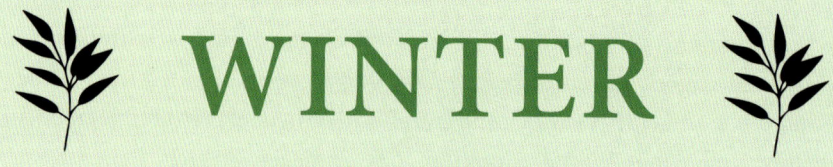

Frosty-white and cold it lies
Underneath the fretful skies;
Snowflakes flutter where the red
Banners of the poppies spread,
And the drifts are wide and deep
Where the lilies fell asleep.

But the sunsets o'er it throw
Flame-like splendor, lucent glow,
And the moonshine makes it gleam
Like a wonderland of dream,
And the sharp winds all the day
Pipe and whistle shrilly gay.

Safe beneath the snowdrifts lie
Rainbow buds of by-and-by;

In the long, sweet days of spring
Music of bluebells shall ring,
And its faintly golden cup
Many a primrose will hold up.

Though the winds are keen and chill
Roses' hearts are beating still,
And the garden tranquilly
Dreams of happy hours to be
In the summer days of blue
All its dreamings will come true.

'The Garden in Winter' by
Lucy Maud Montgomery (1874–1942).

DECEMBER to FEBRUARY

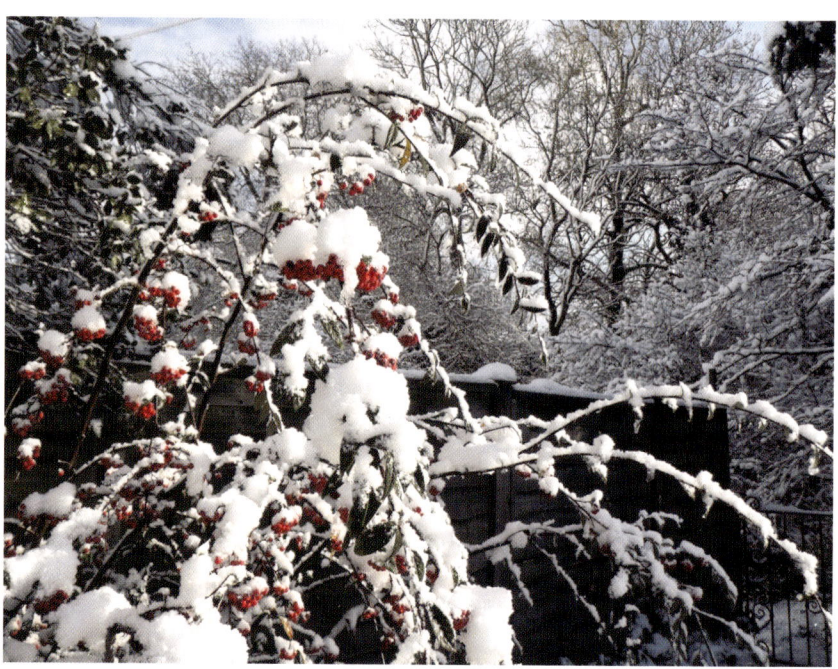

Berries are a vital food source for birds in winter.

Winter is here. Most plants wisely die down during the cold weather and retreat underground for storage of their nutrients or else survive in the form of seeds, awaiting the warmth of spring sunlight and showers to re-awaken the new shoots. Amazingly, some 'weeds' manage to linger on, especially if the weather is mild or if they happen to have planted themselves in a protected corner.

A few can even be found in flower at any month of the year, plants which are truly extraordinary survivors. One such is shepherd's-purse. As a self-pollinator, it has no need to rely on insects, birds, animals or the wind to reproduce itself. Another is groundsel, which establishes itself in our garden in the most unlikely of places, such as cracks between the paving stones. As for chickweed, it has a special liking for our greenhouse and insists on popping up between the winter lettuces. Nutrient dense and tasty, it makes a useful addition to our salads.

The plant which, perhaps, has my greatest admiration goes by the unlovely name of stinking hellebore. It always astonishes me how the flowers manage to open out during the grip of winter while light levels are still very low and the air perishingly cold. Such is nature's ability to defy the elements!

Chickweed (Stellaria media)

Pink family (Caryophyllaceae). Annual. Self-fertile. Propagated by seed. Edible. Medicinal.

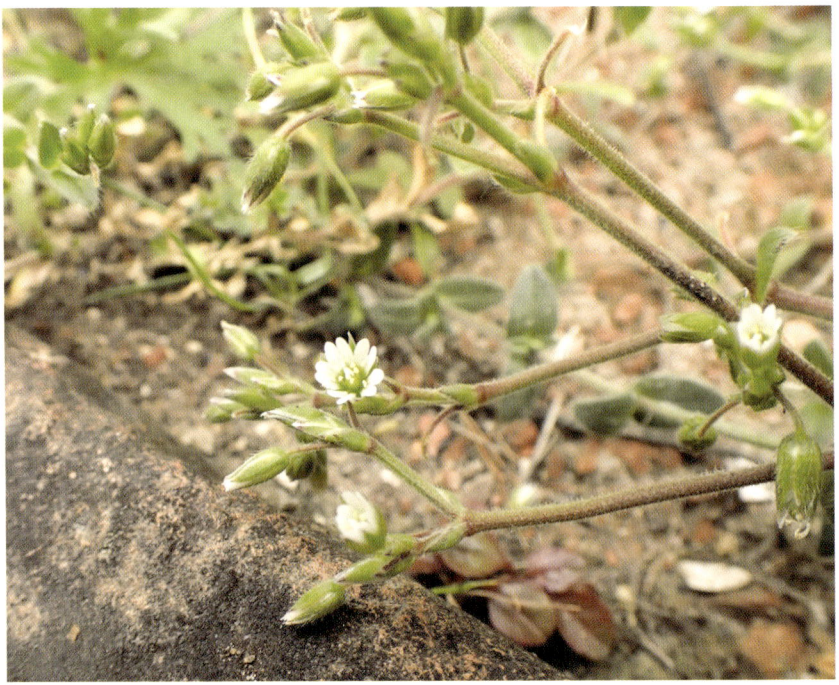

Seeds of chickweed are very long lasting in the soil and known to germinate even after forty years. Chaffinches love to eat them.

We are not entirely sure how chickweed seeds arrive in our greenhouse, but it could simply be that they are already dormant in the soil, brought in to fill our pots. The warmth and moisture quickly bring them to life during any month of the year. We have always avoided buying peat-based compost in our own personal effort to help preserve those ancient habitats, so valuable as carbon sinks and for their unique plant and wildlife species. We make up our own growing medium from a mixture of mole-hill soil enriched with garden compost plus some sand for drainage.

Chickweed has a rather sprawling habit, but closer examination reveals pretty, starry, white flowers. Its long, low-growing stems have light green, pointed, ovate leaves in opposite pairs. It is easily confused with field mouse-ear which has similar flowers, but if you look carefully, you will see that the petals of this plant are twice as long as the sepals and that its leaves are narrower.

Seeds can number as many as 2,500 per plant. When each capsule is mature, it splits open and wind shakes out the contents. Ants may carry them away, or they may attach to passing feet or paws, which ensures further dispersal. They have been known to survive in the soil for up to forty years and still be capable of germinating. Seeds may sprout at any time as long as the temperature is 2^0C or more and under 30^0C. Like our other winter survivors, seedlings are generally frost hardy and the plant's life cycle can be completed very quickly, in as little as five to six weeks. The tiny, brave flowers may appear in any month of the year, even under snowy conditions, although they may not then open. It doesn't matter if there are no insects about as chickweed is a self-pollinator.

Folklore

If you are in need of some good luck, especially in connection with your home, then follow the example of the people of the Fen country. Here it was customary to plant chickweed in pots and bring it into the house for protection and good fortune. Moreover, if a plain woman were to pick the plant while it was sparkling with dew, she would be transformed into a beauty!

It has been noted how this plant tends to grow in clusters and seems to enjoy the companionship of others. For this reason it has become associated with good relationships and loyalty. It was thought that wearing or carrying a posy of chickweed would help to attract the attention of a lover.

Chickweed has often been used to foretell the weather. If its flowers and leaves close up, then this is a warning to put on your great coat. If, however, the flowers are only partly open, then it's likely to rain, but not for long. You can expect sunshine if the flowers and leaves are fully open.

Several plants seem to have this capacity to respond to the weather and even forecast it.

Uses

The plant is extremely nutritious, containing many important minerals and trace elements, including calcium, potassium, magnesium and selenium. In addition, it is particularly abundant in vitamin C and contains useful amounts of vitamin A, as beta-carotene, along with some B vitamins. That said, it also contains oxalic acid, which in large amounts can inhibit the absorption of calcium. So, the plant is not good for anyone suffering from osteoporosis, nor is it recommended during pregnancy or breast-feeding. In any case, it is best taken moderately, perhaps in a mixed side salad. Nevertheless, chickweed is particularly welcome as a winter tonic when fresh greens are less available.

Medicinally, it is one of the best herbs for the relief of dry and itchy skin, including the uncomfortable conditions of psoriasis and eczema. Dab the affected area with a chickweed tea, made simply by pouring boiling water over a couple of tablespoons of the fresh herb then allowing it to cool. To treat a larger area, tie several handfuls of chickweed in muslin and hang under the hot bath tap. When the bath is full, squeeze out the muslin into the bath water and then have a good relaxing soak. This can also help to relieve the pain of rheumatism.

Culpeper knew from experience that chickweed was 'good against scurvy'. This, of course, is true as the disease is the result of a lack of vitamin C, which is replenished by this herb. He also said it would make a healing ointment when 'boyled with Hogs-Greas'. A salve can be similarly made as follows:

Soothing chickweed salve

175 g/6 oz fresh chickweed
275 ml/½ pint almond or olive oil
15 g/¼ oz beeswax

Chop the chickweed finely. Put the oil in a pan and add the chickweed. Cook over a gentle heat for about 20 minutes until the oil has taken on the colour of the plant. Strain. Add the beeswax and stir until it melts, turning up the heat again if necessary. Test the consistency by dripping a spoonful into a bowl of cold water. A firm salve will form small balls. You can adjust by adding more beeswax or oil little by little. ♦ Pour into a wide-mouthed jar and screw on the top when cool.

Keep this salve handy as emergency first-aid for bites, stings and bruises. Use regularly for any itchiness, especially if psoriasis or eczema are involved. It should last a year.

Wildlife

This unobtrusive little plant is surprisingly useful as a wild food once its benefits to us are appreciated. Owners of chickens, geese and pet birds will probably know how much these love chickweed, which is a special treat for them. If you have a feeding station for wild birds, then add chickweed to the breadcrumbs. Chaffinches in particular adore the seeds, as does a species of ground beetle. It has in the past made a very important contribution to the diet of farmland birds, but herbicides have mostly eliminated it from our fields. Unfortunately, it can be the host of several plant viral diseases which can spread to crops, causing damage. For this reason farmers do their best to get rid of it, much to the detriment of the birds.

Several species of moth rely on chickweed as a larval food plant, in particular the pretty yellow shell that flies from June to August. Despite the common name, colours of the wavy-patterned wings can range from bright yellow, through to amber, or even brown. Slightly larger, with a wingspan of about 35 mm/1¼ inches, is the rustic moth. This also flies from June to August, although its patterned wings are more sombre in colour, being a mixture of greys and browns. The larvae feed on several low-growing plants including chickweed.

Groundsel (*Senecio vulgaris*)

Daisy family (Asteraceae). Annual. Self-fertile. Propagated by seed. Contains toxins. Topically medicinal.

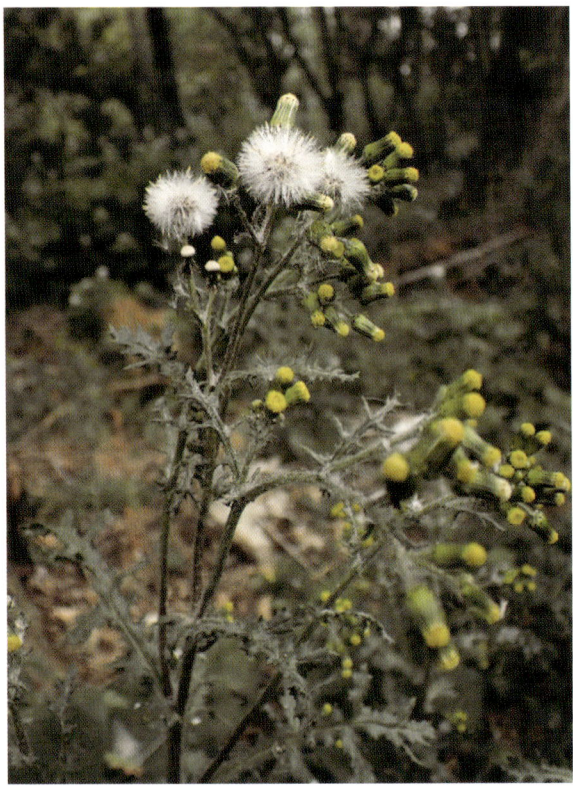

Groundsel can appear at any time. As the seedlings are frost resistant, they can survive the winter cold very well.

All gardeners know of the persistence of this 'weed' as it will readily pop up in any piece of disturbed ground. That said, it is not disliked quite as much as its close relative, ragwort, even though it can harbour rust fungus. In summer or autumn, you may notice the orange-brown pustules on its leaves. This disease can spread to cultivated plants, so it is wise to hoe it up or pull it out.

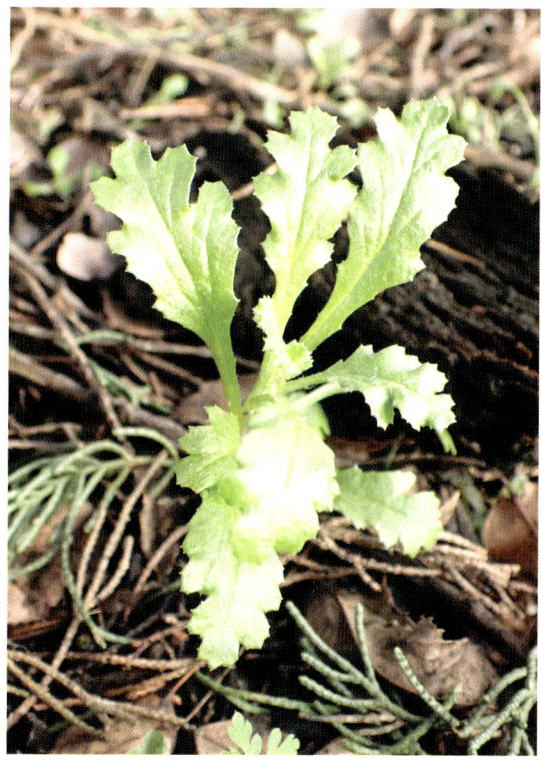

The seedlings are easy to recognise from their lobed and rather ragged-looking leaves.

It is surprising how hardy this rather feeble-looking plant is. With its hollow, fleshy stems, it sometimes seems to have difficulty holding up its flower heads, despite their small size. Seedlings appearing in winter are in fact frost resistant. The plant is also self-pollinating, so the lack of insects at this time of year poses no problem. It can produce as many as 1,700 tiny seeds per plant, each of which is carried on the wind by a silky parachute. When wet, the seeds become sticky and will adhere to animal fur or human clothes or even birds' feet, thus being transported considerable distances. The seeds can then lie dormant in the soil for several years. This amazing plant can complete its entire life cycle in less than six weeks and will produce several generations in a year. Little wonder it is rather unpopular with farmers!

The lemony-coloured flowers are extremely shy, being mostly hidden by black-tipped bracts, thus forming a cylindrical shape at the tip of every branching stem. Each minute floret is tubular with five petals. Occasionally there are outer ray florets with petals curled backwards.

As for the bright green, lobed leaves, these have a distinctive sheen on the upper surface but are a little downy beneath. Generally, they have no stalks and the higher ones tend to clasp the stem.

Folklore

Where does the name *Senecio* come from? It seems to derive from the Latin *senex*, meaning 'old man'. Mrs Grieve in her *Modern Herbal* compares the fluffy seed heads to 'white hair'. She continues, '… and when the wind bloweth it away, then it appeareth like a bald-headed man'.

Yet, despite this association with old men, there is also a long-standing tradition that groundsel signals the presence of witches. In the Fen country, it is said that if you see groundsel growing in thatch, then this means that a witch has been flying nearby on her broomstick and this is where she decided to land. Down on the ground, a cluster of groundsel by the side of a footpath indicates where a witch has stopped to pee! (Perhaps this has something to do with the colour of the flowers.) However, if there is a substantial clump of the plant, then several witches have convened here to plot tactics. So beware!

Uses

Groundsel contains many important minerals and was until comparatively recently grown as animal fodder. However, it is not now recommended for human consumption in significant amounts as it can cause damage to the liver from the pyrrolizidine alkaloids. Goats and sheep have a natural ability to detoxify these alkaloids through particular bacteria resident in their stomachs, so they are not affected. Nevertheless, in Culpeper's day it was frequently used as a remedy.

Even today it has value when applied externally, either to draw a boil out or to soothe chapped hands.

Gypsies' remedy

This is a traditional gypsy remedy to draw out a boil, which is purported to be very effective.

1 large handful groundsel leaves
Piece of gauze or linen, about 30 cm/12 in square
boiling water

Pick a couple of handfuls of groundsel leaves and wash, then chop roughly. Wrap immediately in gauze or linen and tie into a parcel. Place in a bowl and pour on boiling water. ♦ When cool enough to handle, gently squeeze out the parcel, then lay it over the boil. Repeat as necessary.

Easing chapped hands

It is very convenient that you can find groundsel growing in winter, just at the time when you may need relief from sore and chapped hands.

2 groundsel plants, boiling water

Using the plants very fresh, cut or tear them into pieces and place in a large bowl. Pour on the boiling water and allow to steep for 10 minutes. When sufficiently cool, soak your hands in the infusion.

Wildlife

Like ragwort, groundsel is a foodplant of the yellow- and black-striped caterpillar of the beautiful cinnabar moth. It is also important for many other lepidoptera, including the flame shoulder and ragwort plume moths. Finches, as well as canaries, will eat the leaves greedily, while sparrows are partial to the seeds.

Groundsel is very easy to pull out, but do leave some here and there for the moths and birds. Any unwanted plants can be put on the compost heap where they add enriching nutrients.

Stinking Hellebore (*Helleborus foetidus*)

Buttercup family (Ranunculaceae). Perennial. Pollinated by insects, especially ants. Propagated by seed. Irritant. Poisonous.

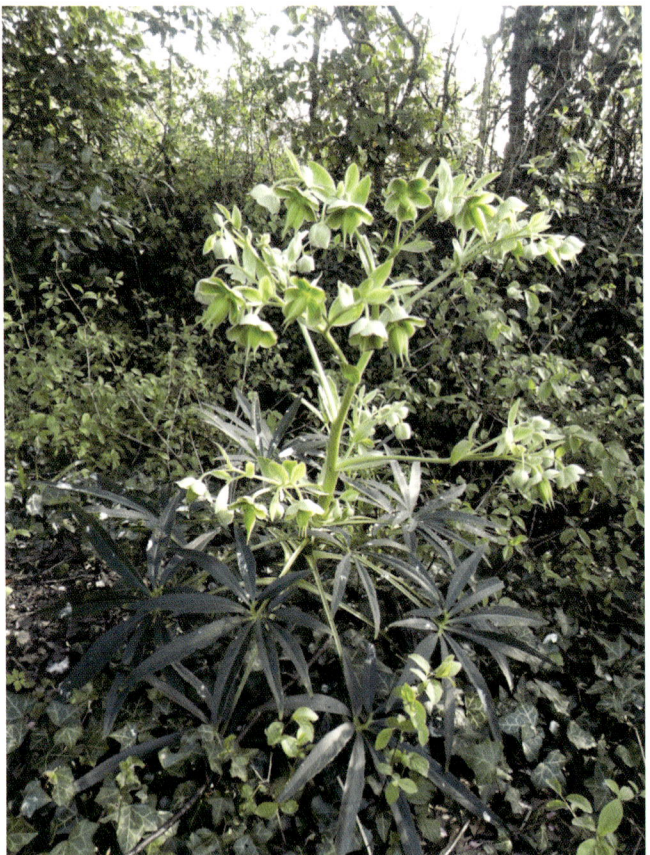

The flowers of our native stinking hellebore cheer up the dark days of February.

It is the very last day of February, the 28th, and our wild hellebore, which has been pushing up all month, is finally in flower. After the long dark days of winter, what could be more magical than this display of pale green, cup-shaped flowers, delicately edged in purple, nodding their heads in the cool breeze and brightened by a patch of pale sunlight! This is truly my most favourite 'weedy' plant of all, a personal herald of spring. What a marvellous lift to the spirits!

I first noticed the striking dark green, deeply divided leaves beside a nearby ditch and wondered what they were. When I later discovered them under some trees in our garden, I watched the plant's development closely. The flowers, when they finally appeared, looked so exotic that I presumed it must be a garden escapee – but no, stinking hellebore can be found wild in many parts of England. It had chanced upon an ideal position in our little woodland where it thrives in dappled shade in the rich, leafy humus. It's a shame that it has such an unattractive name. In fact, on sniffing the plant I was surprised how fresh it smelt, although I could detect a slightly mousy odour. However, if you crush the leaves, they can be quite pungent.

While closely related to the Christmas rose (*Helleborus niger*), the family is in fact that of the buttercup, Ranunculaceae. The five 'petals' are in reality sepals that may remain on the plant for many months, offering a valuable and attractive show from late winter through the spring. The thick, succulent flowering stems can be quite tall, up to 80 cm/2 ft 7 in. After the flowers finally wither, the glossy, evergreen foliage continues to provide interesting texture, with its many long, narrow leaflets finely serrated at the edges.

Seeing how much wild hellebore favours our patch, I decided to try some garden varieties. *Helleborus orientalis* was a good choice, flowering for many weeks and easily surviving the winter chill. Available in white, pink or deep purple, the nodding, cup-shaped flowers rise above the leaves, huddled together in a dense cluster. These have been a real success.

Folklore

The name may come from the Greek *hellos* (fawn) and *bora* (food), in other words 'food of the fawn'. Equally it could be derived from *hele*, meaning to take away, referring to its purging nature.

The plant is referred to by Dioscorides in the 1st century AD. He says that if an eagle should see you digging up hellebore it will bring about your death. Pliny offered a solution: beforehand, make a circle around the plant, turn to the east and pray. In lowland England there is no risk of such a demise as this is not the habitat of eagles! However, the story could have been a superstitious allusion to the plant's poisonous nature.

At any rate, the plant is well known in Greek mythology. The daughters of King Proitos of Argos were scathing about the worship of the god Dionysus. In revenge, he drove them mad and they rushed off into the mountains. Here they were found by the prophet Melampos, who cured them with hellebore root. It is interesting that hellebore grows prolifically in these mountains.

Uses

First, it is important to emphasise the poisonous nature of this plant, and indeed of all hellebores, although *Helleborus foetidus* is thought to be the least toxic of the genus. Today its only use therapeutically is in very minute amounts in homoeopathy to treat depression and kidney infections. In the early part of the 20th century, it was prescribed as a heart stimulant, the active ingredients being the glycosides helleborin and helleborigenin, but later discontinued due to their toxicity.

Like all the buttercup family, hellebore contains protoanemonin which can irritate the skin after prolonged handling. Therefore, it is better to wear gloves if moving or dividing your garden arrivals. There is a story that a driver accidentally sat on some seeds during a long journey, causing unpleasant burning to his posterior!

The 18th-century naturalist Gilbert White prized the plant for its ornamental attractiveness and transplanted it to his garden. In his journal he relates that hellebore leaves were commonly dried and powdered and then administered to children to treat worms. He adds that it was a 'violent remedy'. As an emetic, it was no doubt effective but further doses could prove lethal. Culpeper knew of the risks and described it as 'a very harsh medicine' and warned caution in its use. Gerard seems to have been influenced by the writings of the Ancient Greeks: 'A purgation of Hellebor is good for mad and furious men, for melancholy, dull and heavie persons, and briefly for all those that are troubled with blacke choler.' He does not describe the outcomes of such a prescription.

Wildlife

Within the five 'petals', or more accurately sepals, are minute, cup-shaped nectaries, which are modified petals containing nectar. There may be up to ten of these, along with many stamens. Bees, ants and other insects find the nectar deliciously attractive, an important food source in early spring. Recently there has been a fascinating discovery. It seems that the yeasts which become established in the nectaries have the effect of raising the temperature of the flower, thereby augmenting the evaporation of the volatile organic compounds. This helps the insects to discover the flowers and so the effectiveness of pollination is increased. Nature's varied devices to ensure survival never fail to amaze me.

Even though stinking hellebore is poisonous, I nevertheless adore this plant for its beauty and for its early supply of nectar when there is little else available for insects to feed on. I am therefore delighted to discover some seedlings popping up around the parent plant. These I will cultivate and cherish.

Shepherd's-purse (*Capsella bursa-pastoris*)

Cabbage family (Brassicaceae). Annual/biennial. Self-fertile. Propagated by seed. Edible. Medicinal.

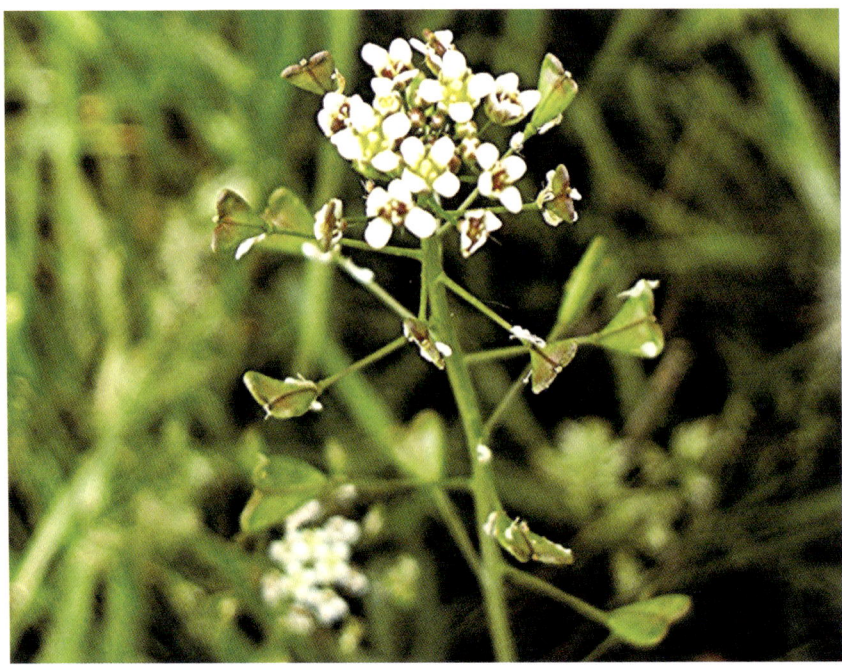

Shepherd's-purse, to ensure its survival, produces around 2,000 seeds per plant and can self-pollinate, so has no need to rely on insects. *Photo © NatureSpot / Graham Calow.*

The size of a shepherd's-purse plant entirely depends on the conditions in which it has planted itself. Ours seem to favour our gravelly parking place, the resilient sinewy stem tolerating even the tyres of cars and footsteps of visitors. This means that it gains little height but produces its tiny, white flowers, nevertheless. If it becomes established in a border, then it can grow to 60 cm/2 ft. It loves disturbed places, so it may well make an appearance if you have recently turned the soil over.

The leaves at the base of the stem form a rosette and are lobed or 'gashed in the edges' as Gerard puts it and are therefore easily recognisable. The higher ones are pointed and wrapped close to the stem. At first the white flowers, each with four tiny petals, are clustered together, forming a flattish top. They then separate as the plant pushes up, so that the 'purses' will ultimately hang individually from the stem. Despite this weed's ability to self-pollinate, minute beetles and other small insects will nevertheless visit the flowers. Like the other year-round germinator groundsel, the seeds become sticky when dampened by rain and will then cling to the feet of birds, animals or even of gardeners, dispersing them widely. The plant is so fertile that during the year several generations can grow. What a survivor!

Folklore

Everyone knows that the name of this 'weed' comes from the distinctive heart-shaped seed capsules, reminding us of those purses that country folk used to wear attached to their belts. Moreover, when the ripe fruit finally splits down the middle, out tumble flat, round, yellowish 'coins'. Children over the centuries have devised games using these. If the seeds are yellow when they open the pod, then they will be rich; if green, they will be poor. Considering that one plant can produce as many as 2,000 seeds, some of these game-players could find themselves very wealthy indeed! A rather callous trick is to persuade a child to pick a ripe pod which will almost certainly split open. This provides the opportunity to say: 'You've broken mother's heart' – hence the other common names of 'mother die' or 'mother's heart'.

In the 17th century, other familiar names were 'pickpurse' or 'pickpocket'. Local people were aware of how this plant seemed to thrive in very poor conditions. This led them to believe that the 'weed' had stolen away the wholesomeness of the farmer's land. A traditional rhyme refers to this:

> Pickpocket, penny nail,
> Put the rogue in jail.

It seems from this that such nasty robbers must be quickly pulled out and discarded.

Uses

As long ago as 1597, the herbalist Gerard says of shepherd's-purse, 'it staieth bleeding in any part of the body', while a century later Pechey confirms: 'Tis outwardly used by Common People, to heal Wounds, with good success.' Indeed, it was so effective that it earned the names of 'stanche' and 'sanguinary'.

The remedy was little used in the 19th century but then re-emerged during World War I when conventional medicines were in short supply and there was a need to turn to traditional methods of treatment. Today it is still recommended by some qualified herbalists for the control of heavy periods. However, it should never be used by women during pregnancy as it is powerful enough to provoke contractions of the uterus.

The leaves, abundant in the vitamins A, B and C, are edible and very good in salads. They are best when picked just before flowering. As for the seeds, they can add welcome piquancy to soups and stews. In 1950, shepherd's-purse was found in the stomach of Tollund Man who lived 2,400 years ago in what is now Denmark. As a green food, they clearly found it appetising.

Today, not everyone finds the tisane appealing, but a tincture made from the leaves is a convenient stand-by for emergency treatment of cuts and grazes, also nosebleeds and bruising.

Tincture of shepherd's-purse

Shepherd's-purse to fill a jar
vodka or brandy
a little water

Pick the herb when it is flowering, wash and chop into small pieces, then put into the jar. Mix the spirit with a little water, then pour it over the shepherd's-purse until well immersed. Put the top on the jar and leave in a dark place for two weeks. You will need to shake the mixture each day. When the liquid has taken on the colour of the plant, strain it off through muslin. Pour into a sterilised storage jar (preferably coloured), put on the top and label clearly. ♦ Dosage for bruising or bleeding: ½ tsp 3 times a day. ♦ The tincture should keep for a year or so. **N.B. Do not use during pregnancy.**

Wildlife

Like other crucifers, or flowers with four petals, shepherd's-purse is very attractive to the orange tip butterfly, which will lay its eggs here, as will the large white.

The common garden carpet moth prefers the suburbs to the countryside, so, as its name implies, you may find that it has taken up residence in your plot. You may spot its larvae any time between April and September. These are pale green with tiny black spots. These also have a liking for cruciferous plants, including shepherd's-purse. The adult is two-tone grey or brown, the distinctive darker patches displayed on the leading edges of the forewings.

Postface

During a conversation with my neighbour in the early spring, I happened to mention that I was writing this book. She immediately asked me which plants were included and reeled off a string of names. I assured her that each of those was featured. Then she enquired about scarlet pimpernel. I explained that the volume comprised only those wild flowers, or 'weeds', that happened to arrive in our garden and that I had never seen it here. She assured me that it made a regular appearance in her garden. How strange!

Some weeks later I was tidying up outside our greenhouse, where used pots had been left, some still containing compost. I was about to empty one out, until I noticed, much to my astonishment, several starry, little, orange-red flowers staring up at me. Scarlet pimpernel! Sadly, it was too late to include it in the main body of this book.

Another recent arrival is toad flax – though I suspect that it may be a garden escapee. Nevertheless, its spikes of deep violet flowers are a magnet to bees. I have decided, therefore, to make it a permanent feature of our summer borders. Last July also saw the appearance, around the base of a rose bush, of the cheerful yellow flowers of creeping cinquefoil. There is no need to encourage this plant as its runners will readily root themselves.

The reality is that wild plants come and go, and a garden is a living, ever-changing place. Next year there will no doubt be yet more new discoveries – perhaps even enough to inspire another volume!

Acknowledgements

I sincerely thank my mother, Margaret Stewart, for all those wonderful wayside walks that instilled in me a love of nature and fascination with plants. It was some years later that my sister, Mary Pratt, a biologist, set me on the path of thinking like an ecologist, with an understanding and appreciation of the inter-connectedness of living species

My husband, John, initially perplexed as to why I would want to write about weeds, nevertheless helped me with the photography by lending me tripods, by fending off the breeze with a glass pane, or by holding up a white screen to reflect more light on to the subject. I am grateful for this practical help.

In addition to my family, my friends and colleagues have been consistently supportive during the creation of this book, checking to see how I was progressing and always willing to discuss ideas.

NatureSpot, a charity set up to educate and inspire the public about the natural world, have been most kind in allowing me to use some of their photographs.

Last but by no means least, I wish to thank Drs Nicola and Hugh Loxdale of Brambleby Books for believing in *A Weed-lover's Calendar* right from the start and for all their input and valuable suggestions which have greatly enhanced the text.

Glossary

Alkaloids Any of a group of compounds containing nitrogen found in plants. They are characterised by their specific physiological action. Most are crystalline solids, others being volatile liquids or gums.

Allantoin A major metabolic intermediate in most organisms, including animals, plants and bacteria, but not humans or higher apes.

Amygdalin A toxic substance often found in plants, especially in the kernels of bitter almonds, apricots, apples, peaches and plums. When macerated or chewed, hydrogen cynide is released, causing cyanide poisoning.

Anodyne Capable of relieving pain or distress.

Anther The terminal part of a stamen, usually consisting of two lobes, each containing two sacs in which pollen matures.

Anthocyanin Water-soluble pigment appearing red, purple or blue. Found in plants, especially fruits such as blackberries and blueberries. Contributes to taste and may have antioxidant activity (*q.v.*).

Antidermatophytic Serves to heal fungal infections of the skin.

Antioxidant Substance giving protection to cells against damaging free radicals (*q.v.*).

Aperient Laxative.

Astringent Causing the contraction of skin cells and other body tissues. As a cosmetic, it makes the skin less oily.

Aucubin Found in plants and functions as a defensive compound. An iridoid (*q.v.*).

GLOSSARY

Axil The angle between the upper surface of a branch, a leaf or its stalk and the supporting stem.

Betonicine A compound produced during a metabolic reaction in certain plants.

Biennial A plant which takes two years to complete its life cycle, to grow to maturity and set seed.

Boron Necessary for the growth of land plants. In industry extracted from borax and used in the preparation of soaps, abrasives and hard alloys.

Bract A specialised leaf, with a flower or cluster of flowers growing in its axil (*q.v.*).

Bulbil A small bulb-like structure, which may be produced in a leaf axil or in place of a flower. It is able to produce a new plant.

Calyx The sepals of a flower collectively, forming the outer floral envelope that protects the developing bud.

Collagen Fibrous part of connective tissue and bones. Yields gelatine on boiling.

Compositae Class of flowering plants distinguished by their multiple petals.

Connective tissue Found in between other tissues everywhere in the body, including the nervous system.

Consumption A wasting away of the tissues of the body, especially as in tuberculosis of the lungs.

Corolla Whorl of petals, forming the inner envelope of a flower.

Cruciferae The plant family in which the flowers have four petals arranged in the form of a cross.

Cyanide In nature, this is found in certain plants and also produced by some bacteria, fungi or algae. Extremely poisonous. In plants cyanides are generally bound to sugar molecules (**cyanogenic glycosides**) and serve to defend the plant against herbivores.

Cyme Arrangement of flowers on a plant, in which the first flower is the terminal bud of the main stem and subsequent flowers are terminal buds of lateral stems.

Decoction The mashing or chopping of herbal or other plant material, then boiling in water to extract oils and other chemical substances. Used to make herbal teas, coffees and tinctures (*q.v.*). It differs from infusion (*q.v.*) due to the method of preparation and higher temperature, thereby resulting in greater extraction of substances.

Dioecious Having the male and female reproductive organs in separate flowers on individual plants.

Diuretic A drug or substance that promotes the loss of water from the body through urine.

Doctrine of Signatures An idea first promoted by Dioscorides (*c.* 40–90 AD), a Greek physician to the Roman army. If part of a herb resembles part of the body, then that's the 'signature' or sign that it can be used to heal that part. Medieval herbalists took up this method of treatment, including Paracelsus (1491–1541), who wrote: 'Nature marks each growth … according to its curative benefit.'

Dropsy An accumulation of watery fluid in the tissues or body cavity, now known as oedema.

Drupe A fleshy fruit with a single seed or stone, as in peach or cherry.

Ellagic acid A natural antioxidant (*q.v.*) found in many fruits and vegetables, and produced by the plant from hydrolysis of tannins.

Emetic Causing vomiting.

Epithelial cells These line the cavities and surfaces of blood vessels and other organs in the body.

GLOSSARY

Essential oil The oil extracted from a plant which contains the essence of the plant's fragrance.

Ethylene An important plant hormone, released as a colourless flammable gas. Used in agriculture to force the ripening of fruits.

Expectorant Promoting the secretion or expulsion of sputum (phlegm) from the respiratory passages.

Falling sickness A former name for epilepsy.

Fibroblast A cell in connective tissue that synthesises collagen (*q.v.*).

Flavonoids Widely available in plants, particularly as pigments for flower colouration, showing as yellow or red/blue petals. These attract pollinators. Some flavonoids protect against plant diseases. They are also health-giving in the human diet.

Free radicals These are toxic molecules often caused when the body is exposed to environmental factors such as pollution, cigarette smoke, radiation or herbicides.

Furanocoumarins Toxic compounds found in certain plant families, which act as potent defences against many aggressors, ranging from bacteria to mammals. In some, the toxicity is enhanced in the presence of ultra violet radiation.

Glyco- Indicating sugar.

Glycoside A molecule in which sugar is bonded to another functional group. Many plants store them in an inactive state. They are activated by an enzyme, causing the sugar to be broken off, thus releasing the chemical for use.

Haemorrhoids Sometimes called 'piles', these are swollen veins around the anus or in the lower rectum, often causing pain and itching. Can be caused by heavy lifting or straining. Plenty of dietary fibre from wholemeal foods may help to prevent or ease the condition.

Haemostatic Retarding or stopping bleeding.

Hermaphrodite The term derives from Hermaphroditus. The son of Hermes and Aphrodite in Greek mythology, who was reputed to have been born with a body containing male as well as female sex organs. In botany it is used to describe a flower that has both male, pollen-producing parts, and female, ovule-producing parts. If there are separate male and female flowers on the same plant, then this is described as monoecious.

Histamine Formed from ammonia and released by the body tissues in allergic reactions, causing irritation.

Inflorescence The arrangement of flowers on their stalks.

Infusion An extract obtained by soaking, as in a herb tea.

Ingenol mebutate Found in plants of the *Euphorbia* genus. Promotes cell death. A gel containing this is used on the skin to treat pre-cancerous cells.

Inulin A soluble fibre occurring naturally in plants, which use it as an energy store. It is typically found in roots and rhizomes. Can help the plant to withstand cold and drought.

Ionone An aroma compound found in various essential oils, including violet or rose oil. An important chemical in the perfumery industry.

Iridoids In plants they act as a defence against herbivores or infection by microorganisms. They taste very bitter.

Lanceolate Narrow and tapering to a point at each end.

LDL cholesterol Low-density lipoprotein, or the 'bad' cholesterol that tends to deposit in the walls of arteries. Over time this can build up and cause blockages.

Lymph nodes Oval or kidney-shaped organs of the lymphatic system and major sites of immune cells. They act as filters of foreign particles or cancer cells.

Lymphocyte A type of white blood cell and part of the immune system which fights diseases.

GLOSSARY

Mucilage Glutinous carbohydrate secreted by some plants. Relieves irritation of mucous membranes by forming a protective film.

Naturalised Adapted successfully to a foreign environment.

Neutrophils White blood cells formed from stem cells in the bone marrow. Important part of the immune system.

Node The point on a plant stem from which the leaves or lateral branches grow.

Oenothein B A tannin, shown experimentally to be capable of modulating and enhancing aspects of the immune system.

Oxalate Occurs in many plants. When eaten in vegetables or drunk in black tea it blocks the absorption of calcium. It also plays a part in the formation of kidney stones.

Petiole The stalk by which a leaf is attached to the rest of the plant.

Phenolic acids Widely available in plant foods and readily absorbed through the walls of the intestine. They work as antioxidants (*q.v.*), preventing cellular damage.

Piles See haemorrhoids.

Plaister Plaster or poultice.

Plethoric Caused by dilation of superficial blood vessels, as in a reddish face.

Pollination The act of transferring pollen grains from the male anther of a flower to the female stigma.

Polyphenols Found widely in plants, these have antioxidant properties (*q.v.*), involved in defence against ultra-violet radiation or aggressive pathogens. It is thought that diets rich in plant polyphenols offer protection against many diseases, including heart disease and cancer.

Polysaccharide A class of carbohydrates with linked monosaccharide units, as in starch or cellulose.

Protoanemonin A toxin found in all plants of the buttercup family, which is released when the plant is cut or macerated. It is a skin irritant and if ingested in large amounts will cause vomiting or, in extreme cases, even paralysis.

Pyrrolizidine alkaloids Produced by plants as a defence mechanism against insect herbivores.

Quercetin A plant pigment that gives certain fruits and vegetables their colour.

Raceme The flowers are borne along the main stem, with the oldest at the base.

Ranunculin An unstable glucoside found in the buttercup family. On maceration or wounding of the plant, this is broken down by enzymes into glucose and the toxin protoanemonin (*q.v.*).

Rhizome A thick horizontal underground stem, whose buds develop into new plants.

Rutin A plant pigment found in certain fruits and vegetables.

Salicylic acid A white crystalline substance used in the manufacture of aspirin, dyes and perfumes, and as a fungicide.

Saponin A substance with foaming, soap-like characteristics when shaken in aqueous solutions. Found in many plants. Often bitter in taste, perhaps serving to protect the plant against herbivores. A few have the opposite effect, actually aiding animal digestion.

Scurvy A disease caused by a lack of vitamin C. Symptoms are swollen and bleeding gums and the opening of old wounds. It was an affliction largely of sailors until the late 18th century.

Scutellarin A flavone, or class of flavonoids (*q.v.*) found mainly in cereals and herbs.

Sepal Collectively, these form the outermost whorl of parts of a flower, serving to protect the bud, then support the petals. Generally green.

GLOSSARY

Silica A hard mineral found mainly in sand and quartz, but also present in many plants, including vegetables, fruit and grains.

Solanine An alkaloid (*q.v.*) base derived from plants of the *Solanum* genus.

Stamen The male part of a flower, consisting of a stalk bearing an anther in which pollen is produced.

Sterol A group of natural steroid alcohols that are waxy and insoluble, with important physiological action.

Stigma A stalk-like projection from the ovary and the part of the female structure in the flower which receives pollen, generally at the tip.

Stipule A small, paired, usually leaf-like outgrowth occurring at the base of a leaf or its stalk.

Stolon A runner sent out from the main plant able to provide fresh roots and new plants.

Stomata Pores present in large numbers in plant leaves, which control the passage of gases in and out.

Styptic Contracting the blood vessels or tissues.

Tannins Widely distributed in many species of plants, to protect against predation, to regulate growth and as a natural pesticide. Has astringent properties (*q.v.*).

Tap root Single root growing vertically downwards with small lateral roots.

Taraxacin A bitter glycoside (*q.v.*) and chief constituent of dandelion root. It stimulates the urinary organs and is thus used as a diuretic.

Thiaminase Enzyme found in some plants and certain sea foods. If ingested, it will split thiamine (vitamin B1) into two and render it inactive. This vitamin is used in energy metabolism.

Tincture A medicinal extract in a solution of alcohol.

Tisane An infusion (*q.v.*) of dried or fresh leaves or flowers.

Trimethylamine An organic compound and product of the decomposition of plants and animals. In humans it is synthesised by microbes in the gut from certain dietary nutrients, especially the vitamin choline. Has a strong 'fishy' odour.

Triterpenes Compounds in plants and animals which are precursors to the hormonal substances known as steroids. They have recently been discovered to have anti-diabetic properties.

Umbel A cluster of flowers arising from the same point in the main stem, with the youngest in the centre.

Umbelliferae A family of herbaceous plants and shrubs with flowers in umbels (*q.v.*).

Vitamins Substances that are essential, in small quantities, for the normal functioning of the body's metabolism. They occur in certain foods.

Bibliography

Bakshi, N., Kumar, P. & Sharma, M. (2008) Antidermatophytic activity of some alkaloids from *Solanum dulcamara*. *Indian Drugs* 45(6):483–4.

Baseley, G. (1977) *A Country Compendium.* Sidgwick & Jackson, London.

BBC News/ Health (2007) *Rose-hip 'remedy' for arthritis*

Beard, M., North, J. & Price, S. (1998) *Religions of Rome.* Cambridge University Press.

Beeton, I. (1907) *Mrs Beeton's Household Management.* 2nd ed. Ward Lock, London.

Bingen, H. von (1998) *Physica: The Complete English Translation of Her Classic Work on Health and Healing.* Healing Arts Press

Bond, W., Davies, G. & Turner, R. (2007) The biology and non-chemical control of Lesser Celandine (*Ranunculus ficaria* L.) www.gardenorganic.org.uk/organicweeds

Brickell, C. (2008) *A to Z Encyclopaedia of Garden Plants.* Royal Horticultural Society & DK, London, UK.

BSBI & BRC (2013) *Online Atlas of British and Irish Flora.* www.brc.ac.uk/plantatlas/

Britten, J. & Holland, R. (1886) *A Dictionary of English Plant-Names.* Trübner & Company

Bruton-Seal, J. & Seal M. (2008) *Hedgerow Medicine: Harvest and Make your own Herbal Remedies.* Merlin Unwin Books, Ludlow, UK.

Buchan, W. (1797) *Domestic Medicine: or, A treatise on the prevention and cure of diseases by regimen and simple medicines.* 15th ed. James Lyon & Co., Waterford

Bullein, W. (1562) *Bulleins Bulwarke of Defence Againste All Sicknes, Sornes, and Woundes.* Thomas Marshe, London

Burrows, I. (2005) *Food from the Wild.* New Holland, London.

Campbell-Culver, M. (2001) *The Origin of Plants: The people and plants that have shaped Britain's history since the year 1000.* Hodder Headline, London.

Cannon, A. (1998) *Garden Birdwatch Handbook.* British Trust for Ornithology, Thetford.

Chambers, R. (1870) *Popular Rhymes of Scotland.* Chambers, Edinburgh.

Chambers, R. (1878/2005) *The Book of Days: A miscellany of popular antiquities in connection with the calendar.* Chambers Harrap, Edinburgh.

Chevallier, A. (1996) *The Encyclopedia of Medicinal Plants.* DK, New York.

Chinery, M. (1977) *The Natural History of the Garden.* Collins, London.

Clare, J. (1827/1964) *The Shepherd's Calendar.* Eds. Robinson, E. & Summerfield, G. Oxford University Press.

Coombes, A.J. (2012) *The A to Z of Plant Names.* Timber Press, Portland, USA.

Cooper, M.R., Johnson, A.W. & Dauncey, E.A. (2003) *Poisonous Plants & Fungi – An illustrated guide.* 2nd ed. TSO, London.

Culpeper, N. (1652/1980) *Culpeper's Complete Herbal.* Foulsham, London & New York.

Cushnie, T.P.T. & Lamb, A.J. (2005) Antimicrobial activity of flavonoids. *International Journal of Antimicrobial Agents.* 26 (5): 343–356

BIBLIOGRAPHY

Darwin, C. (1862) On the two Forms, or Dimorphic Condition, in the Species of *Primula*, and on their remarkable Sexual Relations. *Journal of the Proceedings of the Linnaean Society (Botany)* 6(22): 77–96.

Davidson, A. (1999) *The Oxford Companion to Food*. Oxford University Press.

Dawson, W.R. (1934) *A Leechbook, or collection of medical recipes, of the fifteenth century*. Facsilile ed. 2010 Kessinger Publishing, Montano, USA

Dimbleby, G. (1978) *Plants and Archaeology: The Archaeology of the soil*. 2nd ed. John Baker, London.

Don, M. (25 March 2014) Comfrey for Compost: The superfood for plants. *Mail Online*.

Evelyn, J. (1678) *Sylva: or, A Discourse of Forest-Trees and the propagation of Timber*. John Martyn, London.

Ewen, C. L'Estrange (1929) *Witch-Hunting and Witch-Trials: the indictments for witchcraft from the records of 1373 assizes*. Kegan Paul, London.

Fitter, R., Fitter, A. & Blamey, M. (1996) *Wild Flowers of Britain and Northern Europe*. 5th ed. Collins Pocket Guide. HarperCollins, London.

Flower, B. & Rosenbaum, E. (1958) *The Roman Cookery Book: a critical translation of The Art of Cooking by Apicius*. Harrap, London.

Forey, P. & Fitzsimons, C. (1990) *Letts Pocket Guide to Wild Flowers*. Charles Letts, London.

Foster, S. & Johnson, R.L. (2006) *Desk Reference to Nature's Medicine*. National Geographic Society, Washington.

Genders, R. (1971) *The Scented Wild Flowers of Britain*. HarperCollins, London.

Gerard, J. (1597/1994) *Gerard's Herbal: The History of Plants*, Ed. M. Woodward, Senate, London.

Godwin, Sir H. (1975) *History of the British Flora: A factual basis for phytogeography.* 2nd ed. Cambridge University Press.

Gosling, N. (1985) *Successful Herbal Remedies for Treating Numerous Common Ailments.* Thorson, Wellingborough, UK.

Green, T. (1820) *The Universal Herbal.* Henry Fisher, Caxton Press, Liverpool.

Grieve, M. (1931) *A Modern Herbal.* Harcourt, Brace & Co., New York.

Halliwell, J.O. (1869) *Popular Rhymes and Nursery Tales.* John Russell Smith, London.

Halvorsen, B.L. *et al.* (2006) Content of redox-active compounds (ie, antioxidants) in foods consumed in the United States. *The American Journal of Clinical Nutrition* 84(1):95–135.

Harford, R. (2019) *Edible and Medicinal Wild Plants of Britain and Ireland.* Independently published

Hatfield, A.W. (1969) *How to Enjoy Your Weeds.* Frederick Muller, London.

Hatfield, G. (1994) *Country Remedies: The survival of East Anglia's traditional plant medicines.* Boydell Press, Woodbridge, UK.

Hatfield, G. (1994) *Country Remedies: Traditional East Anglian plant remedies in the twentieth century.* Boydell Press, Woodbridge, UK.

Hatfield, G. (1999) *Memory, Wisdom and Healing: The history of domestic plant medicine.* Sutton, Stroud, UK.

Hatfield, G. (2007) *Hatfield's Herbal – The curious stories of Britain's wild plants.* Penguin, London.

Hedley, C. & Shaw, N. (2002) *Herbal Remedies: A practical beginner's guide to making effective remedies in the kitchen.* Parragon, Bath, UK.

Henry Doubleday Research Foundation/Garden Organic (2012) *Organic weed management*: www.gardenorganic.org.uk/weed-management

Hensel, W. (2008) *Medicinal Plants of Britain and Europe.* Black's Nature Guides. A & C Black, London.

Hills, Lawrence D. (1989) *Month-by-Month Organic Gardening. The green gardener's calendar.* 2nd ed. Thorsons, Wellingborough, UK.

Hole, C. (1976) *British Folk Customs.* Hutchinson, London.

Joseph, J.A., Daniel, A.N. & Underwood, A. (2002) *The Color Code: A Revolutionary Eating Plan for Optimum Health.* Hyperion, New York.

Justesen, U. & Knuthsen, P. (2001) Composition of flavonoids in fresh herbs and calculation of flavonoid intake by use of herbs in traditional Danish dishes. *Food Chemistry* 73(2):245–50.

Keble M. W. (1982) *The New Concise British Flora.* Michael Joseph/Ebury Press, London.

Kemsey, W. (1838) *The British Herbal: or, A Practical Treatise on the Use and Application of the Common Herbs of Great Britain.* Bristol.

Mabey, R. (1996) *Flora Britannica: The definitive new guide to wild flowers, plants and trees.* Sinclair-Stevenson, London.

Mabey, R. (2004) *Food For Free.* 4th ed. HarperCollins, London.

Newland, D., Still, R. Tomlinson, D. & Swash, A. (2010) *Britain's Butterflies: A field guide to the butterflies of Britain and Ireland.* 2nd ed. Wild Guides, Old Basing, UK.

North, P. (1967) *Poisonous Plants and Fungi in Colour.* Blandford, London.

Pechey, J. (1694) *The Compleat Herbal of Physical Plants*. Henry Bonwicke, London. Facsimile ed. Forgotten Books, 2007, London

Pitchford, P. (2002) *Healing with Whole Foods: Asian Traditions and Modern Nutrition.* 3rd ed. North Atlantic Books, Berkeley, California, USA.

Pliny the Elder (AD 77) *Natural History*; trs. Bostock, J. & Riley, H.T. (1855). Taylor & Francis, Tufts University/Perseus Digital Library.

Podlech D. (1996) *Herbs and Healing Plants of Britain & Europe.* HarperCollins, London.

Pratt, M. M. (2005) *Practical Science for Gardeners.* Timber Press, Portland, USA.

Preston, J. (1981) *The Diary of a Farmer's Wife 1796–1797.* Penguin, Harmondsworth, UK.

Reader's Digest Association (2009) *The Ultimate Book of Herbs.*

Rigelsky, J.M. & Sweet, B.V. (2002) Hawthorn: pharmacology and therapeutic uses, *American Journal of Health System Pharmacy* 59(5), 417–422.

Salmon, W. (1693) Seplasium: *The Compleat English Physician or, The Druggist's Shop Opened. Matthew Gilliflower,* London.

Sanders, J. (2003) *The Secrets of Wildflowers: A delightful feast of little-known facts, folklore and history.* Lyons Press, Globe-Pequot, Guilford, USA.

Sanford, M & Fisk, R. (2010) *A Flora of Suffolk.* D.K. & M.N. Sanford, Ipswich.

Scullard, H.H. (1981) *Festivals and Ceremonies of the Roman Republic.* Cornell University Press, Ithaca, N.Y.

Seymour, M. (2002) *A Brief History of Thyme and other herbs.* John Murray, London.

Simmonds, M., Howes, M.-J. & Irving, J. (2017) *The Gardener's Companion to Medicinal Plants: An A-Z of Healing Plants and Home Remedies.* Kew Experts, Royal Botanic Gardens Kew.

Southwood, T.R.E. (1963) *Life of the Wayside and Woodland: A seasonal guide to the natural history of the British Isles.* Frederick Warne, London.

Spedding, C. & Spedding G. (2003) *The Natural History of a Garden.* Timber Press, Portland, USA.

Spence, L. (1948) *The Fairy Tradition in Britain.* Rider, UK.

Stuttaford, T. (2007) Rosehips: a magic ingredient to beat the pain of arthritis. *The Times*.

Sutton, D. (1996) *Field Guide to the Wild Flowers of Britain and Northern Europe*. Larousse, London.

Thomas, J.A. (2007) *Guide to Butterflies of Britain and Ireland*. Philip's/Octopus, London.

Toussaint-Samat, M. & Bell, A. (2008) *A History of Food*. 2nd Ed. Wiley-Blackwell, London.

Turner, B. (1982) *Home Made Wines and Beers*. Park Lane Press, London.

Vedel, H. & Lange, J. (1960) *Trees and Bushes in Wood and Hedgerow*. Methuen, London.

Vickery, R. (1995) *A Dictionary of Plant Lore*. Oxford University Press.

Watts, D.C. (2007) *Elsevier's Dictionary of Plant Lore*. Academic Press, London & New York.

Weise, V. (2004) *Cooking Weeds*. Prospect, Totnes, UK.

White, G. (1789 *The Natural History And Antiquities of Selborne; with observations of various parts of nature; and the naturalist's calendar*. B. & J. White London.

White, G. (1986) *A Selborne Year: The Naturalist's Journal for 1784*. Webb & Bower, Exeter, UK.

Whithering, W. (1785) *An Account of the Foxglove and Some of its Medical Uses*. Robinson, London

Winther, K., Apel, K. & Thomsborg, G. (2005) A powder made from seeds and shells of a rose-hip subspecies (*Rosa canina* |L) reduces symptoms of knee and hip osteoarthritis: A randomized, double-blind, placebo-controlled clinical trial. *Scandinavian Journal of Rheumatology* 34:302–308,

Wong, J. (2009) *Grow Your Own Drugs*. HarperCollins, London.

Index

Aaron's rod 207
abscess 161
Achillea 'coronation gold' 243
acne 66, 118, 189, 236
age spots 47
Alzheimer's disease 236, 283
amygdalin 13
anaemia 47, 214
analgesic 167
angina 94-6
anthocyanin 66, 161, 282, 292
anti-aging 236
antibiotic 89, 167, 221, 292
anti-coagulant 135
anti-fungal 253
antihistamine 167
anti-inflammatory 83, 137, 161, 167, 207, 214, 236, 260, 306
anti-microbial 137, 167, 236
antioxidant 67, 95, 167, 222, 282, 287, 292, 304-6, 338, 340, 343, 350
antiseptic 20, 157, 189, 240, 245, 269, 306
antispasmodic 241, 314
anti-viral 143, 208, 221, 236
ants 2, 44, 53, 192, 233, 321, 328, 331
aphids 37, 69, 80, 87, 144, 162, 219, 226, 294, 296
appetite 47, 103, 118, 153, 302
aroma 18, 28, 86, 93-4, 99, 118, 158, 243, 342 - *see also* odour, smell
arteriosclerosis 94-5
arthritis 24, 260, 283
  osteo- 306
  rheumatoid 305

arum, wild 104, 106 - *see* lords-and-ladies
Ascham, Roger 29
ash 9, 62, 128, 178, 236
asthma 157, 270-1
astringent 52, 68, 137, 236, 238, 282, 338, 345

Bach™ Flower Remedies 13, 113
bacteria, beneficial 47, 188
Bartsia, red **248-50**
Beaumont and Fletcher 23
bees - *see also* bumble bees
  carder 250
  honey 49, 84, 116, 149, 269
  'hotel' for 204
  long-tongued 53
  white-tailed 123
beetles
  leaf 223, 266
  soldier 204
Beeton, Mrs Isabella 48, 284, 347
berries
  edible 140, 143, 280, 291
  poisonous 104, 106, 126, 155, 264-6, 292
  red 105-6, 126, 128, 129, 131, 158, 266, 279, 308
Bindweed, hedge **180-1**
birds
  berries for 128, 137, 145, 158, 289, 291-2, 303, 308-9, 315, 318
  death of 296
  invertebrates for 178
  nests 7, 35, 96, 158, 178, 246, 248, 303, 307, 314

INDEX

seeds for 17, 42, 44, 49, 59, 75, 92, 128, 132, 169, 179, 223, 225, 230, 260, 266, 290, 307, 321, 323, 327
bites, insect 144, 161, 166-8, 260, 273-4, 323
Bittersweet, woody **125-8**, 264 - *see also* nightshade
Blackberry **280-4**
blackbirds 256, 278, 298, 301, 309
Black bryony **129-32**
blackcaps 59, 307
black spot 62
Blackthorn 12, 31, **34-7**, 92, **300-3**
bladder, tonic for 271
blood 35, 48, 95, 99, 135, 188, 215, 240, 244-5, 289, 306
blood pressure 94-5
blue tit 230, 314
boils 83, 161, 167, 189, 208, 218, 260, 282
bones, broken 35, 83 - *see also* fractures
boron 172
bracts 46, 86, 150, 171, 185, 220, 229, 250, 326
  hooks on 187
bramble 247, 280, 282-4, 307 - *see also* blackberry
Bristly oxtongue **184-6**, 279
bronchitis 20, 30, 208, 269
Browning, Robert 4
bruises 43, 44, 83, 131, 161, 168, 246, 322
Buddleja 2, 248, **251-3** - *see also* butterfly-bush
bullfinch 14, 59
bumble bees 8, 50, 53, 84, 158, 223 - *see also* bees
  buff-tailed 11, 99
  red-tailed 11
Burdock, lesser **187-9**
burns 24, 189, 222
burrs 118, 187-9
Buttercup, creeping **72-5**
butterflies
  Apollo 176

blue 192
brimstone 314
brown argus 192
brown hairstreak 37
clouded yellow 135
comma 216, 253, 284
Duke of Burgundy 25, 41
fritillary 30, 230
gatekeeper 284
green-veined white 90, 103, 223
grizzled skipper 75, 119
heath fritillary 69
holly blue 315
large white 223, 335
marsh fritillary 75
meadow brown 178, 230
orange-tip 32-3, 69, 90, 99, 103, 261
painted lady 162, 189
peacock 216, 253, 278, 289
Queen of Spain fritillary 66
red admiral 179, 253, 272, 312, 315
ringlet 230
silver-studded blue 183
skippers 230
small copper 110, 219, 260
small skipper 135
small tortoiseshell 216, 248, 253, 284
small white 90, 99, 223
speckled wood 284
white admiral 158
Butterfly-bush **251-3** - *see also* buddleja

calcium 167, 252, 256, 274, 305, 322
cancer 83, 135, 137, 170, 172, 236, 264, 283, 287, 306
capsule, seed 23, 27, 65, 97, 99, 191, 232, 321, 333 - *see also* pod
cardiovascular system 95-6, 308
carpel 105
catarrh 30, 43, 52, 143
caterpillars 30, 32, 37, 41, 49, 53, 66, 87, 90, 96, 103, 110, 119, 135, 139, 144, 158, 169, 176, 178, 179, 181, 183, 192, 199,

201, 210, 219, 241, 260-1, 263, 272, 284, 287, 314-5 - *see also* larvae
cinnabar 217-18, 219, 327
for birds 218
Celandine
greater 8, 10
lesser **8-11**
chaffinch 320, 323
Chaucer, Geoffrey 43, 156, 290
Cherry plum **12-14**, 248, **254-6**
Chickweed 279, **321-3**
chilblains 130
children 40, 43, 50-1, 53, 156, 160, 237, 259, 305, 330
danger to 86, 106, 130, 232, 265, 310
children's games 43, 46, 62, 73, 147, 165, 181, 188
cholesterol 94-5, 188, 306, 309, 342
chrysalis 158, 218, 260
circulation 94-5, 215
Cleavers **76-80**
climate change 71 - *see also* global warming
Clover 71, 182, 274, 298
red **133-5**
white 72, **133-5**
colds 52, 89, 143-4, 161, 169, 208, 221, 222, 245, 284, 292-3, 306
cold sores 222 - *see also* herpes
colon 47
Comfrey
common **81-4**
rough 81
companion plant 147, 173, 242, 246
complexion 39, 40-41, 143
compost 51, 88, 101, 320, 336
heap 84, 172, 178, 242, 263, 298, 327
compress 52 - *see also* poultice
connective tissue 63, 83, 195, 339
constipation 167, 181, 188
consumption 20, 83, 116, 214, 326, 339
copper 47, 242, 271, 279
coppicing 17

corns 314
corolla 19, 181, 339
corymb 140, 144, 299
coughs 20, 30, 43, 134, 161, 167, 208, 263, 286, 302, 306
Cow parsley **85-7**, 179
Cowslip 25, 32, **38-41**, 102
Crane's-bill, cut-leaved **190-2**
Cuckoo flower 100, 102 - *see* lady's smock
Cuckoo pint **105-7** - *see* lords-and-ladies
cuckoo spit 79, 102
Culpeper, Nicholas 11, 16, 20, 40, 52, 66, 78, 94, 103, 107, 118, 127, 148, 153, 166, 172, 183, 195, 221, 225, 260, 262-3, 265, 271, 283, 286, 301-2, 306, 322, 326, 330
cuts 24, 44, 83, 98, 144, 167, 192, 221, 240, 243, 246, 334 - *see also* wounds
cystitis 63, 78-9, 161, 271

Daffodil 6, 9, 111
Daisy **42-4**, 45, 52, 299
Dandelion **45-9**, 150-1, 185, 225, 268, 279, 295, 296
and burdock 188
Dead-nettle
cultivated 32
red **50-3**
white **50-3**
deafness 20
death 10, 28, 35, 86, 94, 296, 329
omen of 12, 24, 93
decoction 11, 137, 215, 340
dementia 236
depression 330
dermatitis 76, 203, 260
detoxification 78
devil 116, 118, 142, 213, 221, 271, 282
diabetes 188, 215
diarrhoea 52, 138, 167, 192, 236, 265, 283, 292
diet, Neolithic 78, 281
digestion 13, 69, 103, 119, 161, 256

digestive tract 166
digitalis 148-9
dioecious 212, 340
Dioscorides, Pedanius 56, 94, 166, 171, 286, 329, 340
dispersal of seeds 115, 191, 262
    animals (or humans) 54, 77, 118, 165, 187, 229, 266, 268, 321, 325, 333
    ants 44, 53, 233, 321
    birds 44, 92, 128, 132, 137, 227, 266, 333
    water 258
    wind 203, 229, 252, 258, 268
diuretic 17, 37, 47-8, 63, 78, 143, 148-9, 188, 199, 208, 214, 340
Dock 20, 99, 108
    broad-leaved **257-60**
    curled 258-60
Doctrine of Signatures 10-1, 195, 221, 340
Dog's mercury **15-17**
Dog-rose **136-9**, **304-7**
Dogwood 122, **288-90**
douche 52
drying
    flowers 29, 69, 144, 161, 208-9
    herbs 221
    leaves 167, 208, 215, 237
    roots 215
dysentery 166, 167
dye 44, 109, 219, 275, 301

earache 208
eczema 47, 66, 69, 118, 128, 134, 144, 189, 322-3
Elder **140-5**, **291-3**
elderflower 141, 143-5
ellagic acid 283, 340
emetic 143, 330, 340
Euphorbia cyparissias 232
Euphorbia griffithii 'fireglow' 232
Evelyn, John 290
expectorant 207, 314, 341

eyes 172, 232, 292
    tired 144
eyesight 48, 282, 296 - *see also* vision
eyewash 240

fairies 19, 43, 93, 103, 142-3, 147, 156, 218
feet 7, 14, 95, 165, 168-9, 215, 321
female problems 17, 51-2, 244, 245
fertiliser 46, 81, 84, 116, 216
fever 134, 221-2, 245, 265
fibre 84, 213
    dietary 282
    soluble 47, 161, 188, 306
fieldfares 307
field mouse-ear 321
Figwort, common **193-6**, 210
finches 158, 179, 230, 260, 327
flavonoids 43, 95, 137, 143, 161, 167, 208, 292, 306, 308-9, 341
flies 8, 11, 15, 22, 26, 54, 64, 91, 99, 105, 107, 119, 132, 197, 238-9, 275, 308, 311
    drone 269
    fruit 186
flowers
    edible 18, 22, 24, 38, 40, 50, 67, 135, 140, 161, 164, 204
    female 15-16, 101, 105-6, 112, 129, 182, 212, 232
    hermaphrodite 13, 101, 112, 182, 259, 342
    male 13, 16, 101, 112, 129, 182, 212, 232
'flu 143-4, 221, 222, 245, 292-3, 306
Forget-me-not 31, **54-6**, 279
Foxglove 82, 122, **146-9**
fractures 83, 161- *see also* bones, broken
fragrance 23, 85, 181 - *see also* perfume, scent
frog hopper 79, 102
frost 298-9, 301-2, 306, 309, 321, 324-5
fruit, edible 12, 34, 254, 301, 305

gall 186, 226, 286
  red 21
gall midge 132, 226
gall stones 47
gall wasp 21, 186, 226
gargle 43, 69, 118-9, 167, 222, 236-7, 283, 302
Garlic mustard 33, **88-90**, 103 - *see also* Jack-by-the-hedge
gastro-intestinal irritation 265
Gerard, John 20, 30, 58-9, 94, 102, 104, 107, 125, 127-8, 131, 148, 151-3, 157, 166, 198-9, 218, 229, 233, 239, 245, 282, 311, 330, 333-4
gingivitis 283
global warming 1, 123, 299 - *see also* climate change
Goat's beard **150-3**
goldfinch 49, 169, 230
Goosegrass 76, 78, 279 - *see also* cleavers
gout 69, 199-200, 260
greenfinch 307
greenfly 80
Grieve, Mrs Maud 20, 39, 109, 127, 143, 192, 198, 326
ground cover 32, 51, 286, 315
Ground-elder 71, **197-201**
Ground-ivy **18-21**
Groundsel 219, 279, 319, **324-7**, 333

habitat, loss of 32, 116, 176, 191
haemorrhoids 10-11, 195, 341 - *see also* piles
hair 28, 54, 63, 118, 187, 214, 271, 282
hairs
  hooked 54, 185
  stinging 51, 211, 214
hands, chapped 24, 138, 144, 326-7
Hatfield, Gabrielle 78, 127, 143, 195
Hawkbit, autumn 279, **294-6**
Hawthorn 71, **91-6**, 155, 279, **308-10**
hay fever 143, 201

headache 20, 30, 157, 166
heart
  healthy 94, 148, 309
  problems 47, 94-5, 188, 283, 306
Heartsease 64, 66 - *see* pansy, wild
hedgehog 309
Hedge mustard 33, 103, **261-3**, 279
Hellebore, stinking **328-31**
Helleborus orientalis 329
hemlock 86-7
herb, medicinal 20, 51, 68, 97, 163, 220, 238, 242, 245, 285, 322
herbicide 1, 40, 64, 163, 227, 294, 323
Herb-Robert **97-9**, 190, 279
  strewing 28
herpes 221 - *see also* cold sores
hiccoughs 236
Hippocrates 17
histamine 211, 342
Hogweed **202-4**, 299
  giant 209
homoeopathy 330
honesty 32-3, **57-9**
honey 157, 237, 302, 306
Honeysuckle 122-3, **154-8**
  fly 156
Hopkins, Gerard Manley 1
Horehound, black **285-7**, 299
horses 20, 60, 63, 130, 142, 217, 218, 225
Horsetail, field **60-3**
hoverflies 67, 69, 80, 85, 87, 99, 145, 169, 204, 205, 224, 226, 242, 246, 269, 275, 294, 296
hydrocyanic acid 13

immune system 78, 116, 143, 162, 172, 214, 291, 292, 306
indigestion 20
infection
  chest 169
  sinus 292
  urinary tract 48, 161, 214

inflammation 30, 74, 128, 161-2, 207, 218, 265, 271, 306
infusion 29, 37, 79, 143-4, 157, 168, 192, 208, 240, 260, 327, 342
    oil 138, 168, 208
insomnia 29, 265
invasiveness 11, 15, 63, 180, 202, 252
iron, dietary 49, 167, 214, 305
irritant 8, 20, 111, 129-30, 170, 172, 174, 184, 202, 231, 233, 270, 328, 344
itching 166, 305
Ivy, common **311-15**

Jack-by-the-hedge 88 - *see also* garlic mustard
jaundice 47

kidney problems 20, 199, 214, 260, 330
    tonic for 271

Lacnunga 164-5
ladybirds 80, 246
Lady's smock 32, 90, **100-3**
Lamium maculatum 32, 51
larvae 14, 21, 63, 45, 69, 80, 87, 96, 99, 102, 107, 110, 119, 132, 135, 139, 145, 149, 153, 162, 185-6, 189, 196, 216, 223, 226, 246, 250, 257, 260, 266, 272, 287, 290, 294, 296, 314, 323, 335 - *see also* caterpillars
lavender 241
lawn 2, 32, 38, 42-3, 45, 69, 71, 107, 111, 139, 163, 165, 176, 182, 220, 298
Lawrence, D. H. 10
laxative 37, 143, 160, 167, 170, 172, 181
leaf mine 14, 139, 153
leaves
    edible 11, 24, 38, 42, 45, 52, 89, 108, 110, 135, 161-2, 185, 194, 214, 260, 262, 268, 334
    poisonous 13, 17, 83, 144, 265, 292, 313
    rolled 87
leukaemia 172, 287

Linnaeus, Carl 171
lips, dry 138, 222
liver
    damage 83, 218, 326
    tonic for 47
Longfellow, Henry Wadsworth 7
Lords-and-ladies **104-7**
love 24, 28, 35, 43, 55, 64-5, 136, 156, 244
luck
    bad 35, 93, 103, 142, 218
    good 65, 134, 148, 289, 321
lymph 48, 236
    nodes 195, 342
lymphocytes 236

magic
    beneficial 16, 39, 225
    black 35, 140, 142-3
Mallow
    common 124, **154-62**
    marsh 160
    musk 160
manganese 282
meadows 33, 39-40, 101, 223
    damp 9, 33
    loss of 90, 101
menstruation 167, 245 - *see also* periods
mice 265, 309
midges 80, 98, 104-5, 132
mildew 62, 144
minerals, dietary 47, 179, 214, 243, 322
moles 173, 232
moths
    Agonopterix heracliana 87
    angle shades 216, 260
    barred rivulet 250
    barred straw 80
    blood-vein 110
    brimstone 96
    buff ermine 216, 260
    carpet 80
    cinnabar 217-18, 219, 327
    Cochylis hybridella 185

common garden carpet 335
common marbled carpet 260
common swift 287
death's head hawk moth 210
dot moth 201, 216
emperor 37, 260, 290
feathered thorn 139
flame shoulder 327
foxglove pug moth 149
frosted orange 196
garden tiger 53, 158, 260
ghost 260, 287
golden Y 119, 241
goldtail 96
green brindled crescent 139
grey dagger 96, 201
grey tortrix 153
heart and dart 169
herald 315
hummingbird hawk 158
least yellow underwing 162
lesser broad-bordered yellow 107
lesser yellow underwing 260
light grey tortrix 110
metallic coleophora 135
mottled beauty 158, 260
mottled grey 80
mouse 216, 260
mullein 194, 196, 210
plume 99
ragwort plume 327
rose leaf miner 139
rustic 323
shaded pug 223
shark 226
six-spot burnet 183
small fan-footed wave 169
small rivulet 241
spot pinion 110
swallow-tailed 158, 314
tawny speckled pug 219
underwing 107, 162, 260
V-pug 145

white ermine 49
white plume 181
white-spotted pug 145
yellow shell 80, 323
mouse-ear, field 321
mucilage 161, 188, 207, 343
mucous membranes 207
Mullein, great **205-10**
muscles, sore 189

nails, brittle 63
narcotic 37, 127-8, 265, 290
necklace 43, 127, 160, 195
nectar 11, 13, 14, 21, 32, 46, 49, 50-1, 53, 56, 75, 85, 99, 116, 124, 126, 133, 135, 138, 145, 149, 154, 156, 158, 169, 179, 183, 192, 219, 223, 228, 230, 234, 237, 241, 248, 250, 253, 269, 275, 284, 288, 296, 298, 299, 312, 315, 331
nectaries 331
nerves 27, 41, 138
Nettle 20, 162, 166, 178, 259, 272, 279
    common **211-16**
    stinging 49, 51, 212, 259
nightingale 40
Nightshade - see also bittersweet
    black **264-6**
    deadly 126
    woody 126
Nipplewort **267-9**, 299
nitrates 242
nitrogen 73, 116, 134, 183, 213, 216, 269
nosebleed 98, 244-5, 334

odour 28, 105, 176, 204, 285-6, 329, 346 - see also aroma, smell
oils, essential 43, 118, 188, 200, 215, 342
ointment 11, 40, 43, 75, 143-4, 148, 219, 240, 246, 322 - see also salve
Orchid
    bee 111
    pyramidal 32, 70, 71
osteoporosis 322

oxalic acid 109, 260, 274, 322
oxlip 17

pain relief 40, 43, 157, 161, 167, 189, 195, 199, 209, 214, 219, 240, 245, 271, 305-6, 322
Pansy, wild **64-6**
Paracelsus 10, 340
'parachute' 44, 46, 71, 150, 185, 225, 268, 325
Parkinson, John 268
Parkinson's disease 287
Pechey, John 74, 157, 334
Pellitory-of-the-wall **270-2**
perfume 2, 6, 27-8, 31, 39, 123, 138, 154, 156, 194, 252, 253 - *see also* fragrance, scent
periods, heavy 52, 236, 334 - *see also* menstruation
pesticides 32, 116, 124, 149
petiole 115, 343
phosphates 242
photosynthesis 181, 198, 258
piles 11, 52, 195, 208, 246, 341, 343 - *see also* haemorrhoids
pilewort 10
pipistrelle 314
pistil 232
plaister 239-40, 343
Plantain
    greater **163-9**, 279
    ribwort **163-9**
Pliny the Elder 137, 166, 329
pod 32, 54, 58-9, 98, 101, 102, 115, 171, 183, 191, 199, 203, 232, 233, 262, 268, 273, 333 - *see also* capsule, seed
    explosive 97, 171, 191, 233, 273
poison 1, 37, 106, 118, 128, 148, 166, 218, 232-3, 265-6 - *see also* toxin
pollen 73, 99, 105-6, 107, 232,
pollination 343
    ants 328

bees 8, 11, 12, 13, 18, 26, 31, 38, 45, 50, 53, 54, 64, 65, 81, 114, 116, 117, 123, 125, 128
beetles 8, 11, 85, 91, 145, 197, 308
butterflies 38, 67, 133, 223, 227, 242, 261, 280, 288, 294
cross- 23
flies 8, 11, 15, 22, 26, 54, 64, 65, 81, 104, 105, 145, 202, 205, 224, 242, 251, 294, 311
hoverflies 67, 69, 85,
insects 12, 13, 18, 28, 34, 42, 45, 50, 57, 72, 76, 85, 88, 96, 100, 101, 111, 117, 123, 125, 129, 136, 137, 140, 150-1, 159, 170, 174, 180, 184, 187, 193, 202, 205, 217, 220, 223, 224, 231, 234, 242, 249, 254, 261, 264, 267, 273, 285, 288, 291, 300, 304, 328
moths 96, 133, 154
rain 72-3
self- 22, 38, 42, 45, 57, 64, 67, 150-1, 182, 254, 267, 319, 320-1, 324-5, 332-3
wasps 193-4, 242, 311
wind 15, 108, 163, 211, 257, 270
polyphenols 68, 236, 343
potassium 47, 73, 84, 167, 271, 322
poultice 52, 78-9, 83, 161, 167, 169, 189, 199-200, 208, 210, 218, 230, 252 - *see also* compress
Primrose 6, **22-5**, 32, 39, 41, 314
prostate 215-6, 236
prunasin 13
psoriasis 134, 189, 322-3
purgative 17, 233

Queen Anne's lace 86 - *see also* cow parsley

Ragwort, common **217-19**, 324, 327
rain 9-10, 46, 71, 73, 81, 123, 134, 147, 152, 215, 321, 333 - *see also* showers
rash 118, 167, 168-9, 176, 260

RESCUE Remedy® 13 - *see also* Bach™ Flower Remedies
respiratory ailments 13, 52, 157, 265
rheumatism 143, 200, 214, 314, 322
rhizome 15, 50, 61, 117, 180, 197, 199, 211, 212, 238, 242, 344
Ribwort 163, 169 - *see also* plantain
ringworm 143
roots
    in folklore 9, 213, 218
        remedies from 83, 130-1, 143, 153, 181, 199-200, 215, 260
        uses 119, 229, 232, 253
rosehips 178, 297, 304-7
rust fungus 324

salad 24, 40, 47-8, 52, 69, 71, 89, 109, 135, 152, 161, 199, 226, 260, 262, 268, 274, 319, 322, 334
salve 40, 43-4, 52, 138, 168, 218, 222, 322-3 - *see also* ointment
sap 80, 267, 279, 313
    caustic/irritant 74, 113, 172, 176
    milky 46, 150, 185
    therapeutic 47, 167, 170, 172, 181
saponin 11, 40, 106, 207, 344
sawflies 37, 195, 204
scent 27-8, 119, 122, 140, 154, 193, 252 - *see also* fragrance, perfume
scrofula 195
scurvy 11, 103, 322, 344
sedative 40, 244, 265, 287
seed head, 'clock' 46, 150-1
seeds
    down of 227, 229, 235
    ejection of 27, 65, 97, 171, 191, 233, 238, 273
    for birds 42, 49, 59, 75, 169, 223, 230, 260, 266, 290, 307, 323, 327
    for moths 87, 135, 149, 219, 223, 250
    in folklore 46, 213, 259, 305, 333
    long-lasting 181, 206, 258, 262, 321, 325
    numbers of 164, 171, 225, 235, 258, 262, 268, 299, 321, 325, 333
    toxic 13, 134, 144, 154, 232, 292
    uses 78, 116, 167, 204, 232, 260, 262, 281, 309, 334
    with 'parachutes' 71, 185, 225, 325
self-fertile 12, 60, 97, 146, 182, 190, 254, 267, 320, 324, 332
Selfheal **220-3**
sepals 9, 16, 19, 23, 27, 112, 118, 182, 194, 232, 321, 329, 331, 344
shade 26, 51, 101, 109, 117, 329
Shakespeare, William 23, 39, 65, 92, 102, 127
Shepherd's purse 319, **332-5**
showers 33, 70, 298, 318 - *see also* rain
shrub, deciduous 12, 34, 91, 136, 140, 251, 288, 291, 300, 304, 308
sinusitis 43
skin 20, 44, 61, 66, 74-5, 119, 127-8, 134, 138, 141, 167, 168-9, 172, 189, 203, 208, 222, 236, 246, 260, 283, 330
    dry 138, 144, 322
sleep 28-9, 41, 47, 93, 286, 306
sloes 300-3, 309
slugs 66
smell 16, 18, 84, 86, 97, 142, 217, 230, 238, 251, 253, 271, 285-6 - *see also* aroma, odour
soil 161
    acid 147
    heavy clay 33, 137
    nitrogenous 134, 213, 264
    rich 18, 117, 264
    sandy 112, 206
    temperature 173
sore throat 66, 69, 89, 118, 157, 161, 167, 169, 221, 236-7, 263, 283-4, 293, 301
Sorrel 49
    common **108-10**
    procumbent yellow **273-5**
soup 135, 162, 214, 334
Sowthistle, prickly **224-6**

INDEX

sparrow 75
sparrowhawk 96, 295-6
spathe 104-5
Speedwell 32
    germander **67-9**
    heath **67-9**
    slender **67-9**
spider, wolf 53
splinters 52, 167, 169, 208
sprains 83
Sprengel, Christian Konrad 56
Spurge
    caper **231-3**
    petty **170-3**
sores 148, 165, 222, 283, 271
stamens 9, 16, 23, 105, 125, 149, 155, 164, 171, 232, 241, 264, 271, 331, 345
Star-of-Bethlehem **111-13**
starling 246, 303
stiffness 44
stigma 23, 73, 345
stings 52, 56, 161, 166-9, 256, 323
    nettle 20, 166, 213, 259
stomach 263
    cramps 241
    upset 161, 314
stomata 175, 252, 345
Stonecrop
    biting 175-6
    white **174-6**
stress reduction 40
style 323
styptic 192, 240, 283, 345
sun, sunshine 97, 112, 156, 262, 267, 321
sunburn 40, 143
swelling 106, 128, 130, 161, 166, 168, 195, 226
syphilis 17

tannins 11, 52, 68, 118, 134, 137, 161, 167, 181, 188
tea, herbal 214, 282, 300, 345, 340 - *see also* tisane

teeth 63, 271, 290, 302
temperature, of flower 105, 175, 331
tepal 16, 112
terpene 20, 95, 143, 346
Thistle 162, 225, 279, 299
    cotton 229
    spear **227-230**
thorns 35-6, 92-3, 96, 136, 137, 167, 169, 281, 301, 303
Thornton, Robert 37
throat problem 221 - *see also* sore throat
thrush 66, 128, 158, 303
tincture 95, 334-5, 345
tinnitus 20
tisane 20, 30, 40-1, 63, 66, 79, 134, 143, 161, 199, 222, 245, 334, 345 - *see also* tea
tonic 47, 78, 96, 214-15, 236, 271, 322
toothache 161, 167, 245, 250
toxicity 148, 158, 330
toxin 11, 13, 149, 214, 324
tranquillizer 68
tree sparrow 223
Trefoil, bird's foot **182-3**
    hop 298
tuberculosis 195, 208, 221

ulcers 83, 167, 169, 236, 269, 271, 283, 286
    leg 195
    mouth 99, 221, 301
    stomach 161, 169
umbel 199, 203, 346
urinary tract infection 48, 161, 214

vegetables 7, 48, 84, 103, 178
veins, varicose 52, 167
venom 165, 166
verruca 314
Vetch, common **114-16**, 123
Violet 6, 65, 77
    common dog **26-30**
    pudding 29
    sweet **26-30**

vision 47 - *see also* eyesight
vitamins 47, 103, 169, 179, 214, 346
    vitamin A 47, 66, 89, 167, 214, 282, 305, 322, 324
    vitamin B 47, 63, 167, 282, 305, 322, 324
    vitamin C 11, 20, 47, 66, 68, 89, 103, 167, 214, 274, 282, 292, 302, 304-6, 322, 324
    vitamin D 47, 305
    vitamin E 68, 305-6
    vitamin K 68, 167, 282, 305
    vitamin P 137

warts 47, 74, 171, 233, 301
wasps 69, 80, 193, 194, 242, 246, 248, 250, 256, 311, 315
weather, forecasting 46, 301, 321-2
weed killer 1, 298
White, Gilbert 8, 123, 330

Willowherb
    great 177, **234-7**
    rosebay 179, **234-7**, 279
witches 134, 142-3, 207, 218, 326
Withering, Dr William 148
Wood avens **117-19**
Woodbine 156
woodland 2, 9, 16, 17, 22, 26, 67, 69, 106, 110, 147, 156, 158, 235, 315, 329
Wordsworth, William 8, 9-10
worms, intestinal 166, 185, 330
wounds, healing of 20, 43, 78, 83, 98, 148, 161, 167, 183, 221, 222, 243, 245, 252, 334 - *see also* cuts
Woundwort, hedge **238-41**
wren 7
wrinkles 40, 138

Yarrow **242-6**